Basic Structure and Function
in the Central Nervous System

Neural Organization and Behavior:
A Systems Analysis Approach to Brain Function

Basic Structure and Function in the Central Nervous System

DONALD G. STEIN

CLARK UNIVERSITY
WORCESTER, MASSACHUSETTS

JEFFREY J. ROSEN

BOSTON UNIVERSITY
BOSTON, MASSACHUSETTS

MACMILLAN PUBLISHING CO., INC.
New York

COLLIER MACMILLAN PUBLISHERS
London

Acknowledgment

The authors would like to express their appreciation to Darel Stein, who carried out much of the library research, and to Alfhild Bassett, who patiently typed and revised the material for this book.

Macmillan Publishing Co., Inc.
866 Third Avenue, New York, New York 10022

Collier-Macmillan Canada, Ltd.

Library of Congress Cataloging in Publication Data

Stein, Donald G.   comp.
  Basic structure and function in the central nervous system.

  (Neural organization and behavior)
  Includes bibliographies.
  1. Central nervous system. I. Rosen, Jeffrey J., joint comp. II. Title. [DNLM: 1. Central nervous system—Anatomy and histology. 2. Central nervous system—Physiology. WL300 S 819b 1974]
QP370.S73   612.82   73-3895
ISBN 0-02-416500-X

Printing: 1 2 3 4 5 6 7 8   Year: 4 5 6 7 8 9 80

Tell me, where is fancy bred,
Or in the heart, or in the head?
How begot, how nourished?
    Reply, reply.
It is engend'red in the eyes,
With gazing fed; and fancy dies
In the cradle where it lies,
    Let us all ring fancy's knell.
    I'll begin it—Ding, dong, bell.
Ding, dong, bell.

Shakespeare
(*Merchant* of V*enice*, III, 2)

Preface

In general, a book of readings is constructed and used to acquaint the student with what the author considers to be exemplary work in a particular field of study. If the articles are well chosen, the student can often share in the flavor and excitement of the original research—a feeling not often conveyed in reviews of the literature, or as summarized in most textbooks. However, after looking over most of the anthologies available to students of physiological psychology, we have come away with the vague suspicion that these books may be written with a singular intent: to wit, keeping undergraduates out from underfoot in the periodical room of the university library. Rather than be associated with such a "conspiracy" we have attempted in this book to provide a conceptual and organizational framework within which all of the articles can be integrated. Thus, the reader will find that each section builds upon information presented in the preceding section, and that within a section each of the articles is similarly related. The same may be said for each of the volumes that make up this series.

Anyone who has devoted his time to the study of brain–behavior relationship is impressed and often awed by the complexity and magnitude of the problem. Although great strides have been made in the development of research techniques for studying brain function, less consistent progress has been shown in conceptualizing the nature of the problem. The difficulty in arriving at some unified view of brain function is perhaps best represented by the marked difference in thinking about brain processes as reflected in Sherrington's "switchboard" theory of neural circuits and the Gestalt theory of electromagnetic patterns of excitation.

Our particular bias has its roots, in part, in the concept of hierarchic integration as it was formulated by Heinz Werner.* This term implies that

* Heinz Werner: *The Comparative Psychology of Mental Development.* International Universities Press, New York, 1957.

with increasing differentiation of a structure into its constituent parts, there is a corresponding tendency for the parts to become, rather than autonomous, subordinated to the activity of the entire structure. For example, when one looks at the anatomy of the brain, he can discern a mosaic of different structures. However, according to the concept of hierarchic integration, it would be erroneous to assume that each structure, although anatomically differentiated, has an autonomous or unique behavioral function. In contrast to the view of functional localization, we are proposing that the brain must be viewed as a dynamic organization of differentiated, but highly interrelated, structures. A corollary of this position is that just as each subordinate structure or level can exert afferent control over each structure in the hierarchy, each higher level, in turn, exerts efferent control on subordinate structures. Within this view, no level or structure may operate independently of either subordinate or higher levels of activity; input into any one area of the CNS can affect activity in all areas of the brain. Thus, the concept of hierarchic integration provides an organization for the various structures that make up the brain.

This organization is amenable to an investigation of the functions of the CNS as well. One of the fundamental activities of the brain is information processing. This term refers to the ability of the CNS to transduce external energy forms into a neural "language" or "code." The generation, syntax, and utilization of this code by the brain are the focus of this collection of articles.

In a sense, each section of this book represents a different level of analysis of neural organization and its relation to behavior. The first section studies activity and function of the single cell, the second deals with the way in which individual cells interact to produce complex patterns of activity capable of conveying information about various aspects of the environment, and in the third section we study the ways in which the cortex discriminates and differentiates between incoming information.

In the volume on motivation and emotion we move to a structural level of analysis in which the brain is studied as a *system* of interrelated *parts,* each part contributing to the emerging pattern of activity that is represented as behavior.

The volume on learning and memory deals with these more complex processes and provides a multilevel analysis of the problem.

Each group of readings is preceded by a brief introductory statement that we hope will do the following: (a) relate the readings to one another; (b) relate them to the point of view established in the preceding chapters; and (c) relate them to a general systems analysis approach to brain function. To help the process of "integration" by the reader, we have provided some general thought questions that we feel will direct the student to the relevant issues in the field.

D. G. S.

J. J. R.

Contents

Part III

Part I

Neural Function:
Flow of Information in the CNS

The articles in our first section deal specifically with the operations of the basic anatomical unit of the brain, the neuron. It has been estimated that the central nervous system contains billions of nerve cells, all of which have the capacity to interact with one another. In fact, Thompson * has estimated that the number of possible interreactions that could occur within a single human brain is greater than the number of particles in all the universe. Given this enormous potential, it seems reasonable to assume that before we can attempt to understand how the brain mediates or controls behavior, we must first look at how these units initiate and transmit information.

Of course, depending upon one's level of analysis, it may not be important to know anything about how single neurons work; however, one of the most fundamental problems in physiological psychology deals with the question of "what is the neural code?" If we are to discover the mechanisms involved in acquisition, storage, and retrieval of information, i.e., the processes that are critical for all forms of complex behavior such as learning, emotion, and motivation, we must first know something about the "data language" of the nervous system.

Fortunately, recent technological advances have made it possible for neuroscientists to study the mechanics of single nerve cells and thus explore ways in which the nerve impulses are generated and how they are communicated to other parts of the brain and spinal cord.

The readings in this section begin with a historical introduction to the study of neuron function. In the first article, Bullock points out that the history of research on the problem of how nerves work was marked by a number of important controversies that served to generate great excitement and very

* R. F. Thompson: *Foundations of Physiological Psychology*. Harper & Row, New York, 1967, p. 1.

significant discoveries. In a relatively short time, the results of research carried out in a few laboratories led to such important findings that they helped to shape what Bullock refers to as neuron doctrine.

One of the scientists who helped to formulate the "neuron doctrine" was A. L. Hodgkin, and in his article he describes the sequence of experiments on the mechanisms responsible for conduction of the nerve impulse. For his elegant work he was recently awarded the Nobel Prize in physiology.

The article by Wachtel and Kandel explores another domain of neural activity: how information is transmitted from one neuron to another. Their research also delves into the problem of neuronal inhibition, the process by which some information is excluded from further consideration by the CNS.

Finally, the paper by Gonatas provides an excellent account of the hierarchical interdependence inherent in the CNS. His research illustrates how certain kinds of structural changes, even at the level of the synapse, can produce dramatic dysfunction in behavior.

Neuron Doctrine and Electrophysiology

THEODORE HOLMES BULLOCK

Reprinted from *Science*, April 17, 1959, Vol. 129, No. 3355, pp. 997–1002.

The neuron doctrine, which we chiefly owe to Cajal (*1*), was unquestionably a giant stride forward in the understanding of the substratum of nervous function. It forms the basis of all modern work on the nervous system. It asserts that the nerve cell and its processes, together called the neuron, form the cellular units of the nervous system which are directly involved in nervous function; that all nerve fibers are neuronal processes; that the neuron and all its extensions develop embryologically from a single neuroblast; and that the neuron is a trophic unit, all its processes being dependent upon the nucleated cell body for their maintenance and regeneration. Although this is not inherent in the original anatomical concept, the neuron has classically come to be regarded as a functional unit, and it is here that newer information forces a reappraisal.

We can appreciate the significance of the neuron doctrine more fully by visualizing the alternative concepts historically available (*2*). In various forms, these alternatives, as formulated by Gerlach in the '70's and by Golgi, Meynert, Weigert, Held, Apathy, Bethe, and Nissl, among others, during several subsequent decades, assumed a diffuse reticulum of anastomosing dendritic and axonal processes. The "reticularists," as this heterogeneous group came to be called, were united mainly in their conviction that anatomical continuity of fibers and branches was the prevalent condition in the nervous system. But without assuming some kind of discontinuity and a useful, noncapricious lability it was extremely difficult, to say the least, to analyze, in a functionally meaningful way, pathways, connections, and the processing of discrete responses through complex centers, and this difficulty became more acute after the discovery of propagating all-or-none nerve impulses.

Early Evidence of Independent Neurons

Actually, the idea that nerve fibers are the greatly elongated extensions of nerve cells, though by no means generally accepted until after the time Harrison observed the outgrowth of processes in tissue culture (1907), had been clearly stated by workers in the first half of the last century (Kölliker, Wagner, and Remak). The individuality of the nerve cell in degenerative as well as in embryological processes was strongly indicated by the works of Forel and His in the '80's. But a convincing illustration of these principles

3

and of the fact that *axons generally terminate among dendritic ramifications*—but freely and without forming a reticulum—awaited that scientific stellar nova, Santiago Ramon y Cajal. It is one of the ironies of history that his start and all his early work were based on the exploitation of a remarkable silver impregnation method discovered by the Italian Camillio Golgi in 1873 but virtually unknown until 14 years later when Cajal, among others (including the Norwegian Fridtjof Nansen, the future polar explorer), began to use it. Golgi shared with Cajal the Nobel prize of 1906 because of the crucial role his method had played in the 20 formative years of the neuron doctrine. But even at that date he had not given up his reticularism and regarded Cajal as an adversary. Flurries of controversy continued for years, but of all the contributions of neurohistologists none has stood the test of time as well as those of Cajal, as amazing for their quality as for their quantity (*3*).

As a subsidiary doctrine, Cajal made the brilliant inference from the anatomical arrangement of sensory, motor, and internuncial neurons that they are all *dynamically polarized,* usually in such a way that excitation can only be transmitted from the axon of one neuron to dendrites or soma of the next and, within a neuron, must normally spread from dendritic to axonal poles (Fig. 1).

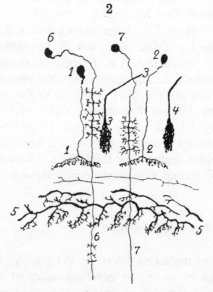

FIGURE 1. Neurons of the optic ganglia (medulla externa) of a crab stained by the Golgi silver impregnation method. Since the eye is above and the brain is below, it is reasonable to assume that most transmission is downward—therefore, from terminals like 3 and 4 to upper (dendritic) processes of 6 and 7. But it is not so easy to say what direction transmission takes in the purely local neurons (1 and 2) or the coarse horizontal fibers (5). (*From Hanström* (*11*).)

Convergence of Physiology and Anatomy

The parallel strides made in electrophysiology during much of the same period, from the time of Helmholz in the middle of the last century to the period just before and after World War I, and the work especially of Keith Lucas, E. D. Adrian, Herbert Gasser, and Joseph Erlanger led to the discovery of the change in electrical potential with action which, in the single nerve fiber, came to be called the nerve impulse. This was found to be an all-or-none event of the order of 1 millisecond in duration and capable of following a preceding impulse only after a short interval. Thus, the concept of a quantum of activity or a *unit of function* came to be emphasized, and the nervous system came to be regarded as a kind of digital computer with a binary—that is, yes-or-no—response. Some would prefer to call it a pulse-coded device, since the intervals between pulses are graded and can introduce noise. We can now recognize four basic tenets which grew out of the impact of electrophysiology on the neuron doctrine during this classical period of the '20's and '30's (classical from the standpoint of present-day textbooks) and which still dominate much of the thinking in the field.

1) We came to think that the all-or-none impulse was synonymous with the neuron in action—that is, that the impulse together with its afterpotentials was the only form of truly nervous activity.

2) We thought that when any part of the neuron was excited this excitation spread to all parts of the neuron as a propagated nerve impulse.

3) We thought that Cajal's doctrine of the dynamic polarity of neurons meant that dendrites propagate impulses toward the cell body.

4) We have thought for many years that the secret of all labile functions must lie in the properties of a junction between neurons. This locus, called the synapse, was supposed to be the only seat of selection, evaluation, fatigue, and facilitation and perhaps of long-persistent changes as well.

Four Main Revisions

The evidence of the last few years has significantly altered all four of these tenets.

1) We now believe that the neuron is a functional unit somewhat in the same sense that a person is in society, in that it speaks with one voice at a time. At least so long as the neuron has but one output path (in terms of the textbook vertebrate neuron, one axon), it will speak with one voice at a time in the all-or-none pulsed code output essential for long-distance propagation. But we know that some neurons have two axons and can deliver two nonidentical pulse-coded outputs at the same time in different directions (*4*). More

important, we believe that this pulsed form of activity—the nerve impulse or *spike*—is only characteristic of a specialized portion of the neuron, the axon, as is explained further below.

2) We now believe that the responses of many or most parts of the neuron to impinging excitation do not spread to become impulses directly but help determine the firing of impulses at some critical region such as the base of the axon—somewhat in the same manner as the impinging sights and sounds act upon the trigger finger of a man with a pistol. These responses we will call *prepotentials* or subthreshold processes, and some of them are enumerated below.

3) We now believe that many parts of the neuron cannot respond in an all-or-none manner and therefore cannot propagate without decrement. The establishment of the conduction of the nerve impulse without decrement was one of the achievements of the '20's and early '30's but apparently applies only to a special portion of the neuron—the axon. *Decremental conduction* is probably characteristic of the great bulk of neuronal surface membrane—that is to say, the cell membrane of the extensive ramifications of dendrites making up much of the gray matter of higher animals and the neuropiles of lower. Decremental conduction requires that all such membranes be within shouting distance of the locus of spike initiation—in other words, within the distance of electrotonic spread—in order to be able to exert a physiological influence on the generation of all-or-none events by the neuron. Many dendrites are so short that we can easily believe this condition is met, but some are so long and fine that it remains seriously open to question whether they can directly influence to any significant degree the initiation of spikes by the cell or whether their main role is quite another one (Fig. 2). In this paragraph we have been traversing a no man's land from areas of more general agreement to areas of less and less agreement, and here we pass definitely into the area of personal speculation. But it has been suggested that much of the activity of dendrites has its significance in an influence upon other neurons, even though the activity is local, graded, and small in amplitude. It seems likely that brain waves are the synchronized subthreshold dendritic potentials of many neurons summed and, further, are perhaps more than a mere by-product like the noise of a car, but are a physiologically significant causal agent (5).

4) We now believe that labile and integrative processes, insofar as they are localizable to the single unit level, are not confined to the synapse but occur as well at other places in the sequence of events preceding the initiation of the propagated spike (6). There may be as many as four or five *different kinds of circumscribed loci* in various parts of the neuron, each of which is integrative in the sense that it does not pass on whatever comes to it in a one-to-one relation but exercises some labile evaluative action (Fig. 3).

These changes in viewpoint add up to a quiet but sweeping revolution. They renew the old hope that we may one day be able to explain complex behavior in terms of neurons—of their patterns and properties. In my opinion

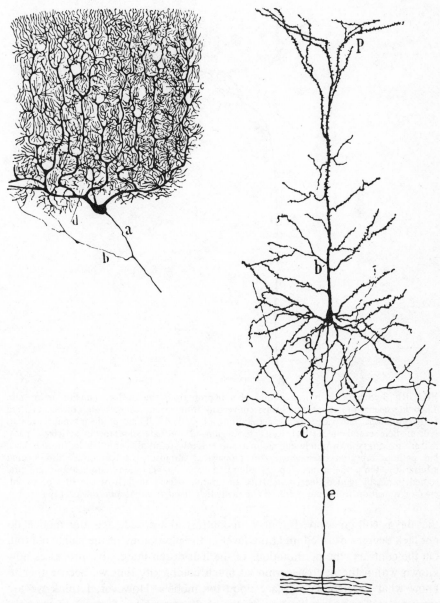

FIGURE 2. (Above) Purkinje cell of the cerebellar cortex of man. (Right) Pyramidal cell of the cerebral cortex of man. Both are shown incompletely; the axon actually extends a long distance downward. (Golgi stain.) The great arborization of dendrites probably does not conduct impulses, and even electrotonic influence from the farthest ones must be very weak in the spike-initiating region, be that soma, or base of the larger dendrites, or axon. (*From Cajal, Histologie du Système Nerveux de l'Homme et des Vertébrés* (12).)

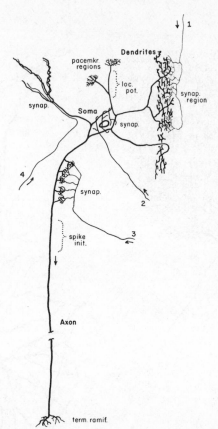

FIGURE 3. Schematic representation of a neuron from the cardiac ganglion of a crab. There are several presynaptic pathways converging from diverse sources—inhibiting, exciting (other followers and pacemakers), accelerating (1, 2, 3, 4). These produce synaptic potentials in their several special loci. Restricted regions also initiate spontaneous activity ("pacemaker" regions, shown purely diagrammatically); local potentials (only labeled in one place but perhaps repeated elsewhere); and propagated impulses ("spike init.," also located arbitrarily). Only the axon supports all-or-none activity. Terminal ramifications are presumed to act by graded, local potentials. Integration occurs at each of the sites of confluence or transition from one event to the next. [*Modified from Alexandrowicz* (13).]

that day is still far away. But now, in contrast to a decade ago, our models do not lack degrees of freedom at the level of the physiology of the single neuron. On the contrary, the permutations of the half dozen integrative processes now known within the neuron permit so much complexity that we need rather to know what restrictions to place upon the models. However, I think we are getting closer to an explanation of one of the most basic features of the neuronal basis of behavior—namely, the mechanism of origin of *temporally patterned impulse sequences*. Such patterns are the coded commands or output of every neuron, high or low, and the problem of how the characteristic sequences within and among neurons of a group are formulated has hardly been investigated heretofore. "Characteristic" means recurrent, and if we state the problem in terms of the mechanism of formulating a meaningful pattern and then retaining or stabilizing that mechanism, we have essentially stated in one form the basic problem of the neuronal basis of instinct as well as of learning.

Capillary Ultramicroelectrode

These drastic changes in viewpoint are almost entirely due to the technical advances made possible by the intracellular electrode, a device introduced by Ling and Gerard in 1949 (7) and perfected by a number of other workers, which makes it possible to record from inside the larger neurons many of the events that occur prior to the initiation of the all-or-none impulse, with but very slight damage. The electrode is a glass capillary tube drawn out to submicroscopic dimensions, of the order of a few tenths of a micron in outside diameter, filled with an appropriate salt solution as conductor and inserted into the cell to measure the electrical potential difference between the inside and a second electrode outside the cell.

The technique is not extraordinarily difficult, but under the best of conditions it presents problems. The electrodes are of high resistance—from several to many tens of megohms—and require special circuits for reasonable fidelity of recording of rapid events. They introduce many microvolts of noise. The capillary pipettes have to be drawn again and again to the same shape, carefully filled, and frequently replaced, for they break not only under the stress of a little connective tissue but of their own accord, presumably from internal stresses. While the tips are quite visible in air, they are beyond the limits of ordinary microscopy under water, and in most experiments the penetration is made blindly. A rather satisfactory sign that the tip has penetrated into a cell is provided by the sudden appearance of a negative potential of several score millivolts. The main limitation, however, aside from uncertainty about exactly where the tip is located, is the intolerance of small cells and processes—below about 10 microns—of even the finest electrodes thus far produced. Our knowledge is based on sampling from a rather small number of types of large neurons, and even here only from the axon, the cell body, and perhaps the bases of the larger dendrites.

Let us now look a little more closely at the major evidence for the main conclusions stated above.

Subthreshold Activity

Every neuron so far penetrated gives at least one output of all-or-none spikes, and a few have been encountered which can give two different rhythms of spikes and which have two axons or major processes going in different directions (*4*). But it would probably occasion less surprise today than ever before were someone to find a neuron which gave no all-or-none impulses but whose axon carried only graded and decrementally spreading activity. This may well be the primitive property, and it may well be retained in the many very short axoned neurons in the highest centers of both invertebrates and vertebrates. This is to say that the possibility remains with us that in the most complex and finely textured higher centers, made up largely of very small neurons, perhaps much of the normal functioning is carried out *without nerve impulses*—that is without all-or-none, propagated spikes but by means of graded and decrementally spreading activity. Perhaps the first direct demonstration that subthreshold events in one neuron can increase the activity in another neuron has recently been supplied by experiments of Watanabe and myself on the nine-celled ganglion of the lobster heart (*8*). Here, relatively long-lasting pulses of current repeatedly applied through the intracellular electrode into one of the five large anterior cells increased the pace of firing of small posterior cells many millimeters away, even when the applied currents were below threshold or were in the wrong polarity for spike production. (The internally anodal stimuli caused the distant small cells to tend to fire during the long pulse, while the internally cathodal currents caused the small cells to tend to fire their impulses just after termination of the current.) These effects, obtained without the intervention of nerve impulses, are not due to escape of current but occur only if the stimulated cell is penetrated.

The Several Forms of Activity

Like the multiplication of the fundamental particles of physics, the known forms of activity of nerve cells have multiplied from a single one—the all-or-none impulse or spike—which was all that was known up to 1938. In that year Hodgkin, using the giant fiber of the squid, and very soon thereafter Katz, using the sciatic nerve of the frog, discovered the local potential, which can be graded and which spreads essentially passively—"electrotonically"—declining to half amplitude about every millimeter. Later work has shown several more kinds, the exact number depending on the distinctions one wishes to make.

The scheme proposed in Fig. 4 indicates the relations between most of these. The first two, the *spike* potential and the *local* potential, are regarded as responses to antecedent activity within the same cell (when physiologically activated, not artificially stimulated); both are mediated by the local electric currents across the membrane as the result of the change in resistance of the already active regions and the standing "batteries" or electromotive forces between the two sides of the membrane. The one is regenerative, all-or-none, and propagated; the other is graded and decremental. In contrast, *generator* potentials of receptor neurons and *synaptic* potentials are responses of cells to impinging external events of specific kinds—sensory stimuli and junctional

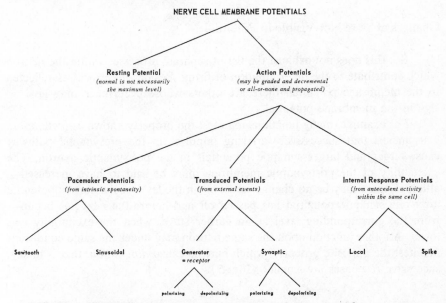

FIGURE 4. The types of nerve cell membrane potentials.

transmitters. There are two subdivisions of each of these categories based on the polarity of the response. On the basis of other differences, further subdivisions can be defined. There are also prepotentials resulting from no impinging environmental change but occurring under normal steady-state conditions and therefore properly called *spontaneous*. These can be manifested in more than one form: one is more or less sinusoidal (the time course is relatively independent of the occurrence of spikes); another is more or less saw-tooth-like (the time course is dependent on the intervention of a spike or local potential to reset the starting condition; a relaxation oscillation).

It is highly probable that some if not all of these different kinds of activity represent specialized kinds of cell surface membranes (9). This is suggested by the striking differences in properties and by the localization of each of these processes to restricted regions of the neuron. The circumscribed loci may recur at more than one site on the surface of a given neuron. Any one of the prepotentials is probably capable of causing spike initiation, at the restricted locus where this occurs, but commonly two or more prepotentials will act in sequence to this end. Perhaps any of the potentials can interact with any of the others to alter its rate of development or amplitude. But besides these sources of complexity a still more important source may prove to be the anatomical distribution of these different kinds of cell membrane over the neuron, their spatial separation, and the possibilities of interaction, of attenuation, and of invasion by the explosive all-or-none spike process. Only some regions of the cell are capable of supporting such a process, and perhaps it is just those which cannot support it that are most integrative.

Changes of State Not Visible in Potential

But this does not exhaust the list of separate processes within the neuron which contribute to the determination of firing. Besides the processes reflected in the membrane potential, there are others whose occurrence may give no sign in the membrane potential.

For example, many junctions manifest the property known as *facilitation*. This means that successively arriving impulses in the presynaptic pathway cause larger and larger synaptic potentials in the postsynaptic neuron. The excitability of the postsynaptic membrane may be said to have increased— although there may be no change whatever in the level of membrane potential after one synaptic potential has passed off and before the next has begun— from the corresponding level at an earlier stage, when the excitability was lower. Another junction upon the same neuron may under the same conditions manifest the opposite property, which may be called *diminution;* that is to say, successive responses are smaller (Fig. 5).

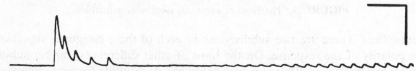

FIGURE 5. Facilitation and diminution. An ultramicroelectrode inside a nerve cell (of the cardiac ganglion of a lobster) recorded first the synaptic potentials resulting from a burst of five arriving impulses from one presynaptic pathway (from posterior small cells) and then those responding to a series of impulses arriving in another pathway (from the central nervous system). The former responses show diminution—the amplitude declines; the latter show facilitation—the amplitude grows. (Calibration, 100 msec, 21 mv.) [*Courtesy of Dr. Carlo Terzuolo.*]

Aftereffects provide still other indications of differences in excitability not predictable from the membrane potential. Some cells under certain conditions continue to fire for a considerable time after the input has ceased; others show the opposite response—namely, a prompt rebound or overshooting return after input has ceased. Thus, if the response to the input is an increase in the level of activity, then there may occur after the cessation of this input a continued afterdischarge—a maintained high level of activity for some time; or there may occur a rebound, which would mean in this case a period of decreased activity even below the previous background level. If on the other hand, the given input has for its effect an inhibition of ongoing activity, upon its cessation there may continue for a period an afterinhibition, or there may occur a rebound increase in activity above the previous ongoing level.

Whereas the classical concept of the neuron has recognized the importance of excitability, this has been measured or thought of in terms of the spike threshold. The spike threshold is certainly important, although only at one point in the neuron—namely, the point where spikes are initiated. After this initiation has occurred, the spike excitability elsewhere is relatively unimportant, because the margin of safety is usually quite large for the activation of each successive point along the axon. What the newer knowledge has added is understanding that prior to initiation of the spike there are critical forms of excitability not measured by thresholds, because they determine the responses of subthreshold, graded and local events as a function of what came before them.

Spontaneity

Still further increasing the complexity of the combination of processes possible is the tendency to spontaneous activity in some neurons. By means of penetrating microelectrodes, spontaneity has now been examined from within in a number of cells—central neurons, receptors, and pacemakers of the heart. The observed voltages are enormously greater than in the usual arrangement of two electrodes outside the cell shunted by extracellular fluids, and this has permitted new insight into the intimate events that occur prior to each spontaneous discharge.

As a consequence, we can see the *continual change of state* at the sub-threshold level, at least insofar as it is reflected in the potential of the cell body and nearby cell membrane (Fig. 6). We can infer also from the observations

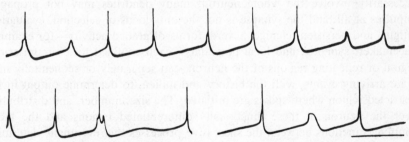

FIGURE 6. Spontaneous activity in a ganglion cell as revealed by an electrode inside the soma (nerve cell body). The spikes are about 10 mv here (electrotonically spread from the axon) and are followed by a repolarization, then a gradual depolarization—the pacemaker potential, which at a critical level sets off a local potential. This, in turn, usually rises high enough to trigger a spike but is seen here several times by itself. Once (in the first half of the bottom row) the local potential fails to be set off. (Time, 0.5 second.) [*Courtesy of Dr. Carlo Terzuolo.*]

that the tendency to spontaneous change of state inheres in certain restricted regions of the neuron (the pacemaker loci), which influence the rest in turn indirectly. Furthermore, there is evidence that, at least in some neurons, more than one locus of spontaneity can exist at the same time in different parts of the cell, each with a different rate of change of state. The continual change of state of parts of the neuron under steady conditions of its environment may have significance not only in generating spontaneous activity but also in altering the responsiveness of the cell to any input impinging upon it. In addition, the spontaneous subthreshold potential changes of one neuron may influence other neurons, perhaps by electrotonic spread over short processes and perhaps by less specific mass field effects—for example, when many cells "beat" in unison, as in brain waves (*10*).

Conclusion

In sum, anatomically the neuron doctrine has never been more firm. The classical controversy gradually focused upon the issue of protoplasmic or neurofibrillar continuity between neurons. Today, while a number of exceptional cases of nerve cell syncytia are commonly accepted (for example, giant fibers of earthworm and squid), the weight of evidence from silver impregnation and, especially in recent years, from electron microscopy is against any such continuity. Physiologically, however, we have a new appreciation of the complexity-within-unity of the neuron. Like a person, it is truly a functional unit, but it is composed of parts of very different function not only with respect to metabolism and maintenance but also in the realms of processing diverse input and determining output—that is, of integration. The impulse is not the only form of nerve cell activity; excitation of one part of the neuron does not necessarily involve the whole neuron; many dendrites may not propagate impulses at all; and the synapse is not the only locus of selection, evaluation, fatigue, and persistent change. Several forms of graded activity—for example, pacemaker, synaptic, and local potentials—each confined to a circumscribed region or repeating regions of the neuron, can separately or sequentially integrate arriving events, with the history and milieu, to determine output in the restricted region where spikes are initiated. The size, number, and distribution over the neuron of these functionally differentiated regions and the labile coupling functions between the successive processes that eventually determine what information is transferred to the next neuron provide an enormous range of possible complexity within this single cellular unit.

In the face of this gradual but sweeping change in functional concepts, any statement but the most diffuse about expectations for the future must be very dangerous. Nevertheless I will venture to suggest that in the near future we will gain significant new insight at this unitary level of neurophysiology with respect to the functions and differentiations among dendrites, the chemical and perhaps ultramicroscopic specification of different kinds of surface membrane, additional labile processes, sites of possible persistent change, and the normal functional significance of intercellular reactions mediated by graded activity without the intervention of all-or-none impulses.

References and Notes

1. S. Ramon y Cajal, *Neuron Theory or Reticular Theory?* (Consejo Superior de Investigaciones Cientificas, Madrid, 1954), English translation.
2. A. T. Rasmussen, *Some Trends in Neuroanatomy* (Brown, Dubuque, Iowa, 1947).
3. For a complete bibliography, see S. Ramon y Cajal, *Recollections of My Life;* English translation by E. H. Craigie, *Mem. Am. Phil. Soc.* **8** (1937).
4. T. H. Bullock and C. A. Terzuolo, *J. Physiol.* (*London*) **138**, 341 (1957).
5. F. Bremer, *Physiol. Revs.* **38**, 357 (1958).
6. T. H. Bullock, *Revs. Modern Phys.,* in press; *Exptl. Cell Research* **5**, suppl. 323 (1958).
7. G. Ling and R. W. Gerard, *J. Cellular Comp. Physiol.* **34**, 383 (1949).
8. The study by Watanabe and Bullock was aided by a grant from the National Institute of Neurological Diseases and Blindness, National Institutes of Health, and by a contract (NR 101-454) between the Office of Naval Research, Department of the Navy, and the University of California.
9. H. Grundfest, *Physiol. Revs.* **37**, 337 (1957).
10. See further: *Ciba Foundation Symposium, Neurological Basis of Behavior* (Churchill, London, 1958); J. C. Eccles, *The Physiology of Nerve Cells* (Johns Hopkins Press, Baltimore, Md., 1957); H. Fernandez-Moran and R. Brown, *Exptl. Cell Research* **5**, suppl. (1958); A. Fessard, *Proc. Intern. Physiol. Congr. 20th Congr. Brussels* (1956).
11. B. Hanström, *Arkiv. Zool.* **16**, 10 (1924).
12. S. Ramon y Cajal, *Histologie du Système Nerveux de l'Homme et des Vertébrés* (Maloine, Paris, 1909–11).
13. J. S. Alexandrowicz, *Quart J. Microscop. Sci.* **75**, 182 (1932).

The Ionic Basis of Nervous Conduction

A. L. HODGKIN

Reprinted from *Science*, Sept. 11, 1964, Vol. 145, pp. 1148–1154. Copyright 1964 by the American Association for the Advancement of Science.

Trinity College, Cambridge, which I entered in 1932, has a long-standing connection with neurophysiology. As an undergraduate I found myself interested in nerve and was soon reading books or papers by Keith Lucas (*1*), Adrian (*2*), Hill (*3*), and Rushton (*4*), all of whom are, or were, fellows of Trinity. I had a particular reason for looking at Lucas's papers because my father and Lucas had been close friends and both lost their lives during the first world war. My reading introduced me to Bernstein's membrane theory (5), in the form developed by Lillie (6), and I thought it would be interesting to test their assumptions by a simple experiment. A central point in the theory is that propagation of the impulse from one point to the next is brought about by the electric currents which flow between resting and active regions. On this view, the action potential is not just an electrical sign of the impulse, but is the causal agent in propagation. Nowadays the point is accepted by everyone, but at that time it lacked experimental proof. By a roundabout route I came across a fairly simple way of testing the idea. The method depended on firing an impulse at a localized block, and observing the effect of the impulse on the excitability of the nerve just beyond the block. It turned out that the impulse produced a transient increase in excitability over a distance of several millimeters, and that the increase was almost certainly caused by electric currents spreading in a local circuit through the blocked region (7). More striking evidence for the electrical theory was obtained later, for instance when it was shown that the velocity of the nerve impulse could be changed over a wide range by altering the electrical resistance of the external fluid (8). But this is not the place to describe these experiments, and I would like to take up the story again in 1938, when I had the good fortune to spend a year in Gasser's laboratory at the Rockefeller Institute in New York. Before leaving Cambridge I had found, by a lucky accident, that it was quite easy to isolate single nerve fibers from the shore crab, *Carinus maenas*. This opened up several interesting lines of investigation, and I became increasingly impressed with the advantages of working on single nerve fibers. *Carcinus* fibers are very robust, but they are at most $\frac{1}{30}$ millimeter in diameter and for many purposes this is inconveniently small. There was a good deal to be said for switching to the very much larger nerve fibers which J. Z. Young (9) had discovered in the squid and which were then being studied by Cole and Curtis (10) in Woods Hole. Squids of the genus *Loligo* are active creatures, 1 or 2 feet long, which can swim backward at high speed by taking water into a large cavity and squirting out a jet through a funnel in the front of the animal. The giant nerve fibers, which may be as much as a millimeter in diameter, run in the body wall and supply the muscles that expel water from the mantle cavity. Although these fibers are unmyelinated, their large size makes them conduct rapidly, and this may be the teleological reason for their existence. It should be said that large nerve fibers conduct faster than small ones (11) because the conductance per unit length of the core increases as the square of the diameter, whereas the electrical capacity of the surface increases only as the first power.

You may wonder how it is that we get along without giant nerve fibers. The answer is that vertebrates have developed myelinated axons in which the fiber is covered with a relatively thick insulating layer over most of its length, and the excitable membrane is exposed only at the nodes of Ranvier. In these fibers, conduction is saltatory and the impulse skips from one node to the next. I regret that shortage of time does not allow me to discuss this important development, with which the names of Kato, Tasaki, and Takeuchi (*12*) are particularly associated.

Early in 1938, K. S. Cole asked me to spend a few weeks in his laboratory at Woods Hole where squid are plentiful during the summer. I arrived in June 1938 and was greeted by a sensational experiment, the results of which were plainly visible on the screen of the cathode-ray tube. Cole and Curtis (*13*) had developed a technique which allowed them to measure changes in the electrical conductivity of the membrane during the impulse; when analyzed, their experiment proved that the membrane undergoes a large increase in conductance which has roughly the same time course as the electrical change (Fig. 1). This was strong evidence for an increase in ionic permeability, but

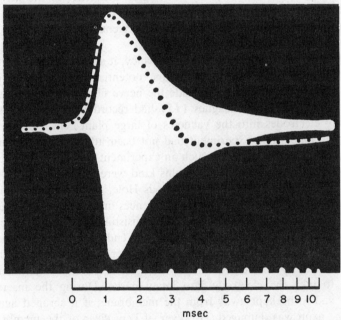

FIGURE 1. Action potential (dotted curve) and increase in conductance (white band) in squid axon at about 6°C [*From Cole and Curtis* (*13*).]

the experiment naturally did not show what ions were involved, and this aspect was not cleared up until several years after the war. At first sight, Cole and Curtis's results seemed to fit in with the idea that the membrane broke down during activity, as Bernstein and Lillie had suggested. However, there was one further point which required checking. According to Bernstein, activity consisted of a momentary breakdown of the membrane, and on this view the action potential should not exceed the resting potential. Huxley and I started to test this point early in 1939. We measured external electrical changes from *Car-*

cinus fibers immersed in oil with a cathode-ray tube, direct-current amplifier, and cathode followers as the recording instrument. The resting potential was taken from the steady potential between an intact region and one depolarized by injury or by isotonic potassium chloride. To our surprise we found that the action potential was often much larger than the resting potential—for example, 73 millivolts for the action potential as against 37 millivolts for the resting potential. [Although I was not aware of it until much later, Schaefer (*14*) had previously reported a similar discrepancy in the sartorius and gastrocnemius muscles of the frog.] Our results did not give the absolute value of the membrane potentials because of the short-circuiting effect of the film of sea water which clings to a fiber in oil. However, there is no reason why short-circuiting should affect one potential more than another, and the discrepancy seemed much too large to be explained by some small difference in the way the two potentials were recorded. Nevertheless, we were extremely suspicious of these results with external electrodes, and before they could be published both of us were caught up in the war.

Before going further with the discrepancy, it seemed important to establish the absolute value of the membrane potentials by recording potential differences between an electrode inside the nerve fiber and the external solution. Osterhout and his colleagues (*15*) had recorded internal potentials by introducing electrodes into the vacuoles of large plant cells, but for obvious reasons the comparable experiment had not been attempted with nerve. The best preparation on which to try such an experiment was the giant axon of the squid, and the first measurements of this kind were made during the summer of 1939 by Curtis and Cole (*16*) at Woods Hole, and by Huxley and myself (*17*) at Plymouth. There were minor differences in technique, but the general principle was the same. A microelectrode consisting of a long glass capillary, filled with saline or metal, was inserted at one end of the fiber and pushed in for a distance of 10 to 30 millimeters. The fiber was damaged at the point where the capillary entered it, but an insertion of 10 to 30 millimeters was sufficient to take the electrode into intact nerve. During the insertion the electrode had to be kept away from the membrane; if it scraped against the surface the axon was damaged. However, if kept clear of the membrane, the electrode did no harm, and it has since been shown that axons will conduct impulses for many hours after being impaled in this way. Figure 2*A* * shows an electrode inside an uncleaned axon; Figure 2*B* is similar, but the small nerve fibers round the giant axon have been removed and dark ground illumination has been used.

In 1939 both the Woods Hole and Plymouth groups found that large action potentials could be recorded between an internal electrode and the external solution, thus providing strong evidence for the idea that the action

* Editor's note: Figure 2 has been omitted.

potential arises at the surface membrane. With this technique Huxley and I again obtained the disturbing result that the action potential was much greater than the resting potential (*17*). Figure 3, which illustrates one of these experiments, shows an action potential of 86 millivolts and a resting potential of 45

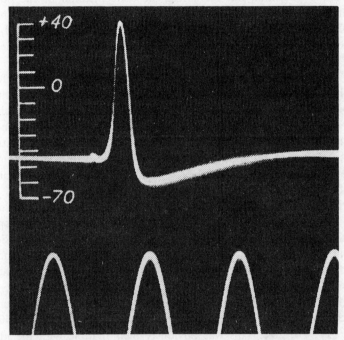

FIGURE 3. Action potential and resting potential recorded between inside and outside of axon with capillary filled with sea water. Time marker, 500 cy/sec. The vertical scale indicates the potential of the internal electrode in millivolts, the sea water outside being taken as at zero potential. [*From Hodgkin and Huxley* (17); *see also* 23.]

millivolts. In their 1939 experiments Curtis and Cole (*16*) recorded the action potential with a condenser-coupled amplifier; later measurements with a d-c amplifier gave an average action potential of 108 millivolts and an average resting potential of 51 millivolts (*18*). Curtis and Cole also showed that the resting potential could be abolished, reversibly, by increasing the external potassium concentration until it was about the same as that in the axoplasm; at high concentrations the membrane behaved like a potassium electrode, as predicted by Bernstein's theory.

The small size of most nerve or muscle fibers made it difficult to extend the technique employed for the giant axon to other preparations. However, another very convenient and powerful method was developed by Graham, Gerard, and Ling, who showed that extremely small glass capillaries could be inserted transversely into muscle fibers without causing appreciable damage

(*19*). In order to obtain consistent results it is desirable that the electrodes should have an external diameter of less than 0.5 micron. This small diameter means that the electrodes have a high resistance, and special precautions must be taken with the recording system. Initially the electrodes were used to measure the resting potential, but increasing the concentration of the potassium chloride in the electrode to 3 molar enabled the action potential to be recorded as well (*20*). Many types of excitable cell have now been examined, and in nearly every case it has been found that the action potential exceeds the resting potential, often by 40 to 50 millivolts.

Yet another method is required for myelinated nerve fibers, which do not take kindly to impalement. A useful way of eliminating external short circuiting was introduced by Huxley and Stämpfli in 1950 (*21*), and their method has been refined in a very elegant way by Frankenhaeuser (*22*). The values found by applying these methods to amphibian nerve fibers are: action potential, 120 millivolts; resting potential, 70 millivolts. Absolute values for mammalian nerve fibers are not known, but they are probably not very different from those reported for frog.

At the end of the war, the position was that several of Bernstein's assumptions had been vindicated in a striking way, but that in one major respect the classical theory had been shown to be wrong. By 1945 most neurophysiologists agreed that the action potential was propagated by electric currents, and that it arose at the surface membrane; it was also clear that the resting potential was at least partly due to the electromotive force of the potassium concentration cell. On the other hand, there was impressive evidence that in both crab and squid fibers the action potential exceeded the resting potential by 40 to 50 millivolts (*17, 18, 23*). This was obviously incompatible with the idea that electrical activity depended on a breakdown of the membrane; some process giving a reversal of electromotive force was required.

The Sodium Hypothesis

There were several early attempts to provide a theoretical basis for the reversal, but most of these were speculative and not easily subject to experimental test. A simpler explanation, now known as the sodium hypothesis, was worked out with Katz and Huxley and tested during the summer of 1947 (*24*). The hypothesis, which undoubtedly owed a good deal to the classical experiments of Overton (*25*), was based on a comparison of the ionic composition of the axoplasm of squid nerve with that of blood or sea water. As in Bernstein's theory, it was assumed that the resting membrane is selectively permeable to potassium ions and that the potential across it arises from the tendency of these ions to move outward from the more concentrated solution inside a nerve or muscle fiber. In the limiting case, where a membrane which is permeable only to potassium separates axoplasm containing 400 mM K from plasma containing 20 mM K, the internal potential should be 75 millivolts negative to the external solution. This value is obtained from the Nernst relation

$$V_K = \frac{RT}{F} \ln \frac{[K]_o}{[K]_i} \tag{1}$$

where V_K is the equilibrium potential of the potassium ion defined in the sense internal potential minus external potential and $[K]_o$ and $[K]_i$ are potassium concentrations (strictly, activities) inside and outside the fiber. Resting potentials of 70 millivolts have been observed in undissected squid axons (26); the smaller values found in isolated axons may be explained by a leakage of sodium into fiber. If the permeability to sodium were 1/12 that to potassium, a potential of about 50 millivolts is predicted for an isolated axon in sea water (350 mM K, the mM Na in axoplasm 10 mM K, 450 mM Na in sea water).

From Bernstein's theory it might be assumed that when the membrane broke down, the ratio of the permeabilities to Na and K would approach that of the aqueous mobilities of these ions, about 0.7 to 1. In that case, the action potential could not exceed the resting potential and would in fact be less by at least 8 millivolts. However, it is simple to rescue the hypothesis by assuming that the active membrane undergoes a large and selective increase in permeability to sodium. In the extreme case, where the membrane is much more permeable to sodium than to any other ion, the potential should approach that given by the Nernst formula; that is,

$$V_{Na} = \frac{RT}{F} \ln \frac{[Na]_o}{[Na]_i} \tag{2}$$

This gives a limiting value of + 58 millivolts for the tenfold concentration ratio observed by Steinbach and Spiegelman (27) and accounts satisfactorily for the reversal of 50 millivolts commonly seen in intact axons.

A simple consequence of the sodium hypothesis is that the magnitude of the action potential should be greatly influenced by the concentration of sodium ions in the external fluid. For the active membrane should no longer be capable of giving a reversed electromotive force if the concentration of sodium is equalized on the two sides of the membrane. The first quantitative tests were made with Katz, in the summer of 1947. They showed that the action potential, but not the resting potential, was reduced by replacing external sodium chloride with choline chloride or with glucose. If all the external sodium was removed the axon became reversibly inexcitable, in agreement with Overton's experiment on frog muscle. Figure 4 illustrates one of the experiments. In the physiological region, the overshoot varied with external sodium concentrations in the same manner as a sodium electrode (24).

It was also shown that a solution containing extra sodium increased the overshoot by about the amount predicted by Eq. 2. This is a particularly satisfactory result, because it seems most unlikely that an increase beyond the

normal could be brought about by an abnormal solution. Figure 5 illustrates
one of these experiments. Later Stämpfli (*28*) showed that at the node of
Ranvier an increase of about 35 millivolts in the overshoot is brought about
by a fourfold increase of external sodium.

The effect of varying external sodium concentration has now been
studied on a number of excitable tissues: for example, frog muscle (*20*),
myelinated nerve (*29*), Purkinje fibers of the heart (*30*), and crustacean
nerve (*31*). In all these cases the results were very similar to those in the
squid axon.

There are at least two cases where the mechanism is thought to be
basically different. These are crab muscle, in which an entry of calcium, or
other divalent cations, provides the inward current (*32*), and the plant cell,
Chara, where an exit of chloride ions from the vacuolar sap may be the primary process (*33*).

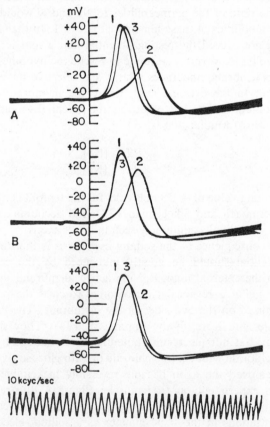

FIGURE 4. Effect of sodium-deficient external solutions on the action potential of a giant
axon. Records labeled 1 and 3 were with the axon in sea water; a2, with 0.33 sea water,
0.67 isotonic dextrose; b2, with 0.5 sea water, 0.5 isotonic dextrose; c2, with 0.7 sea
water, 0.3 isotonic dextrose. [*From Hodgkin and Katz* (24).]

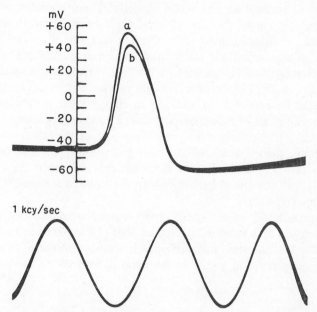

FIGURE 5. Effect of sodium-rich external solution on the action potential of a giant axon. Record *a*, in sea water; record *b*, 50 seconds after applying sea water containing additional NaCl (Na concentration, 1.56 times that in sea water). [*From Hodgkin and Katz* (24).]

Ionic Movement During Activity

During the period 1947–51 several investigators started to measure the effect of stimulation on the movements of labeled sodium across the surface membrane of giant axons. As often happens, work proceeded independently and more or less simultaneously on the two sides of the Atlantic, the principal investigators being Keynes (*34*) in England and Rothenberg (*35*) and Grundfest and Nachmansohn (*36*) in America. In 1949 Keynes reported that stimulation of *Sepia* axons at 100 per second caused a 15-fold increase in the rate of uptake of ^{24}Na. There was also a substantial increase in the outflow of labeled sodium, and at first it was difficult to decide whether activity was associated with a net uptake of sodium. Keynes and Lewis (*37*) resolved the difficulty by measuring the sodium concentration in axoplasm by activation analysis, and there is now general agreement that at 20°C the net entry of sodium in one impulse amounts to 3 to 4×10^{-12} mole per square centimeter. Other experiments showed that a similar quantity of potassium ions leave the fiber during an impulse (*38*). It is perhaps easier to get an idea of what these quantities mean by saying that one impulse is associated with an inward movement of 20,000 sodium ions through 1 square micron of surface.

An entry of 4×10^{-12} mole of sodium per square centimeter is more than enough to account for the action potential. From the work of Cole and his colleagues it is known that the electrical capacity of the membrane is about 1 microfarad per square centimeter (*10*). The quantity of charge required to change the voltage across a 1-microfarad condenser by 120 millivolts is 1.2 $\times$ 10^{-7} coulomb; this is equivalent to 1.2×10^{-12} mole of monovalent cation, which is only one-third of the observed entry of sodium. A discrepancy in this direction is to be expected. In addition to charging the membrane capacity during the rising phase of the action potential, a good deal of sodium exchanges with potassium, particularly during the early part of the falling phase. From the quantitative theory which Huxley and I developed, the size of the ionic movements can be predicted from electrical measurements. As Huxley describes (*39*), the theoretical quantities turn out to be in reasonable agreement with experimental values.

The quantity of sodium which enters a myelinated axon during an impulse is much less than in an unmyelinated fiber of comparable size (*40*). This is presumably because the ionic exchange is confined to the node of Ranvier and the capacity per unit length of the axon is reduced by the thick myelin sheath.

Analysis of Membrane Currents:
Voltage Clamp Experiments

In pursuing the evidence for the ionic theory I have departed from the strict order of events. During the summer of 1947 Cole and Marmont (*41, 42*) developed a technique for impaling squid axons with long metallic electrodes; with this technique they were able to apply current uniformly to the membrane and to avoid the complications introduced by spread of current in a cable-like structure. Cole (*41*) also carried out an important type of experiment in which the potential difference across the membrane is made to undergo a steplike change and the experimental variable is the current which flows through the membrane. In Cole's experiments a single internal electrode was used for recording potential and passing current; since the current may be large, electrode polarization introduces an error and makes it difficult to use steps longer than a millisecond. However, the essential features of the experiment, notably the existence of a phase of inward current over a range of depolarizations, are plainly shown in the records which Cole obtained in 1947 (*41*). It was obvious that the method could be improved by inserting two internal electrodes, one for current, the other for voltage, and by employing electronic feedback to supply the current needed to maintain a constant voltage. Cole, Marmont, and I discussed this possibility in the spring of 1948, and it was used at Plymouth the following summer by Huxley, Katz, and myself (*43*). Further improvements were made during the winter, and in 1949 we obtained a large number of records which were analyzed in Cambridge during the next 2 years (*44*). Huxley describes these results in more detail (*39*); here all that need be said is that by varying the external ionic concentrations it was possible to separate the ionic current flowing through the membrane into components carried by sodium and potassium, and hence to determine how the ionic permeability varied with time and with membrane potential.

To begin with, we hoped that the analysis might lead to a definite molecular model of the membrane. However, it gradually became clear that different mechanisms could lead to similar equations and that no real progress at the molecular level could be made until much more was known about the chemistry and fine structure of the membrane. On the other hand, the equations that we developed proved surprisingly powerful, and it was possible to predict much of the electrical behavior of the giant axon with fair accuracy. Examples of some of the properties of the axon which are fitted by the equations are: the form, duration, and amplitude of the action potential; the conduction velocity, impedance changes, ionic movements; and subthreshold phenomena, including the oscillatory behavior.

Experimental Work on Giant Axons Since 1952

In the last part of this lecture I should like to mention some of the more recent developments in the ionic theory of nervous conduction. One major problem, which has interested a number of physiologists and biochemists, is to find out how cells use metabolic energy to move sodium and potassium ions against concentration gradients. In excitable tissues this process is of particular interest because it builds up the ionic concentration differences on which conduction of impulses depends. When a nerve fiber carries an impulse it undergoes a rapid cycle of permeability changes which allow first sodium and then potassium ions to move down concentration gradients. In giant axons, the changes associated with an impulse are exceedingly small, as can be seen from the fact that a 500-micron axon loses only one-millionth of its internal potassium in a single impulse. Large fibers can therefore conduct many impulses without recharging their batteries by metabolism. Nevertheless, if they are to be of any use to the animal, nerve fibers must be equipped with a mechanism for reversing the ionic exchanges that occur during electrical activity. The necessity for such a system was foreseen by Overton in 1902 when he pointed out that human heart muscle carried out some 2.4×10^9 contractions in 70 years, yet, as far as he knew, contained as much potassium and as little sodium in old age as in early youth (*25*). Forty years later Dean introduced the idea of a sodium pump and showed that the distribution of potassium and chloride in muscle might be a passive consequence of an active extrusion of sodium, but that active transport of potassium or chloride ions would by themselves be inadequate (*45*). The concept was developed further by Krogh (*46*) and

Ussing (47) and is now supported by experiments on a wide range of animal tissues.

Giant nerve fibers provide excellent material for studying ion pumping. One approach is to inject radioactive sodium ions and to collect the labeled ions which emerge from the fiber. Such experiments show that if the fiber is poisoned with cyanide or dinitrophenol it stops pumping, and sodium ions gradually accumulate inside. The fiber remains excitable for many hours because sodium and potassium can still move downhill during the impulse. But any sodium which gets into the fiber remains there and is not extruded as it would be in an unpoisoned axon. The ability to extrude sodium depends on the presence of adenosine triphosphate (ATP), and with an axon in which all the ATP has been broken down, sodium extrusion can be restored by injecting energy-rich phosphate in the right form (48). Figure 6 illustrates one of these experiments. It shows that the outflow of sodium is reduced to a low value by

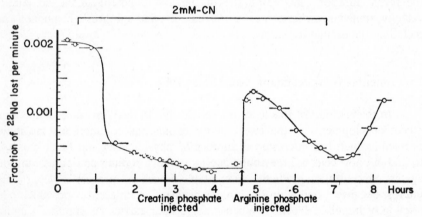

FIGURE 6. Effect on outflow of sodium of (i) poisoning with cyanide; (ii) injecting creatine phosphate; (iii) arginine phosphate; (iv) removal of cyanide. The mean concentrations in the axon after injection were 15.3 mM creatine phosphate and 15.8 mM arginine phosphate. [From Caldwell et al. (48).]

cyanide and can be restored by the molluscan phosphagen, arginine phosphate, but not by the vertebrate phosphagen, creatine phosphate. This is a satisfactory result since it is known that creatine phosphate is not handled by the enzyme which catalyzes the transfer of phosphate from arginine phosphate to adenosine diphosphate (49).

The molecular nature of the pumping mechanism is unknown, but there is much evidence to show that in most cells it is driven by compounds containing energy-rich phosphate, such as ATP or phosphagen. Recent interest in this field has been focused by Skou on an ATP-splitting enzyme which is present in the membrane and has the interesting properties of being activated by sodium and potassium and inhibited by substances which interfere with sodium transport (50).

Perfusion of Giant Axons

In conclusion I should like to mention an interesting new method which has been developed during the last few years. Since the action potential of a nerve fiber arises at the surface membrane it should be possible to replace the protoplasm inside the fiber with an aqueous solution of appropriate composition. Methods for perfusing axons were worked out by Tasaki and his colleagues at Woods Hole (51) and by Baker and Shaw at Plymouth (52). The technique used at Plymouth is based on the observation (53) that most of the axoplasm in giant nerve fibers can be squeezed out of the cut end. This has been known since 1937, but until fairly recently no one paid much attention to the electrical properties of the thin sheath which remained after the contents of the nerve fiber had been removed. Since extrusion involves flattening the axon with a glass rod or roller it was natural to suppose that the membrane would be badly damaged by such a drastic method. However, in the autumn of 1960 Baker and Shaw (52) recorded action potentials from extruded sheaths which had been refilled with isotonic solution of a potassium salt. On further investigation (54) it turned out that such preparations gave action potentials of the usual magnitude for several hours, and that these were abolished, reversibly, by replacing potassium with sodium in the internal solution. As can be seen from Figures 7 and 8, the resting potential and action potential vary with the internal concentrations of potassium and sodium in a manner which is consistent with the external effect of these ions.

A point of some general interest is that, although about 95 percent of the

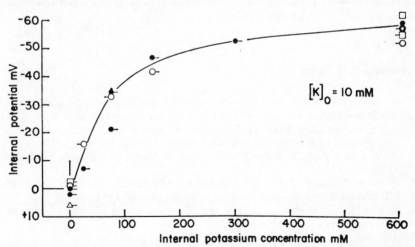

FIGURE 7. Effect of varying internal potassium concentration on the resting potential. External solution, sea water containing 10 mM K; internal solution, NaCl-KCl solutions isotonic with sea water. Note that the resting potential reaches a limiting value of about -55 millivolts at potassium concentration greater than 150 mM. [*From Baker et al. (54).*]

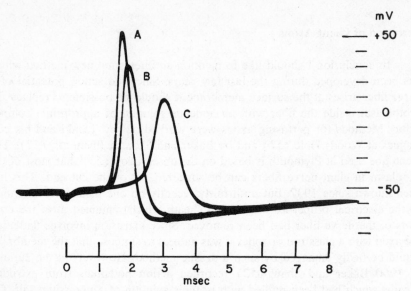

FIGURE 8. Effect on action potential of replacing internal potassium with sodium ions. (A) Isotonic potassium sulfate; (B) 0.25 K replaced by Na; (C) 0.5 K replaced by Na. The records were obtained in the order B, A, C. [From Baker et al. (54).]

axoplasm had been removed, axon membranes perfused with isotonic potassium solutions were able to carry some 300,000 impulses. This reinforces the idea that chemical reactions in the bulk of the axoplasm are not essential for conduction of impulses and that ionic concentration gradients provide the immediate source of energy for the action potential. Huxley (*39*) tells more about the way in which this is done.

References and Notes

1. K. Lucas, *The Conduction of the Nervous Impulse* (Longmans, London, 1917); collected papers (mainly in *J. Physiol. London*) 1904–14.
2. E. D. Adrian, *The Basis of Sensation* (Christophers, London, 1928); *The Mechanism of Nervous Action* (Oxford Univ. Press, Oxford, 1932).
3. A. V. Hill, *Chemical Wave Transmission in Nerve* (Cambridge Univ. Press, Cambridge, 1932).
4. W. A. H. Rushton, *J. Physiol. London* **63**, 357 (1927); *ibid.* **82**, 332 (1934).
5. J. Bernstein, *Elektrobiologie* (Wieweg, Braunschweig, 1912).
6. R. S. Lillie, *Protoplasmic Action and Nervous Action* (Chicago Univ. Press, Chicago, 1923).
7. A. L. Hodgkin, *J. Physiol. London* **90**, 183 (1937); *ibid.*, p. 211.
8. A. L. Hodgkin, *ibid.* **94**, 560 (1939).
9. J. Z. Young, *Quart. J. Microscop. Sci.* **78**, 367 (1936); *Cold Spring Harbor Symp. Quant. Biol.* **4**, 1 (1936).
10. H. J. Curtis and K. S. Cole, *J. Gen. Physiol.* **21**, 757 (1938).
11. H. S. Gasser and J. Erlanger, *Am. J. Physiol.* **80**, 522 (1927).

12. G. Kato, *The Microphysiology of Nerve* (Maruzen, Tokyo, 1934); I. Tasaki, *Am. J. Physiol.* **125**, 380 (1937); I. Tasaki, *ibid.* **127**, 211 (1939); I. Tasaki and T. Takeuchi, *Arch. Ges. Physiol.* **244**, 696 (1941); I. Tasaki and T. Takeuchi, *ibid.* **245**, 764 (1942).
13. K. S. Cole and H. J. Curtis, *J. Gen. Physiol.* **22**, 649 (1939).
14. H. Schaefer, *Arch. Ges. Physiol.* **237**, 329 (1936).
15. W. J. V. Osterhout, *Biol. Rev. Cambridge Phil. Soc.* **6**, 369 (1931).
16. H. J. Curtis and K. S. Cole, *J. Cellular Comp. Physiol.* **15**, 147 (1940).
17. A. L. Hodgkin and A. F. Huxley, *Nature* **144**, 710 (1939).
18. H. J. Curtis and K. S. Cole, *J. Cellular Comp. Physiol.* **19**, 135 (1942).
19. J. Graham and R. W. Gerard, *ibid.* **28**, 99 (1946); G. Ling and R. W. Gerard, *ibid.* **34**, 383 (1949).
20. W. L. Nastuk and A. L. Hodgkin, *ibid.* **35**, 39 (1950).
21. A. F. Huxley and R. Stämpfli, *J. Physiol. London* **112**, 476 (1951); *ibid.*, p. 496.
22. B. Frankenhaeuser, *ibid.* **135**, 550 (1957).
23. A. L. Hodgkin and A. F. Huxley, *ibid.* **104**, 176 (1945).
24. A. L. Hodgkin and B. Katz, *ibid.* **108**, 37 (1949).
25. E. Overton, *Arch. Ges. Physiol.* **92**, 346 (1902).
26. A. L. Hodgkin and R. D. Keynes, reported in A. L. Hodgkin, *Proc. Roy. Soc. London* **B148**, 1 (1958); J. W. Moore and K. S. Cole, *J. Gen. Physiol.* **43**, 961 (1960).
27. H. B. Steinbach and S. Spiegelman, *J. Cellular Comp. Physiol.* **22**, 187 (1943).
28. R. Stämpfli, *J. Physiol. Paris* **48**, 710 (1956).
29. A. F. Huxley and R. Stämpfli, *J. Physiol. London* **112**, 496 (1951).
30. M. H. Drafer and S. Weidmann, *ibid.* **115**, 74 (1951).
31. J. C. Dalton, *J. Gen. Physiol.* **41**, 529 (1958).
32. P. Fatt and B. Katz, *J. Physiol. London* **120**, 171 (1953); P. Fatt and B. L. Ginsborg, *ibid.*, **142**, 516 (1958).
33. C. T. Gaffey and L. J. Mullins, *ibid.* **144**, 505 (1958).
34. R. D. Keynes, *Arch. Sci. Physiol.* **3**, 165 (1949); *J. Physiol. London* **109**, 13P (1949); *ibid.* **114**, 119 (1951).
35. M. A. Rothenberg, *Biochim. Biophys. Acta* **4**, 96 (1950).
36. H. Grundfest and D. Nachmansohn, *Federation Proc.* **9**, 53 (1950).
37. R. D. Keynes and P. R. Lewis, *J. Physiol. London* **114**, 151 (1951).
38. R. D. Keynes, *ibid.* **107**, 35P (1948); *ibid.* **113**, 99 (1950); *ibid.* **114**, 119 (1951); A. M. Shanes, *Am. J. Physiol.* **177**, 377 (1954).
39. A. F. Huxley, *Science,* **145**, 1154 (1964).
40. T. Asano and W. P. Hurlbut, *J. Gen. Physiol.* **41**, 1187 (1958).
41. K. S. Cole, *Arch. Sci. Physiol.* **3**, 253 (1949).
42. G. Marmont, *J. Cellular Comp. Physiol.* **34**, 351 (1949).
43. A. L. Hodgkin, A. F. Huxley, B. Katz, *Arch. Sci. Physiol.* **3**, 129 (1949).
44. A. L. Hodgkin, A. F. Huxley, B. Katz, *J. Physiol. London* **116**, 424 (1951); A. L. Hodgkin and A. F. Huxley, *ibid.*, p. 449; A. L. Hodgkin and A. F. Huxley, *ibid.*, p. 473; A. L. Hodgkin and A. F. Huxley, *ibid.*, p. 497; A. L. Hodgkin and A. F. Huxley, *ibid.* **117**, 500 (1951); A. L. Hodgkin and A. F. Huxley, *ibid.* **121**, 403 (1953).
45. R. B. Dean, *Biol. Symp.* **3**, 331 (1941).
46. A. Krogh, *Proc. Roy. Soc. London* **B133**, 140 (1946).
47. H. H. Ussing, *Physiol. Rev.* **29**, 127 (1949).
48. P. C. Caldwell, A. L. Hodgkin, R. D. Keynes, T. I. Shaw, *J. Physiol. London* **152**, 561 (1960).
49. A. H. Ennor and J. F. Morrison, *Physiol. Rev.* **38**, 631 (1958).

50. J. C. Skou, *Biochim. Biophys. Acta* **23,** 394 (1957).
51. T. Oikawa, C. S. Spyropoulos, I. Tasaki, T. Teorell, *Acta Physiol. Scand.* **52,** 195 (1961).
52. P. F. Baker and T. I. Shaw, *J. Marine Biol. Assoc.* **41,** 855 (1961).
53. R. S. Bear, F. O. Schmitt, J. Z. Young, *Proc. Roy. Soc. London* **B123,** 505 (1937).
54. P. F. Baker, A. L. Hodgkin, T. I. Shaw, *Nature* **190,** 885 (1961); *J. Physiol. London* **164,** 330 (1962); *ibid.,* p. 355.
55. A. L. Hodgkin and R. D. Keynes, *J. Physiol. London* **131,** 592 (1956).
56. A more complete bibliography can be found in A. L. Hodgkin, *Conduction of the Nervous Impulse* (Liverpool Univ. Press, Liverpool, 1963); also in *Biol. Rev. Cambridge Phil. Soc.* **26,** 339 (1951) and *Proc. Roy. Soc. London* **B148,** 1 (1958). From the bibliography it is evident that the development of the ionic theory has been very much a cooperative effort, and I wish to thank all those who have contributed to it. For more direct help, my particular thanks are due to W. A. H. Rushton, K. S. Cole, H. J. Curtis, A. F. Huxley, B. Katz, and R. D. Keynes. I am very grateful to the professors of physiology at Cambridge, Sir Joseph Barcroft, Lord Adrian, and Sir Bryan Matthews, and to the director and staff of the laboratory at Plymouth. I should record my gratitude to R. H. Cook for the design and construction of apparatus and for his unfailing help.

A Direct Synaptic Connection Mediating Both Excitation and Inhibition

HOWARD WACHTEL AND
ERIC R. KANDEL

Reprinted from *Science,* Dec. 1, 1967, Vol. 158, No. 3805, pp. 1206–1208. Copyright 1967 by the American Association for the Advancement of Science.

Direct synaptic connections between two nerve cells have been assumed to mediate either postsynaptic excitation or inhibition, but not both. We have found a connection between two identified cells in the abdominal ganglion of the marine mollusc *Aplysia californica* which mediates both excitation and inhibition. The sign of the synaptic action is determined by the firing rate of the presynaptic element. This finding is of further interest because it contributes to an understanding of the topographical determinants of synaptic action in this ganglion.

The abdominal ganglion can be divided into quarters, each of which contains a number of cells that can be identified on the basis of morphological and electrophysiological criteria (Fig. 1*A*) (*1*). One identified cell, L10, is an interneuron which innervates many other identified cells. This interneuron produces inhibitory postsynaptic potentials (IPSP's) in identified cells in the left rostral quarter ganglion (LRQG) and excitatory postsynaptic pontentials (EPSP's) in cells in the right caudal quarter ganglion (RCQG) (2). In the left caudal quarter ganglion (LCQG) the interneuron produces IPSP's in some cells and EPSP's in others. Cell L7, which receives both EPSP's and IPSP's from L10, lies in this quarter ganglion.

Figure 1B shows a simultaneous recording from L7 and L3, two follower cells of L10. Cell L10 generates a burst of postsynaptic potentials which is synchronous in both follower cells. When the frequency of the postsynaptic potentials in the burst is low, the unitary IPSP's in L3 are synchronous with

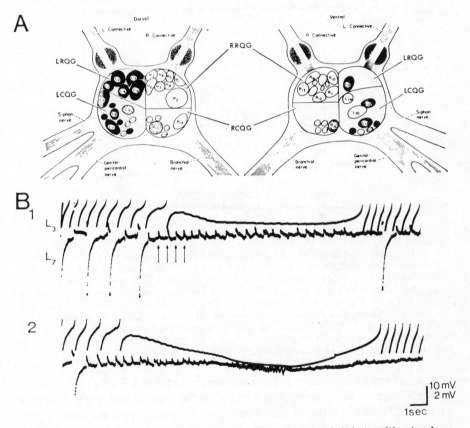

FIGURE 1. A. Schematic drawing of the abdominal ganglion of *Aplysia californica* showing the typical position of the 30 identified cells and of several cell clusters. Cells receiving an inhibitory connection from L10 are shown in black, those receiving an excitatory connection from L10 are stippled. Cell L7 receiving the dual connection is shown half black and half stippled. B. Simultaneous intracellular recordings from L3 and L7, showing common postsynaptic potentials from the interneuron (L10) firing in bursts. The arrows in the upper pair of records indicate several EPSP's in L7 occurring simultaneously with IPSP's in L3. In the lower pair of records a very fast burst from the common interneuron causes the IPSP's in L3 to summate into a smooth hyperpolarization, while the EPSP's in L7 invert to IPSP's.

EPSP's in L7 (Fig. 1, *B1*). Occasionally the burst reaches a higher frequency (Fig. 1, *B2*); when this occurs the IPSP's in L3 summate into a smooth hyperpolarization, whereas the EPSP's in L7 show a progressive decrement and finally invert to IPSP's.

To study the inversion more directly, we impaled L10 and controlled its firing by passing current through the microelectrode (Fig. 2). When the inter-

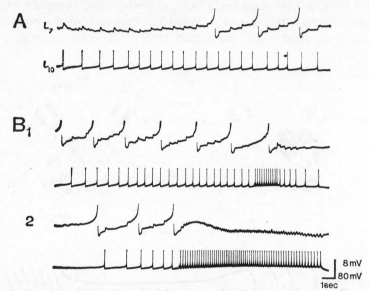

FIGURE 2. Simultaneous intercellular recordings from the follower cell L7 and the interneuron L10 showing a direct, double action, connection between them. A. L10 is firing at a slow rate (about one per second), and every action potential produces an EPSP in L7. B. B1 and B2 are continuous records. L10 is initially firing at a slow rate, producing EPSP's in L7, but when it is briefly speeded (B1) the EPSP's grow smaller and soon invert to IPSP's. For a short time after L10 returns to a slow rate the IPSP's persist, but gradually the initial EPSP state is restored (beginning of B2). When L10 is again speeded up (middle of B2) the EPSP's at first summate to depolarize L7 but then invert to IPSP's, which in turn summate to hyperpolarize L7. The IPSP amplitude remains stable as long as the high firing rate of L10 is maintained.

neuron is fired slowly, every spike produces an EPSP in L7 (Fig. 2*A*). When the interneuron is fired rapidly, the EPSP's diminish in size and invert to IPSP's (Fig. 2, *B1*). If the firing of the interneuron is again slowed, the IPSP's persist for a number of spikes before the initial EPSP state is restored (beginning of Fig. 2, *B2*). A second and maintained increase in the firing rate of the interneuron produces a summated postsynaptic potential which is diphasic, consisting of an early and brief depolarization followed by a sustained hyperpolarization (end of Fig. 2, *B2*). The EPSP's produced by L10 can summate to increase the firing rate of L7, and the IPSP's inhibit firing (Fig. 2*B*).

The postsynaptic potentials in L7 follow the maximum firing frequency of L10. The EPSP does so initially; the IPSP, indefinitely. These data suggest that the double action is mediated monosynaptically. This was further examined with latency measurements. When we superimposed records (taken at high sweep speeds) of the action potentials of L10 and the postsynaptic potentials of L7 before and after their inversion we found that the latency for the two postsynaptic potentials was equal (Fig. 3*A*). However, the latency for the postsynaptic potentials is at the upper limit of that generally encountered for presumed monosynaptic connections in this ganglion (*2*), and the possibility of two tightly interposed interneurons, one for excitation and the other for inhibition, could not be excluded from these findings alone. We tested whether the dual action results from the release of one or of more transmitters. If the connection is monosynaptic the dual action is likely to be mediated by one transmitter in accordance with Dale's principles (*3*). The demonstration of a single transmitter in turn strengthens the arguments for a monosynaptic connection.

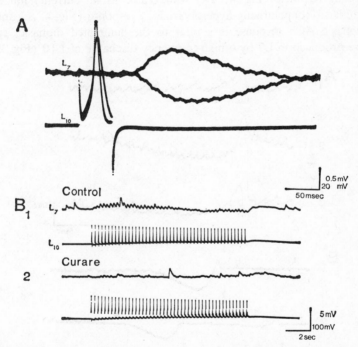

FIGURE 3. A. Simultaneous high-speed recordings photographically superimposed to show a comparison of the latency of the EPSP and IPSP from L10 on L7. The IPSP is associated with the shorter and broader of the two action potentials in L10. The change in the configuration of the action potential of L10 results from the high firing rates needed to produce the inversion of the postsynaptic potentials in L7. B. Simultaneous recordings from L7 and L10 showing the effect of curare. The control record shows both EPSP's and IPSP's in L7, produced by firing L10 at four spikes per second for 10 seconds. In the lower pair of records, taken 15 minutes after the application of *d*-tubocurarine (10^{-4} g/ml), both the EPSP and IPSP have been blocked. Some other postsynaptic potentials produced in L7 by different interneurons are not blocked by curare.

Anatomically verified monosynaptic connections between L10 and other follower cells (for example, L3, R15, and so forth) can be blocked by curare and appear to be cholinergic *(2, 4)*. When we bathed the ganglion in a solution of 10^{-4} g of curare per milliliter of seawater, both the excitatory and inhibitory phases of the dual response in L7 were blocked (Fig. 3*B*). This finding suggests that both the EPSP's and the IPSP's result from cholinergic synaptic transmission and implies a single transmitter.

To further examine the possibility that one transmitter could produce opposite actions on a single follower cell, we applied acetylcholine (ACh) iontophoretically to the cell body of L7 with an external microelectrode. Iontophoretic application has the advantage of limiting the action of ACh to an area probably less than 50 μ in diameter *(5)* and provides the best experimental approximation of a single synaptic knob. Figure 4*A* shows the responses of L7 to pulses of ACh of increasing duration. A brief pulse gives a pure depolarizing response (Fig. 4, *A1*) while (at constant current) longer ones give a diphasic (depolarizing-hyperpolarizing) response (Fig. 4, *A2* and *A3*). The diphasic ACh response is similar to the summated diphasic, synaptic response produced in L7 by a high-frequency discharge of L10 (Fig. 2, *B2*);

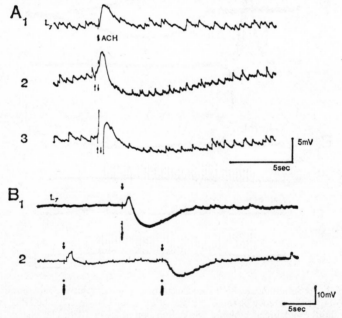

FIGURE 4. A. Recordings from L7 showing the effects of iontophoretic applications of ACh. A very brief pulse of ACh (arrows) results in a pure depolarization (A1). A longer pulse of ACh produces a diphasic response consisting of an early, brief depolarization followed by a longer hyperpolarization (A2). The early depolarization is effective in producing an action potential (A3). B. Recordings from L7 showing desensitization of the D component following repeated iontophoretic application of ACh. In B1 a single, strong application of ACh produces a diphasic response (D-H), whereas in B2 two consecutive weaker applications produce first a D response and then an H response. The separate responses (in B2) are similar to the constituent components of the diphasic response (B1).

the depolarizing phase of the ACh response causes L7 to fire, whereas its hyperpolarizing phase inhibits it. This response to ACh is quite distinct from the monophasic responses shown by other identified cells receiving single actions from L10. For example, L3, which receives only IPSP's from L10, responds to ACh by pure hyperpolarization; whereas R15, which receives only EPSP's from L10, responds with a pure depolarization. Indeed, diphasic responses have not been previously reported in surveys of the cells in this ganglion which categorized the response to ACh as being either purely depolarizing (D) or hyperpolarizing (H) (6). Our finding implies the existence of a new pharmacological cell type (D-H) with dual receptor properties (7). The ability to produce the dual response with highly localized applications of ACh also suggests that the two receptor types are spatially closely related.

With iontophoretic application of ACh we were also able to explore two alternative mechanisms—one presynaptic, the other postsynaptic—which could account for inversion of the postsynaptic potential: (i) The EPSP and IPSP might be mediated by independent branches of L10 ending separately on the two receptor patches, and the decrement of the EPSP could be caused by a presynaptic failure of the excitatory branch due to blocking at high rates of stimulation. Alternatively (ii) the EPSP and IPSP might be mediated by a single branch of L10 which ends on both receptors, and the decrement could represent a rapid desensitization of the excitatory receptor. With repeated iontophoretic application of ACh, the depolarizing component invariably decreased rapidly, providing support for the desensitization hypothesis. In addition, the hyperpolarizing component of the ACh response often increased with repeated applications. In the extreme case, we could demonstrate that the response properties of the two receptors were sufficiently different that the first of two closely spaced ACh pulses produced a pure depolarizing response, whereas the second pulse produced a pure hyperpolarizing response (Fig. 4, B2).

The simplest model to account for the diphasic response of L7 is that of a single branch ending on two separate (perhaps overlapping) postsynaptic receptors for ACh, one giving rise to excitation and the other to inhibition. The excitatory receptor has a low threshold and a rapid risetime and is quickly desensitized; the inhibitory receptor has a higher threshold and a slower risetime and is not readily desensitized. The existence of two different receptors to ACh is consistent with the recent finding of Chiarandini, Stefani, and Gerschenfeld (8) that the depolarization and hyperpolarization produced by ACh in different molluscan cells (H and DILDA) involve different receptor mechanisms producing permeability changes to Na^+ and Cl^-, respectively. It is likely that L7 has both the Na^+ and Cl^- permeability mechanisms to ACh and that these generate the separate components of the dual response.

Cell L7 therefore appears to combine, in a single cell, the receptor properties of cells receiving either purely excitatory or purely inhibitory branches from the same interneuron (L10). These findings provide additional support for the hypothesis (4, 6, 9) that in this ganglion the sign of the synaptic action is determined, not by the chemical nature of the transmitter substance released by the presynaptic neuron, but by type of receptor and the number of receptor types of the follower cell. The presence of L7 in the only quarter ganglion to contain both excitatory and inhibitory follower cells of L10 also suggests that the distribution of the two types of receptors among different follower cells and the permissible combinations of receptors on a given cell are specified regionally within each quarter ganglion.

References and Notes

1. W. T. Frazier, E. R. Kandel, R. Waziri, R. E. Coggeshall, *J. Neurophysiol.*, in press.
2. E. R. Kandel, W. T. Frazier, R. Waziri, R. E. Coggeshall, *ibid.*, in press.
3. H. H. Dale, *Proc. Roy. Soc. Med.* **28**, 319 (1935); J. C. Eccles, *The Physiology of Synapses* (Springer-Verlag, Berlin, 1964).
4. E. R. Kandel, W. T. Frazier, R. E. Coggeshall, *Science* **155**, 346 (1967).
5. L. Tauc and J. Bruner, *Nature* **198**, 33 (1963).
6. L. Tauc and H. M. Gerschenfeld, *ibid.* **192**, 366 (1961).
7. We have recently heard (L. Tauc and M. Kehoe, personal communication) of the discovery of a cell in the pleural ganglion of *Aplysia* that has a compound hyperpolarizing response to ACh; one phase is blocked by curare, but the other is not.
8. D. J. Chiarandini and H. M. Gerschenfeld, *Science* **156**, 1595 (1967); D. J. Chiarandini, E. Stefani, H. M. Gerschenfeld, *ibid.*, p. 1597.
9. F. Strumwasser, *Int. Congr. Physiol. Sci. 22nd* (1962), vol. 2, No. 801.
10. Supported in part by grant R-214-67 from the Cerebral Palsy Foundation, by PHS training grant 5 TO1 HE05608-05 (to H.W.) and by PHS career program award MH 18.558-01 (to E.R.K.). We thank Alden Spencer for his comments on an earlier draft of this manuscript and M. V. L. Bennett for helpful discussions.

Axonic and Synaptic Lesions in Neuropsychiatric Disorders

NICHOLAS K. GONATAS

Reprinted from *Nature*, April 22, 1967, Vol. 214, No. 5086, pp. 352–355.

The part played by the synapse in establishing functional contacts between nerve cells or nerve cells and muscle has been well substantiated.[1] The initiation of the postsynaptic potential by neurotransmitters (neurohumours) is also established beyond any reasonable doubt in the case of several types of synapse.[2] Uncertainties about the structure of the synapse have been clarified by examining this important segment of the neuron under the electron microscope.[3-5] Mitochondria and vesicles containing acetylcholine or other neurotransmitters have been seen in the presynaptic axon terminals (boutons terminaux).[6-8] It is believed that the synthesis of neurotransmitters takes place at the terminal from substrates and enzymes transported from the perikaryon by axoplasmic flow.[9,10] Energy and probably certain substrates and co-enzymes are provided at the presynaptic ending by mitochondria. The site of actual contact between axon and axon, axon and dendrite or axon and soma is characterized by slight thickening of the apposed membranes; the interstitial space between the pre- and postsynaptic terminals (intersynaptic cleft) is filled with linear or spherical osmiophilic material which probably serves as a cohesive matrix between the pre- and postsynaptic membranes.[11,12] The fine structure of the postsynaptic element has also been the subject of a number of investigations.[13-15]

Information is not available about neocortical synapses in neuropsychiatric disease because it is difficult to obtain fresh specimens and because this vital segment of neocortical neurons is inaccessible to histological methods.[16] It is generally assumed that the synapse plays a secondary part, and degenerates in a nonspecific manner after any type of lesion of the perikaryon. Recent evidence suggests that this assumption may not be correct.[17,18] Abnormalities of synaptic fine structure consisting of enlargement of the presynaptic terminal, reduction of the number of synaptic vesicles, and accumulation of fibrillar or vesicular material were observed in biopsy specimens of frontal cortex from patients with psychomotor retardation and Alzheimer's presenile dementia.[17,18] In one case,[17] the synaptic lesions were the only recognized changes by light or electron microscopy. These changes are significant in view of the importance of the synapse in establishing functional contacts between neurons [1] and the current belief that the synaptic transmission is an integral part of learning and memory processes.[19,20]

This article describes axonic and synaptic changes observed in the frontal cortex of a 30-month-old boy with severe psychomotor retardation; the significance of synaptic "lesions" in neuropsychiatric disease will be discussed.

The patient, a Negro male, 30 months old, was admitted to the Hospital of the University of Pennsylvania for evaluation of psychomotor retardation. He was the product of an essentially normal, full-term pregnancy. Development was normal during the first year, but gradually deteriorated and, at the present time, he cannot sit or stand by himself and can only "slur monosyllables unintelligibly." The two siblings, girls 11 and 7 years old, are normal. Physical examination showed this boy to weigh 25 lb. with hypotonia of trunk muscles and spasticity of biceps, hamstrings and quadriceps groups. His deep tendon reflexes were normal. There was generalized motor weakness. He seemed to recognize people around him. Routine laboratory tests of blood, urine and cerebrospinal fluid were within normal limits. Metachromatic granules were not found in the urine. The electromyogram was interpreted as showing a possible neurogenic pattern. A biopsy of the right gastrocnemius showed neurogenic atrophy of muscle and endoneural fibrosis of muscle nerves. A pneumoencephalogram and myelogram carried out in another hospital were reviewed and found normal. The electroencephalogram was normal. The clinical impression was that of a diffuse degenerative disease of the central nervous system. A definite diagnosis could not be established.

A biopsy of the right middle frontal gyrus and underlying white matter was obtained through an open craniectomy. Tissue was immediately fixed in formol calcium,[21] formalin, and glutaraldehyde followed by osmic acid.[22]

Neuropathological examination of the specimen revealed little. The cell structure was normal. There was no cell loss, cellular infiltrates, demyelination, evidence of storage, or deposits of metachromatic material. The leptomeninges and the blood vessels were unremarkable. Silver impregnation stains (Bodian) were within normal limits. Cytochemical stains for lysosomes (acid phosphatase),[23] Golgi apparatus (thiamine pyrophosphatase),[24] and mitochondria (nicotinamide adenine dinucleotide) [25] were normal.

Electron microscopic examination of the specimen revealed no apparent abnormalities in neuronal perikarya, dendrites, glial cells, blood vessels or myelin sheaths. The only abnormalities noted were numerous distended non-myelinated segments of axons and presynaptic terminals (Fig. 1). In contrast with normal presynaptic terminals which measure about $1 \cdot 5\mu$ in greatest diameter, the abnormal terminals measured $5–15\mu$. On a thin section, normal presynaptic terminals contain between ten and forty synaptic vesicles and one or two mitochondria; the enlarged endings contained few or no synaptic vesicles, and mitochondria were not noted in many of the enlarged endings. Instead, the enlarged axons and terminals were filled with haphazardly arranged branching tubular or vesicular profiles with smooth walls 60–70 Å thick. Unlike neurotubules which measure about 270–300 Å in diameter,[26] these tubular or vesicular structures measured 165–550 Å. Neurofilaments and neurotubules were sparse or absent. When present, the neurotubules had a haphazard course instead of a parallel direction to the long dimension of the axon. The apposed plasma membranes at the synapse and the intersynaptic cleft were normal. The postsynaptic element was also normal. Although enlarged presynaptic axon terminals were noted in contact with neuronal perikarya and dendritic trunks, synaptic contacts were definitely identified only between enlarged presynaptic terminals and dendritic spines. These changes were ubiquitous. They were seen in more than sixty sections of the tissue; usually a field at a magnification of 4,000 contained four to six enlarged processes.

The subcortical white matter was normal and only a rare myelinated axon contained similar vesicular structures with few or no mitochondria, neurofilaments and neurotubules (Figs. 2 and 3). The axolemma of these rare abnormal axons was intact; the axon was not enlarged and the surrounding myelin sheath was normal (Fig. 3). It was estimated that only one out of two or three hundred axons showed these abnormalities (Figs. 2 and 3).

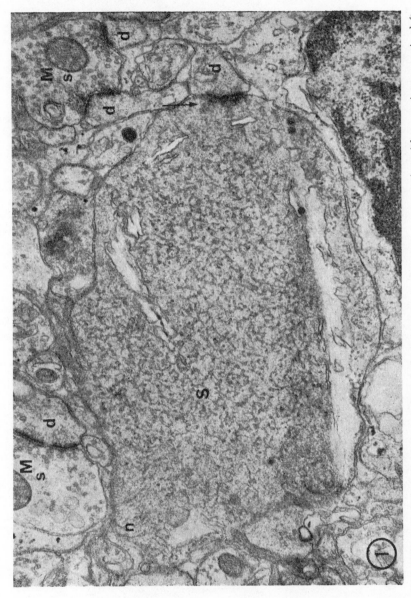

FIGURE 1. *S*, Enlarged presynaptic terminal. Arrow points to one or two synaptic vesicles near intersynaptic cleft. Note absence of mitochondria from abnormal terminal. *d*, Dendritic spine; *n*, neurotubules; *s*, normal presynaptic terminals, note synaptic vesicles filling terminal; *M*, mitochondria. (× 24,000.)

39

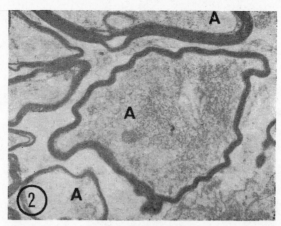

FIGURE 2. Axon (A) in centre of figure contains vesicular structures. Axons in lower left and upper right corners are normal. (× 11,000.)

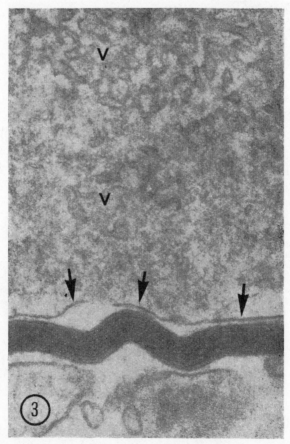

FIGURE 3. Enlargements of Figure 2. V, Branching vesicular structures. Arrowheads indicate intact axolemma with adjacent normal myelin sheath. (× 55,000.)

The following two hypotheses could be advanced as to the significance of the enlarged axons and presynaptic terminals: (a) they are "degenerating" terminals of a destroyed perikaryon or severed axon; (b) the axon and presynaptic swellings either reflect an abnormality localized at the terminal segment of the axon, or are secondary to a disturbance of the metabolism of the perikaryon unassociated with morphological changes detectable by light or electron microscopy.

Enormous enlargements of axons and presynaptic terminals or the peculiar vesicular structures have not been observed in experimental degenerations of nerve endings; [27-35] furthermore, in most experiments the presynaptic terminal disintegrated and became phagocytosed by adjacent glial cells. Also, ultrastructural data in Wallerian degeneration of peripheral nerves bear no resemblance to the findings in this case.[36-42] Wallerian degeneration is characterized by early disappearance of axons and fragmentation of myelin sheaths. In this case, on the other hand, the myelin sheaths are intact and the axons do not undergo lysis.

The axon and its presynaptic terminal may be the sole morphological index of neuronal disease. Examples of experimental conditions or spontaneous disease may support this hypothesis. Experimental vitamin E deficiency in rats is associated with "dystrophic" terminal segments of axons.[43] Axons appear to be extensively involved in the human disease, infantile neuroaxonal dystrophy.[44,45] Electron microscopy studies in infantile neuroaxonal dystrophy are not available for comparison with the present and reported cases; [17] the case reported here may represent an early stage of neuroaxonal dystrophy.

An isolated structural and metabolic defect in axons and presynaptic terminals could cause severe psychomotor retardation or arrest of development. The reduction or absence of synaptic vesicles could represent a decreased synthesis of neurotransmitter substances, increased rate of their release, or both. This would result in an altered function of the presynaptic terminal with direct effects on synaptic transmission, that is, altered intercellular communication and transfer of information. The paucity or absence of mitochondria from the enlarged presynaptic terminals and axons could deprive the synthetic processes of neurotransmitters of essential energy and substrates. Energy provided by mitochondria is also essential for ionic movements associated with the passage of impulses,[46] and it is reasonable to assume that the conduction of nervous stimuli in swollen axons without mitochondria and filled with an unusual material (Figs. 1–3) is altered. The peculiar vesicular structures (Fig. 3) may be precipitates of a normally soluble substance, or products of the breakdown of mitochondria, plasma membrane, neurofilaments or neurotubules; or they could represent abortive attempts for formation or packaging of neurotransmitter substances. Since the peculiar vesicular structures are seen in myelinated segments of the axon, a relationship of the vesicular structures (Fig. 3) to mitochondria, axolemma or neurofilaments and neurotubules, rather than to synaptic vesicles, may be more plausible.

Axonic and synaptic swelling may be due to disturbance of axoplasmic flow.[10] The existence of axoplasmic flow as a mechanical phenomenon is fairly well established.[10] The structural entities and biochemical events contributing to the axoplasmic or cytoplasmic streaming are not, however, known. It has been suggested that microtubules and neurotubules may serve as cytoskeletal elements, and cytoplasmic flow may be due to interactions at the surface of these stationary structures, or that cytoplasmic streaming may be accomplished by undulating motions of the tubules.[47] The homology between the morphological nature of neurotubules and mitotic spindle tubules [26] which are involved in chromosomal motion suggests that neurotubules may be instrumental in cytoplasmic motion. The absence of neurotubules and the swelling of the axons and presynaptic terminals may therefore be related. An impaired axoplasmic flow could interfere with the availability of essential metabolites for neurotransmitter synthesis.

The axonic and synaptic changes described in this 30-month-old child with severe psychomotor retardation constitute the only anatomical substrate of the pathological process. The recognition of similar ultrastructural changes in axons and synaptic endings in other human diseases characterized by disturbance of memory and learning [17,18] justifies the hypothesis that a causal relationship between synaptic "lesions" and some forms of psychomotor retardation or dementia could exist.

This work was aided by grants from the U.S. Public Health Service, and the Widlyer Fund.

References

1. Eccles, J. C., *The Physiology of Synapses* (Academic Press, Inc., New York, 1964).
2. Koells, G. B., in *Evolution of Nervous Control* (edit. by Bass, A. D.), 87 (American Association for the Advancement of Science, Washington, 1959).
3. DeRobertis, E., and Bennett, H. S., *Fed. Proc.*, **13**, 35 (1954).
4. Palay, S. L., *Anat. Rec.*, **118**, 193 (1954).
5. Palade, G. E., *Anat. Rec.*, **118**, 335 (1954).
6. DeRobertis, E. Lores Arnaiz, G. R., Salganicoff, L., Pellegrino De Iraldi, A., and Zieher, L. M., *J. Neurochem.*, **10**, 225 (1963).
7. Whittaker, V. P., and Sheridan, M. N., *J. Neurochem.*, **12**, 363 (1965).
8. Richardson, K. C., *Amer. J. Anat.*, **114**, 173 (1964).
9. DeRobertis, E., in *Histophysiology of Synapses and Neurosecretion*, **1**, 27 (The Macmillan Company, New York, and Pergamon Press, Oxford, New York, 1960).
10. Weiss, P., *Fourth Intern. Neurochem. Symp.*, **2**, 220 (Pergamon Press, New York, 1960).
11. Van der Loos, H., *Z. Zellforsch.*, **60**, 815 (1963).
12. Pappas, G. D., and Purpura, D. P., *Nature*, **210**, 1391 (1966).
13. Palay, S. L., *J. Biophys. Biochem. Cytol. Suppl.*, **2**, 193 (1956).
14. Gray, E. G., *J. Anat. London*, **96**, 420 (1959).

15. Pappas, G. D., *Exp. Neurol.,* **4,** 507 (1961).
16. Boycott, B. B., Gray, E. G., and Guillery, R. W., *J. Physiol.,* **152,** 3P (1960).
17. Gonatas, N. K., and Goldensohn, E. S., *J. Neuropath. and Exp. Neurol.,* **24,** 539 (1965).
18. Gonatas, N. K., Anderson, W., and Evangelista, I., *J. Neuropath. and Exp. Neurol.,* **26,** 25 (1967).
19. Hebb, D. W., *Organization of Behavior. A Neuro-physiological Study* (John Wiley and Sons, Inc., New York, 1957).
20. Elul, R., *Nature,* **210,** 5041 (1966).
21. Baker, J. R., *Quart. J. Micros. Sci.,* **87,** 441 (1946).
22. Sabatini, D. D., Bensch, K., and Barnett, R. J., *J. Cell Biol.,* **17,** 19 (1963).
23. Gomori, G., *Microscopic Histochemistry, Principles and Practice,* **182** (University of Chicago Press, 1952).
24. Novikoff, A. B., and Goldfisher, S., *Proc. U.S. Nat. Acad. Sci.,* **47,** 802 (1961).
25. Novikoff, A. B., Shin, N. Y., and Drucker, J., *J. Biophys. Biochem. Cytol.,* **9,** 47 (1960).
26. Gonatas, N. K., and Robbins, E., *Protoplasma,* **59,** 25 (1964).
27. Smith, C. A., and Rasmussen, C. L., *J. Cell Biol.,* **26,** 63 (1965).
28. Dowling, D. E., and Cowan, W. M., *Z. Zellforsch.,* **71,** 14 (1966).
29. Gray, E. G., and Hamlyn, L. H., *J. Anat. Lond.,* **96,** 309 (1962).
30. Colonnier, M., and Guillery, R. W., *Z. Zellforsch.,* **62,** 333 (1964).
31. Colonnier, M., and Gray, E. G., *Degeneration in the Cerebral Cortex,* **3,** 2 (edit. by Breese, S. S.) (Academic Press, New York, 1962).
32. Colonnier, M., *J. Anat. Lond.,* **98,** 47 (1964).
33. Walberg, F., *Exp. Neurol.,* **8,** 112 (1963).
34. Walberg, F., *J. Comp. Neurol.,* **122,** 113 (1964).
35. Smith, J. M., O'Learny, J. L., Harris, A. B., and Gay, A. J., *J. Comp. Neurol.,* **123,** 357 (1964).
36. Webster, De F. H., *J. Cell Biol.,* **12,** 361 (1962).
37. Thomas, P. K., and Sheldon, H., *J. Cell Biol.,* **22,** 715 (1964).
38. Barton, A. A., *Brain,* **85,** 799 (1962).
39. Lee, J. C.-Y., *J. Comp. Neurol.,* **120,** 65 (1963).
40. Nathaniel, E. J. H., and Pease, D. C., *J. Ultrastruct. Res.,* **9,** 511 (1963).
41. Terry, R. D., and Harkin, J. C., in *The Biology of Myelin,* **303** (edit. by Korey, S. A.) (Paul B. Hoeber, New York, 1959).
42. Ohmi, S., *Z. Zellforsch.,* **54,** 39 (1961).
43. Lambert, P., Bluemberg, T. M., and Pentschew, A., *J. Neuropath. Neurol.,* **23,** 60 (1964).
44. Gowan, D., and Olmstead, E. V., *J. Neuropath. Exp. Neurol.,* **22,** 175 (1963).
45. Seitelberger, F., in *Proc. First Intern. Cong. Neuropath.* (Rome, September 8–13, 1952), **3,** 323 (Rosenberg and Sellier, Turin, 1952).
46. Hodgkin, A. L., *The Conduction of the Nervous Impulse. The Sherrington Lectures VII* (Charles C Thomas, Springfield, 1964).
47. Ledbetter, M. D., and Porter, K. R., *J. Cell Biol.,* **19,** 239 (1963).

Study Question for Part I

Certain characteristics of nervous activity are, by now, well established. They are: (a) all-or-none activity in the nerve axon; (b) excitation and inhibition at the synapse; and (c) graded activity along the dendrites and cell body. From your reading of the preceding articles, consider how the interplay of these three variables could provide the basis for the neural "code." What would activity in the nervous system be like in the *absence* of any one of these variables (for example, ask yourself what would happen if, instead of synapses, there were a continuous "net" of cells)?

Part II

Transduction and Integration
of Sensory Input:
Coding, Decoding, and Scanning
Mechanisms in the CNS

In the previous section we investigated the way in which the basic language of the nervous system is generated and communicated from neuron to neuron. The following articles will deal with the syntax, or patterning, of this neural code. "Syntax" refers to the way in which the elements of a language are put together to communicate a coherent message.

Since we are primarily interested in behavior, we want to know how we can discriminate between qualitatively different sensations: discern differences in taste or distinguish between straight and curved lines. When energy impinges upon our exteroceptive (e.g., eyes and ears) or interoceptive (proprioceptive, kinesthetic) organs, some of it is immediately lost through the process of graded activity or inhibition, and some of it may be amplified through spatial and/or temporal summation. This interplay of excitation and inhibition and the *sequence* of neural impulses provide the basic mechanisms for the development of the neural code. You will see that the energy impinging upon the sense organ is not information, and cannot be utilized, until it is first transduced, transmitted, and received by appropriate target cells.

The first paper, by Kennedy, provides an outline of how physical energy, reaching sensory receptors, is changed into "data language" that the brain is capable of using. However, it should be recognized that this transduction is only the first stage in what amounts to a series of abstraction processes as information is channeled throughout the nervous system. In Erickson's article, we begin to see how impulse activities in different receptor cells, through their temporal and spatial interrelations, provide the basis for an *interpretable* pattern of activity that becomes the physiological correlate of taste.

Whitfield's article is closely related to the preceding material as he discusses how receptor mechanisms in the ear serve to change physical energy into a complex pattern of neuronal activity that we interpret as sound.

If we are to have a "code" then there must be some kind of device to interpret the "message." The article by Hubel describes how patterns of neural impulses arising in the retina are modified as they ascend to the cortical receiving areas. The activity that occurs is more than just amplification or reduction of message content. In reading this article, you will begin to get a better understanding of how the neural code is actually formed and modified. You will read about cortical mechanisms responsible for synthesis and interpretation of patterns arriving from layers of cells in the lateral geniculate nucleus. Lateral geniculate cells, in turn, synthesize and abstract activity arising from receptor cells in the retina.

The final two articles, by Robinson and Sprague, respectively, serve to reintroduce the concept of hierarchic integration on a structural level. In these papers, the authors demonstrate how information processing in the CNS is influenced by a reciprocal feedback system that operates between anatomically distinct structures in the brain. We interpret these articles to suggest that the way in which an organism finally utilizes information, and, indeed, the very selection of stimulus energy that will be transduced to information, is the result of interdependent sensory and motor feedback loops. This interaction of intra- and intercellular events is so delicately balanced that change in either of the systems will result in marked disruption of sensory capacity.

The Initiation of Impulses in Receptors

DONALD KENNEDY

Reprinted from *American Zoologist*, 1962, Vol. 2, pp. 27–43.

The three preparations which have taught us most about the generation of impulses by receptor cells come from crayfish, frog and cat. Obviously, sense organs are appropriate targets for the comparative approach; yet the very diversity of receptor systems makes difficult the task of reviewing them from this point of view. Comparative analysis yields, on the one hand, an emphasis on those common properties of biological systems which we choose somewhat optimistically to call "basic." On the other hand, it also shows that though these properties may have fundamental similarities they are coupled and modified to serve an astonishing variety of adaptive ends.

It will be the purpose of this article to define some of the important steps in the sensory process, and to review what is known of them in a variety of receptors. I hope it will lay stress upon some basic mechanisms which unify the behavior of sensory systems, and equally upon the variety of adaptive modifications which equip them to fulfill the special behavioral requirements of their owners. The treatment will necessarily be incomplete, and for many of the examples used, others could have served as well.

The Nature of Sensory Discharge

Receptors are the peripheral outposts which initiate most of the impulse traffic in the central nervous system. From our own experience, we know that such receptors can signal not only the existence of a stimulus, but its intensity as well. The pioneering studies of Adrian (1928), which were among the earliest applications of modern recording techniques to sensory nerves, showed that receptors communicate differences in intensity level by producing trains of impulses in which the frequency of discharges is some function of intensity. Later studies on a variety of sensory systems have revealed, in agreement with psycho-physical conclusions reached earlier, that the increase in discharge frequency is approximately linear with respect to the *logarithm* of the stimulus intensity over much of the dynamic range. The means by which sense organs accomplish this logarithmic transformation are obscure, but the adaptive advantage of the situation is obvious. Neurons are limited to frequencies of about a thousand impulses per second by their refractory periods, and any sensory channel which responded linearly with increasing intensity would rather quickly reach a maximal discharge rate. Since the dynamic range with which most sensory systems must contend is enormous (about 10^{12} for human vision and hearing), a logarithmic response contour is a practical necessity, even though the whole range may not be covered by a single element.

The properties of sensory endings were, in a sense, brought into logical relation to those of the neuron by analyses of the repetitive responses of some nerve fibers to direct current stimulation. In certain crustacean motor axons, for example, the frequency of these repetitive discharges depends upon the current strength, and declines ("adapts") with varying rapidity during passage of a given stimulating current. Experiments on such neurons (see Hodgkin, 1948) made possible the prediction that "natural" currents, perhaps generated by permeability changes in the sensory cell, could produce discharges in un-myelinated sensory endings by analogous means. A basis was thus established for interpreting the frequency of sensory discharge as a product of membrane time-constants and the displacement of membrane potential in the receptor, rather than as a product of limits imposed by refractoriness.

Events in the Receptor Process

The observations mentioned above, and others, have gradually led to the specification of a series of events which takes place in sensory cells and links the reception of stimulus energy to the production of impulses in their afferent nerve fibers. The process involves (1) the absorption of stimulus energy; (2) its conversion or *transduction* into some kind of electrical energy; (3) the production of a slow "generator" potential which subsequently (4) initiates repetitive impulse discharge in the axon. These steps will be considered in turn.

Absorption of Energy

It is axiomatic that energy, in order to produce an effect, must first be absorbed. The functional selectivity of a given sense organ in responding to one particular type of stimulus energy is thus partially determined by the absorption mechanisms which couple it to its environment. It is here that some of the most interesting and complex adaptations of sense organs occur. Their very variety is testimony of the continuous adaptive challenge to improve and adjust mechanisms for energy absorption.

1. MECHANORECEPTORS.   The basic architecture of all mechanorecep-tive endings involves arrangements for the production of a membrane deformation in response to some mechanical stimulus. In muscle receptors, the arrange-ment may involve deformation of a nerve ending by compression (vertebrate muscle spindles) or of a set of dendrites by stretch (crustacean muscle receptor organs, see Fig. 6). Some endings sensitive to touch may be encapsulated with connective tissue layers, which increase the area of response, though not neces-

sarily the absolute sensitivity (vertebrate Pacinian corpuscles, see Fig. 5). Other mechanoreceptors employ articulated hairs which bend the dendrite of a sensory neuron (arthropod exoskeletal hairs), or ciliated hair cells of epithelial origin which make synaptic contact with the afferent neuron proper (lateral-line neuromasts, cochlear hair cells, and other derivatives of the vertebrate acoustico-lateralis system, see Fig. 2).

Overlying these fundamental differences in receptor cell structure, a host of more complex variations in coupling systems is found. For example, in mammalian muscle two types of stretch-sensitive receptors exist; the difference in their reactions depends on different coupling, and was first worked out by Matthews (1933). The muscle spindle is placed in the belly of the muscle, in parallel with its fibers. Stretch applied to the muscle compresses the spindle, and produces a sensory discharge from its primary ending; but reflex contraction of the muscle releases this compression, and the discharge ceases. The Golgi tendon organ, on the other hand, is spoken of as being in series with the muscle fibers because of its location in the tendon. Like the spindle, it fires on stretching. But contraction of the muscle merely increases pressure in the tendon region, and so augments discharge from the receptor. This simple case,

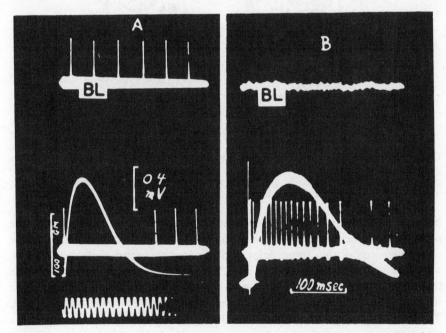

FIGURE 1. Differing responses to contraction in muscle receptors. A. Recording from primary ending of muscle spindle; the baseline discharge (top record) is interrupted by contraction (bottom record). B. Recording from Golgi tendon organ afferent, which was inactive at this level of stretch; contraction (bottom record) produces a sensory discharge. Contraction of the muscle in bottom records of A and B indicated by second oscilloscope trace, which measures tension. (*From Hunt, 1952, Cold Spr. Harb. Sympos. Quant. Biol.*)

illustrated in the records of Figure 1, demonstrates as well as any other the
way in which altered physical arrangement can differentiate the responses from
deformation-sensitive cells.

A more complex series of coupling mechanisms is found among derivatives of the acoustico-lateralis system in vertebrates. Hair cells belonging to this
group are all morphologically quite similar (Fig. 2). The cellular mechanism

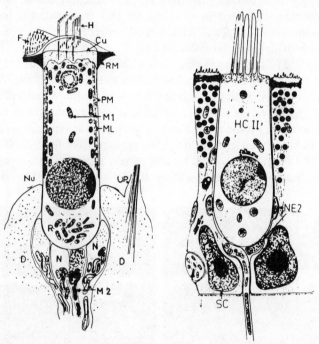

FIGURE 2. Vertebrate hair cells; drawings based on reconstructions from electron
photomicrographs. *Left,* cell from ampullar crista of semicircular canal; *right,* cochlear hair
cell (Type II). Note especially the junctions between the epithelial hair cell and the
sensory neurons in each case. (*From Engström and Wersäll, 1958,* Exp. Cell Research.)

of excitation in all is probably dependent upon shearing forces applied to the
hairs. Yet such cells in the cochlea of some bats can indicate specifically to the
central nervous system frequencies of a hundred thousand cycles per second,
while the lateral line receptors of most fish are limited to about a hundredth
that frequency. The frequency response of cochlear receptors depends upon
their location along a stretched membrane which divides a fluid-filled column.
The mechanics of the column are such that applied pressure variations produce
a traveling wave along the membrane, exciting the hair cells upon it in different
zones depending on the frequency (von Békésy, 1956). Coupling between air
and the internal fluid is achieved by the three middle ear bones, which concentrate pressure from the large tympanic membrane onto the smaller area of the
round window which forms part of the entrance to the cochlea. The increase

in force achieved by this concentration of pressure onto a smaller area effectively matches the acoustical impedance of air to that of the fluid. Cochlear receptors can indicate high frequencies because of the unique mechanical arrangements which produce vibrations of the membrane bearing them, and because it is actually the *position* of the excited receptor which indicates to the brain what the frequency is. But lateral-line receptors cannot analyze frequency by place-representation. Instead, they must respond to the direct stresses placed upon them by molecular motion in the medium.

Receptors of the vertebrate semicircular canals are very similar to the previous two; but these cells have their sensory hairs embedded in a gelatinous cupula which extends like a swinging door across the swollen ampulla of each canal. Its movement is heavily damped by the fluid which fills the canals, and when acceleration occurs in the plane of a canal the inertia of fluid and cupula places a shearing stress on the hairs, which is the effective stimulus for discharging impulses in the sensory axons. Direct visualization (Steinhausen, 1931) and measurement of the duration of after-discharge following rotation (Lowenstein and Sand, 1940) have both yielded estimates that the period of the damped system is about 20 seconds. Thus in the labyrinth, the same basic receptor type is coupled in an entirely different way, producing a sensory system with extremely low frequency response. In the sensory cristae of the sacculus, utriculus and lagena of fish, Lowenstein and Roberts (1949, 1951) have found a variety of hair receptors which may respond either to gravity or to vibrations. Again, the frequency response of the cells depends upon whether they are loaded or not; those whose hairs are embedded in an otolith organ are gravitation receptors, but those with free hairs respond to vibrations. In fact, the high frequency response of the latter type is itself dependent upon secondary coupling: high-frequency sensitivity in cyprinoid fishes is achieved by a chain of bones (the Weberian ossicles) which contact the utriculus, whereas in clupeid fishes it is managed by association of the sacculus with the swimbladder wall.

Frequency-response variation dependent upon loading has also been demonstrated for hair receptors in crustacean statocysts by Cohen (1960); and an especially interesting example from another arthropod mechanoreceptor has been reported by Walcott and Van der Kloot (1959). They have shown that the lyriform organ of the spider tarsus is a vibration receptor: sensory units from it respond to very narrow frequency bands. The sensitivity peaks of individual receptors, however, can be adjusted from one frequency to another by changes in tension of the leg. Thus in some situations the coupling between receptor and environment is labile, and allows for reflex adjustment of frequency sensitivity.

2. PHOTORECEPTORS.   The problem of energy absorption in visual cells has received especial attention. Among the reasons for this is the fact that light is a uniquely satisfactory energy variable in respect to the precision with

which it can be controlled and measured. Furthermore, the photosensitive pigments employed by such receptor cells are frequently present in sufficient concentration to encourage their extraction and biochemical characterization. Photoreceptors therefore offer a particularly complete case history in the adjustment of absorption mechanisms to environmental requirement.

Visual cells with a wide assortment of phylogenetic origins are characterized by a remarkable similarity in their structure. All of them feature a lamellar ultrastructure, consisting of a set of membranes derived from cilia (vertebrates, molluscs) or a honeycomb-like array of hexagonal tubules (arthropod rhabdomeres). A variety of evidence suggests that the visual pigments are organized in or among the lamellae in a highly oriented fashion. The latter point is particularly strongly supported for vertebrate rods, in which Denton (1959) has shown that visual pigment derivatives exhibit strongly polarized fluorescence. Visual pigments may constitute a large fraction of the dry weight of the sensory cell (40% in frog rods) and thus absorb a very high proportion of light impinging along the long axis of the receptor (density about 0.5 at 500 mμ in frog rods).

In all photoreceptors so far examined, the primary photosensitive pigment has turned out to be a carotenoid protein in which the carotenoid chromophore is retinene (vitamin A aldehyde). The biochemistry of such pigments has been reviewed by Wald (1959), in whose laboratory many of the important advances have taken place. The retinene molecule shows isomer specificity: of five known isomeric configurations, only the ll-*cis* form will combine with the protein to make functional visual pigment. Hubbard et al. (1959) have shown that the bleaching of such visual pigment in solution depends upon a photo-isomerization of the retinene molecule to the all-*trans* (straight) form, followed in vertebrates by its separation from the protein. In cephalopod molluscs, however, the retinene remains permanently attached. This situation has led to the prediction that the initial isomerization of retinene, or a partial denaturation of the protein which appears to follow it, is responsible for initiating the electrical activity of the receptor cell, and that subsequent hydrolysis of the retinene from the protein is probably not involved. There is, however, no direct evidence for this view in vertebrates.

The molecular similarity of visual pigments still permits considerable variation in the spectral band covered by the receptors—which is, of course, primarily determined by the absorption characteristics of the pigment. Rhodopsin, the visual pigment of rods in most marine and terrestrial vertebrates, usually has an absorption maximum near 500 mμ, whereas the rod pigments of fresh-water fish and reptiles are based upon a slightly different retinene and have absorption maxima near 522 mμ. In the cones of these two groups of vertebrates, the visual pigments consist of the same chromophores combined with a very different protein from that found in rods. These cone pigments have absorption maxima at 562 mμ (iodopsin from chickens, and probably many other vertebrates in which rhodopsin is the rod pigment) and 620 mμ

(cyanopsin, the cone pigment of reptiles and fresh-water fish). A more sensitive series of adaptive variations within these broad categories is made possible through adjustment of the properties of the protein moiety. Deep-sea fish (Denton and Warren, 1957) and cephalopods (Brown and Brown, 1958) have rhodopsins in which the absorption maximum is displaced to values around 480 mμ, corresponding to the center of the spectral band best transmitted through sea water.

Variations in the short-wavelength extent of visual sensitivity in fishes also exist, and have ecological correlates; they depend upon the presence of intra-ocular color filters, especially in the lens (Kennedy and Milkman, 1956). The shift to longer-wavelength sensitivity in the rod and cone pigments of fresh-water fish, which is achieved through the substitution of a chemically different retinene, may be an adaptation to the relatively greater transparency of fresh-water to long-wavelength radiations. Marine arthropods, like marine fish, have rhodopsins absorbing maximally near 500 mμ; but at least one fresh-water arthropod, the crayfish, shows a 60 mμ displacement of its spectral sensitivity maximum toward longer wavelengths (Kennedy and Bruno, 1961). The shift in this instance is achieved by utilization of a different protein, not a different carotenoid.

The family of visual pigments is constantly being expanded, especially as a result of investigations on groups with known color vision abilities. Rushton (1958) has applied an extraordinary technique of reflection photometry to the living human fovea, where he has characterized two cone pigments and studied the kinetics of their bleaching and resynthesis. Several receptor types, differing in spectral sensitivity, have recently been found through microelectrode studies on insect retinula cells (Autrum and Burkhardt, 1961). Previously, Goldsmith (1958) had obtained evidence for receptor types with differing spectral sensitivities in the bee's eye, and succeeded in extracting a visual pigment (the only one to date from an insect) which matched one of them.

3. CHEMORECEPTORS.   Nowhere is the specificity of absorption mechanisms more apparent than in chemoreceptors, but in vertebrates these have proven among the most difficult of sensory systems to analyze and interpret. For example, the receptors of the olfactory system have tenaciously resisted single-unit analysis at the first order level. Farther upstream, some recording has been done—with mitral cells in the olfactory bulb; these have revealed some faint suggestions of peripheral differentiation into specific receptors sensitive to classes of stimulating molecules, but the embarrassing fact is that very few substances can produce sensory adaptation to others. This lack of cross-adaptation leaves one in the awkward position of having to assume thousands of receptor types, each sensitive to a very few closely similar molecules, and each with specific absorption systems for its own stimulant. The gustatory receptors of the tongue are more easily divisible into submodalities, and absorption theories therefore are somewhat easier to develop.

The only chemoreceptors for which a really thorough analysis at the receptor cell level has been made are those of certain insects, especially flies (Hodgson and Roeder, 1956; Wolbarsht and Dethier, 1958). The organ consists of a hollow exoskeletal spine which contains the dendrites of two chemoreceptor neurons (and sometimes a third, mechanically-sensitive unit). The cell bodies of these neurons are at the base of the hair; spike activity in them can be recorded by means of an ensheathing capillary microelectrode placed over the hair. The electrode can be filled with various solutions and thus used to stimulate as well as record. One neuron produces impulses in response to a variety of chemicals, including acids, salts and organic compounds, whereas the other responds only to sugars. This combination of one specific and one relatively unspecific channel is well-adapted for the use of the fly, since stimulation of only a single receptor can evoke acceptance behavior to sugars or rejection to nearly anything else.

Insects as a group present a remarkable set of behavioral responses triggered by specific molecules, in many cases at extremely low concentrations. Not many of these have been investigated; one which has, is the response of male Saturniid moths to volatile sex attractants released by the female. Schneider (1957) has located the responsible chemoreceptors in male antennae, and shown that they are specifically sensitive to female odorant. The threshold concentrations are fantastically low; but it is never possible to express such thresholds in terms of molecules per receptor cell with any degree of confidence because of the uncontrollable possibility that the stimulating molecules may clump by adsorption onto particles. It nevertheless seems likely that some chemoreceptors of this sort approach the exquisite sensitivity of retinal rods or cochlear hair cells.

Mechanisms for the combination of stimulating chemicals with receptor sites on the surface membrane of the chemoreceptor have been difficult to demonstrate. There is no qualitative difference between this problem and the one presented by the chemical sensitivity of sub-synaptic membranes to transmitter substances. In the latter case uncoupling of the transmitter molecule from its receptor may be achieved by its splitting through the action of hydrolytic enzymes; but it is somewhat difficult to suppose that each chemoreceptor surface has a specific enzyme to accomplish dissociation of stimulating chemical from receptor. Some workers in olfaction have hypothesized (e.g., Moncrieff, 1955) that a loose, reversible adsorption between stimulating molecule and receptor surface takes place. Any such union must, however, be intimate enough to produce a permeability change in the membrane of the receptor cell.

4. TEMPERATURE RECEPTORS.   One tends to think of thermal receptors as perhaps the least specific of all sensory channels, and it is true that temperature sensitivity, often quite well developed, is frequently a property of endings whose primary response is to other modalities (see below). The problem of assigning a mechanism for thermal stimulation becomes a very specific

and challenging one, however, in receptors such as the pit organ of rattlesnakes, where Bullock and Diecke (1956) have shown that a temperature rise of around one-thousandth of a degree centigrade is sufficient to produce altered discharge in the ending. This corresponds to a Q_{10} of approximately 10^{30}! With receptors in the tongue, Hensel and Witt (1959) have shown that a thermal gradient in the skin is unnecessary for the production of impulses, and so *exchange* of thermal energy across the receptor is not a necessary condition for stimulation. Endings specifically sensitive to a *decrease* in temperature are found both in fish (Sand, 1938) and mammals (Zotterman, 1936), and their action clearly cannot be interpreted as a simple acceleration of temperature-sensitive chemistry in the receptor.

5. SUMMARY.   The emphasis of the foregoing section has been that although for a particular class of receptors the basic mechanism of energy absorption may be similar, the means of coupling the sensory ending to its environment produces vast differences in sensitivity (and often the frequency response) of the ending. It is in this realm that the greatest evolutionary differentiation of receptor endings has occurred. In the later stages of the receptor process, to be described below, a less variable set of mechanisms intervenes, and the following discussions will emphasize some properties in which many receptor endings appear to be quite similar.

Transduction

This term is applied, by analogy with certain physical devices, to the process by which the form of energy characteristic of the mode of stimulation is converted into electric currents which lead to the production and propagation of impulses. It is agreed that this is a most crucial problem in receptor physiology; yet it is the step in the process about which we have the least information. In the following section, it will be shown that in most receptors, a depolarizing slow potential follows the event of transduction, and is the direct cause of the initiation of impulse activity. The transduction problem thus centers about the question of how stimulus energy, once absorbed by the sensory ending, triggers the current flow associated with this slow depolarization. It is generally assumed that this process must involve an alteration in the permeability of some portion of the receptor membrane. Such membranes are, in general, electrically polarized just as are neural membranes. The result of such a permeability change would be a depolarizing current, carried primarily by entering sodium ions.

It need not be assumed, however, that the membranes across which such potentials exist are in every case like neural membranes, or even that they are single ones. For example, in the cochlea, a resting potential exists between scala media and scala tympani; in other words, across the sensory hair cells themselves. Excitatory currents in this system could thus be produced by changing the total resistance between these two compartments by some means not precisely analogous to the change in potential across a single membrane between the inside and outside of a cell.

The suggestion that a change in sodium permeability is involved in the origins of the electrical activity of receptors is based upon the generalization that depolarizing currents in excitable cells are carried primarily by the inward movement of cations, among which sodium is by far the likeliest candidate. Gray and Sato (1955) have shown that in the Pacinian corpuscle of the cat, perfusion with sodium-free solutions reduces nearly to zero the amplitude of the "generator" potential in that ending. Even if it could be shown, however, that all sensory transductions involve the alteration of membrane permeability (either to sodium or to all ions generally), we would still not have a satisfactory explanation for the mechanism of transducer action itself; for the same question would have to be asked again at the next level, i.e., "How does stimulus energy act upon the membrane to produce such permeability changes?" Here, of course, the receptor physiologist and the neurophysiologist are up against the same question, for the nature of the physical changes affecting membrane permeability are not known for any excitable system.

Generator Potentials

The notion that receptors produce, upon excitation, slow potentials which are responsible for generating impulse discharge is by now a very general one. Such slow potentials have been recorded from isolated sensory endings in several preparations in such a fashion as to leave no doubt that they are indeed, in these cases, responsible for triggering impulse discharge. However, studies on "generator" activity have been fraught with problems of interpretation, frequently related to the difficulty of being sure that a given slow potential is the product of pure receptor activity. Slow potentials from multi-unit receptor systems are familiar from the vertebrate retina (the electroretinogram, see Granit, 1947), insect eyes (Autrum, 1950), the olfactory epithelium (Ottoson, 1954) and others. Microphonic potentials, assumed to have the function of generator potentials, have been observed in the other derivatives of the acoustico-lateralis system in addition to the cochlea. In each of these cases there is some ambiguity, either concerning the origin of the slow potentials recorded, or their relation to neural discharge. It is almost certain, for example, that in the retina much of the electroretinogram is actually generated by structures belonging to the neural retina (Brown and Wiesel, 1958). In insect eyes, doubts of the same kind exist, though Autrum and Gallwitz (1951) have claimed that a monophasic potential attributable to receptors alone remains when the optic ganglion is removed from insect eyes. And while the cochlear microphone is an appropriate candidate for a generator potential because of its phase relationship to discharge in the auditory nerve, we have at this point no absolute assurance that it is not an accessory product of the events of excitation.

Even where microelectrode recordings from single receptor cells are possible, some ambiguities may exist in the interpretation of generator potential activity. A case in point is the ommatidium of *Limulus*. This preparation, in the hands of Hartline and his collaborators (e.g., Hartline et al., 1952), has had an illustrious history as one of the most thorough applications of the single fiber recording technique to sensory axons. The primary receptors are the retinula cells, organized in a circular array about a central rhabdome made up of individual rhabdomeres secreted by each retinula cell (Fig. 3). A second type of cell, the eccentric cell, sends its dendrite up amongst the retinula cells through the center of the rhabdome, and its axon passes to the central nervous system via the optic nerve. The retinula cells are also neurons, and do send axons centrally. However, from a single ommatidium in *Limulus* only a single fiber is electrically active; it is that from the eccentric cell. The retinula cell axons have not yet been shown to conduct impulses. Microelectrode penetrations of units within the ommatidium have given rise to records like that shown in Figure 3 (Fuortes, 1959). Spikes are superimposed on a slow depolariza-

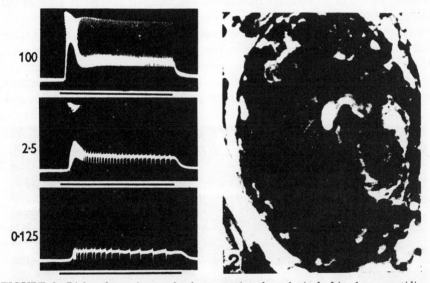

FIGURE 3. *Right*, photomicrograph of cross-section through single *Limulus* ommatidium. The rosette is formed of retinula cells, whose inner borders collectively form the rhabdome. The eccentric cell is seen at right, its dendrite curving into the rhabdome. The black material surrounding the sensory cells is screening pigment. (*From Miller, 1957*, J. Biophys. Biochem. Cytol.) *Left*, intracellular records from eccentric cell of *Limulus*, showing generator potentials with superimposed spikes. Figures at left give relative light intensity; duration of illumination indicated by bars beneath records. (*From Fuortes, 1959*, J. Physiol.)

tion, which reaches an early maximum and then subsides to a constant amplitude which is maintained during the period of stimulation. The difficulty is that this probably does not represent the activity of the first-order cell in this receptor system. It now seems quite certain that the visual pigment is located in the rhabdomere portions of the retinula cells, but that the slow potentials with superimposed spikes are recorded from the eccentric cell. The "generator potential" is thus analogous to a synaptic potential in that it is produced by presynaptic influence, possibly neurohumoral, emanating from the retinula cells. In a recent review, Davis (1961) has attempted to revise the terminolgy to suit such situations. He would restrict the term "receptor potential," often used synonymously with "generator potential," to those situations in which the spike-generating currents are produced in the receptor itself. The term "generator potential" would then apply to those cells, like the eccentric cell of *Limulus*, in which the spike-generating current is produced in a second-order neuron as the result of receptor activity.

To date, unambiguous receptor potentials responsible for generating repetitive impulses have been found in only a few sense organs. These are the muscle spindle of frog, shown in Figure 4 (Katz, 1950b), the Pacinian corpuscle (Gray and Sato, 1953) and the muscle receptor organs of decapod Crustacea (Eyzaguirre and Kuffler, 1955); a recent addition to this now-familiar trio is the hair mechanoreceptor of insects studied by Wolbarsht (1960). In the first two cases mentioned, the receptor potentials arise in the fine terminations of the nerve fiber involved—the portions from which the myelin sheath is absent. In the crustacean stretch receptor cells, the receptor potential originates in the dendrites. The potentials are in each case graded, and propagate decrementally in the same fashion as do synaptic potentials. And in all cases the region of spike initiation in the fiber is at some distance from the endings in which current sinks for the receptor potential are located.

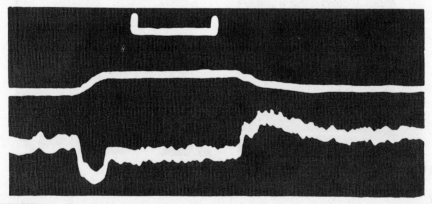

FIGURE 4. Generator potential recorded from frog's spindle, in response to a stretch indicated by the upper beam. Note static and dynamic phases of response, and hyperpolarization at "off." Time marker indicates 0.1 sec. (*From Katz, 1950b, J. Physiol.*)

Spike Initiation

At the heart of the problem of spike initiation in receptors is a recent generalization which concerns the initiation of impulses in neurons by natural means, whether these means are involved with neurohumorally-mediated synaptic action or with sensory excitation. This generalization was first made by Grundfest (1957); it has recently been applied to sensory endings in reviews by Gray (1959) and Davis (1961), and is discussed extensively in this volume by Hoyle. According to this view, the process of excitation involves the action of two fundamentally different kinds of excitable membrane. The first kind, termed "electrically inexcitable" membrane, is capable of undergoing graded depolarization (and decremental conduction) in response to specific chemical or other stimuli. It is not, however, capable of supporting a full action potential of the regenerative type, nor of being activated by electric current. The second type, called "electrically excitable" membrane, is characteristic of the conductile regions of axons. It typically supports over-shooting action potentials which propagate without decrement by successive electrical excitation of adjacent regions of the same kind of membrane. Evidence for this concept was first adduced by Grundfest from data on electric organs in a variety of fishes, and extended to a number of other types of excitable cells. Similar behavior is now thought to be shown by many kinds of sensory endings. In particular, evidence from the three types of mechanoreceptors described in the preceding paragraph suggests that the endings which produce receptor potentials of a graded kind are electrically inexcitable; that is, that they will not support a full spike either when activated by normal means or when stimulated antidromically. In all three of the systems mentioned, the site of impulse initiation appears to be appropriately distant from the ending itself:

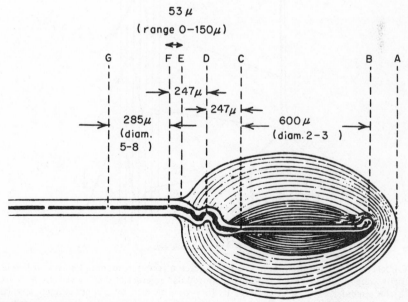

FIGURE 5. Diagram of the cat's Pacinian corpuscle giving various significant dimensions. The central core between B and C is occupied by the unmyelinated terminal of the receptor neuron: D indicates the first and F the second node of Ranvier. Impulses are initiated at D. (*From Quilliam and Sato, 1955, J. Physiol.*)

in the Pacinian corpuscle, for example, excitation of spikes takes place at the first node of Ranvier near the point of exit of the sensory fiber from the capsule (Fig. 5). In crustacean stretch receptors, the slow potential produced in the dendrites initiates spikes first at a point several hundred microns down the axon from the cell body (Edwards and Ottoson, 1958). In the latter case, the spike propagates not only centripetally along the axon, but also invades the soma of the receptor cell in a retrograde fashion (Fig. 6). The evidence suggests, however, that it does not invade the terminal portions of the dendrites where the stretch-induced depolarization is initiated. If all-or-none impulses did invade the very terminations of the receptor cell, the spikes would repolarize the membrane in those regions, and make it necessary for the entire depolarization cycle to be initiated over again. It is doubtful whether, under

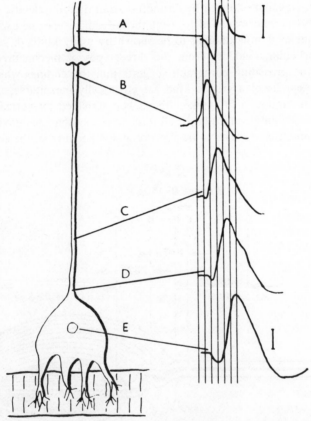

FIGURE 6. Impulse initiation in crustacean stretch receptor neuron. The action potentials at right were recorded by an exploring extracellular microelectrode moved from A to D, with the second lead fixed at position E; they were evoked by a quick stretch applied to the muscle. The response at B (0.5 mm down the axon) has the shortest latency and no initial positivity, indicating that B is the normal site for spike initiation. (*From Edwards and Ottoson, 1958*, J. Physiol.)

such circumstances, most receptor cells could maintain the high rates of discharge known to be characteristic of them. One perhaps hypothetical exception should be noted, however, to this generalization: reinvasion would be no handicap to an ending for which the normal stimulus is brief, especially if the response is typically a single impulse. In fact, reinvasion and consequent repolarization of any remaining generator potential might even safeguard the accuracy of its response to repeated, temporally discrete stimuli.

Special Problems

Poise of Excitability

While many sensory endings, like most neurons, are silent unless specifically stimulated, others show a resting discharge. This is characteristic, for example, of many mechanoreceptor endings when they are in the "normal" position, and of some temperature receptors (both warm and cold). In addition, second- or third-order neurons in other systems are active in the absence of sensory input, and discharge may be inferred to occur in the primary endings which they serve. It is clear that in many such cases so-called "spontaneous" activity may not be spontaneous at all, but the result of constant low-level stimulation of the ending which the experimenter is unable to detect. But in other systems it seems probable that "resting" discharge actually represents a poise towards excitation of the spike-generating portion of the sensory cell, possibly achieved through the existence of potential differences between different regions of the receptor unit.

Such resting discharges may be irregular, as in the case of statocyst hairs in crustaceans (Cohen, 1960) and thermal receptors in the pit organ of vipers (Bullock and Diecke, 1956); or they may be constant in frequency as in semicircular canal receptors (Lowenstein and Sand, 1940), or photoreceptor neurons in molluscs (Kennedy, 1960). Irregularities in the discharge of the former class may arise because of multiple, branching endings, with a number of out-of-phase sites of spontaneous excitation.

Constant-frequency spontaneous activity may have a number of functions. First of all, it provides a sensitive background against which appropriate central receiving stations may measure excitability changes. As Bullock (1959) has recently emphasized, modulation of ongoing discharge may require much less current than that necessary to excite a silent ending. A second function of regular spontaneous discharge may be in the opportunity it gives for bi-directional responsiveness. In vertebrate semicircular canals (Lowenstein and Sand, 1940), resting discharge from ampullar receptors is increased by ipsilateral and depressed by contralateral acceleration. Without spontaneous discharge, a single ending would be unable to inform the central nervous system of angular acceleration in both directions.

Related to this problem, but somewhat different from it, is the opportunity that spontaneous firing gives for "off" as well as "on" responses. An illustration of this comes from a photoreceptor neuron in the siphonal nerve of a lamellibranch mollusc (Kennedy, 1960). The afferent axon shows constant-frequency spontaneous activity in the dark. This is inhibited by illumination at low levels, but the cessation of illumination is followed by a high-frequency off-discharge (Fig. 7). In this case, it has been shown that inhibitory and

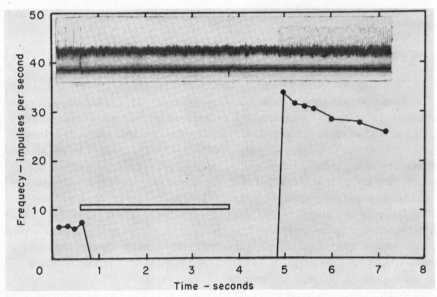

FIGURE 7. Inhibition by light in a molluscan photoreceptor neuron. The inset shows the oscilloscope tracing; duration of the stimulus is indicated by deflections on the second beam, and by the open bar on the graph. Points on the graph show discharge frequency, averaged over the preceding 0.2 sec. during the off-discharge. Stimulus wavelength 550 mμ, intensity 6×10^{-3} watts/cm^2. Longer wavelength stimuli produce a stronger and shorter-latency off-discharge than this; shorter wavelength stimuli produce a much longer inhibitory pause. (*From Kennedy, 1960, J. Gen. Physiol.*)

excitatory processes (the balance between which depends upon the wavelengths used to stimulate) occur simultaneously during illumination. The inhibitory process terminates abruptly at the end of the stimulus, releasing the off-response. This has the greatest importance for the behavior of the animal, which shows withdrawal responses to shadows. And, as in the previous case, the resting discharge allows for primary inhibition in response to stimulation. In another system, the insect ocellus (Ruck, 1961), the spontaneous discharge of a second-order neuron, which is suppressed or inhibited by the action of light-induced impulses in the sensory axons which synapse with it, apparently serves a similar function. Off-responses in the vertebrate retina (see for example Kuffler, 1953) may also arise through a mechanism involving secondary inhibition.

Accommodation and Receptor Time-Constant

Just as the crustacean motor axons studied by Hodgkin (1948) could be divided into classes according to their tendency to maintain firing rate during constant-current stimulation, so sensory endings show varying time-constants of accommodation. Those in which the discharge adapts quickly have usually been called phasic, the slowly-adapting ones tonic. Related to this differentiation is the question of what properties in the receptor ending determine its ability to support continued firing during a constant stimulus.

Many mechanoreceptor systems have now been found to consist of such dual channels, one tonic and the other phasic. Usually, the phasic channel tends to be served by thick-fibered, relatively high-threshold afferents. This problem was discussed some years ago by Bullock (1953). Since then, examples have multiplied: similar duality has been shown to exist for muscle receptor organs in crustacea (Eyzaguirre and Kuffler, 1955), for tactile receptors in mammalian skin (Hunt and McIntyre, 1960a), for mammalian joint receptors (Boyd and Roberts, 1953), and for proprioreceptors in the appendages of *Limulus* (Pringle, 1956; Barber, 1960) and decapod Crustacea (Burke, 1954; Wiersma and Boettiger, 1959).

The question of what makes a sensory ending quickly- or slowly-adapting is thus of great importance, and it is likely that the answers will differ from one case to the next. In many mechanoreceptors, for example, the deformation produced at the ending by a steadily applied force may decrease owing to visco-elastic properties of the coupling system. This explanation has been applied to frog tactile receptors (Lowenstein, 1956b). It appears to account satisfactorily for the change from "dynamic" to "static" firing in mammalian muscle spindles (Lippold et al., 1960a) and for adaptation in the Pacinian corpuscle (Hubbard, 1958). The reflection of these changes in receptor potential from the frog spindle is demonstrated in Figure 4; not only is there a "dynamic" phase followed by a "static" maintained depolarization, but a rebound hyperpolarization occurs upon relaxation. The differing adaptation rates between "fast" and "slow" muscle receptor organs in Crustacea may have the same basis (Eyzaguirre and Kuffler, 1955). Even though this sort of explanation may be satisfactory in most cases, it must be borne in mind that (1) the spike-initiating regions of neurons may show considerable variation in their ability to generate iterative responses to constant currents, and (2) non-linear process may intervene in the transduction of stimulus energy to depolarizing receptor potential. Either of these mechanisms is capable of affecting the overall time-constant of the receptor.

Central Control of Receptor Sensitivity

The central nervous system of an organism is much like a decision-making device into which a number of amplified input channels, the sensory pathways, are fed. The relative importance of these channels to the ultimate decision varies from moment to moment. We are beginning to learn of a number of mechanisms by which central "attentiveness" may be directed specifically at one or another of these channels. But this is not the only way in which their balance can be regulated: the central nervous system can, in some cases, adjust the gain of sensory channels by reflex outflow.

While this is usually done upstream of the primary ending, two cases are well known where it is accomplished at the very periphery. Though both of the receptors involved serve analogous functions, the mechanisms of central control are quite different, one operating directly upon the ending and the other indirectly. The first involves the motor nerve supply to the intrafusal muscle fibers of mammalian muscle spindles. These fibers, much smaller than those innervating ordinary extrafusal fibers, produce a tonic, facilitating excitation of the intrafusal muscle fibers; and this in turn affects the spindle's response to stretch (Hunt and Kuffler, 1951). By this means the sensory ending is enabled to produce discharges in response to stretch at any given muscle length, so that in effect the activity of small motor nerves increases spindle sensitivity by "taking up the slack." This is especially important when the spindle is suddenly decompressed during an active contraction of the extrafusal fibers around it. A complex central regulation of small motor nerve discharge exists, and has been recently reviewed by Hunt and Perl (1960).

Both "fast" and "slow" muscle receptor organs in decapod Cructacea are also centrally controlled. In this case, however, the centrifugal nerve supply is inhibitory, and reduces the sensitivity of the receptor instead of increasing it (Kuffler and Eyzaguirre, 1955). The inhibitor neuron ends in the vicinity of the receptor dendrites, and acts upon them through the liberation of a transmitter substance presumably identical to that liberated at the peripheral inhibitory endings upon muscle. The reflex role of these inhibitor neurons has recently been analyzed by Eckert (1961); other changes in sensitivity may be caused by central motor outflow of the receptor muscles themselves.

Other instances of centrifugal control include some more indirect effects, e.g., that of sympathetic stimulation upon the sensitivity of tactile receptors in frog skin (Lowenstein, 1956a). But it seems safe to predict that further cases of direct influence will come to light in other systems.

Modality Purity

Many sensory endings have now been shown to respond to more than one form of energy in apparent violation of the principle of receptor specificity which has been a traditional part of the sensory physiologist's doctrine. This issue has been reviewed by Rose and Mountcastle (1959) with respect to cutaneous receptors in mammals, and will not be treated extensively here. The inventory of endings which show lack of modality purity, however, is becoming impressive: it now includes touch receptors in mammals (Witt and Hensel, 1959; Hunt and McIntyre, 1960b), muscle spindles (Lippold et al., 1960b), lateralis organs and ampullae of Lorenzini in fish (Murray, 1956, 1959), and others. In each case, temperature sensitivity is combined with mechanoreceptive function; and in some of the cases it is difficult indeed to decide which is the *primary* modality served.

An odd variation on this theme is represented by the photosensory nerve cells of the sixth abdominal ganglion in the crayfish first discovered by Prosser (1934). These cells play a functional role in the regulation of motor activity, and their discharge upon illumination can be recorded from single units in the ventral nerve cord (Kennedy, 1958). Recent experiments (Kennedy, unpublished) have shown that each of the primary photoreceptor afferents which passes anteriorly in the nerve cord also acts as a second order inter-neuron relaying phasic tactile stimuli from the tail. Electrical stimuli delivered to the ipsilateral afferent roots of the ganglion produce postsynaptic responses in the photosensory neuron, and these are identical to those elicited by natural stimulation of tactile hairs. Contralateral afferents are inhibitory, and repetitive stimulation can inhibit both ipsilaterally-evoked discharges and the response to illumination of these cells. These relationships are illustrated in the records of Figure 8. Thus these units, too, have a dual functional sensory character,

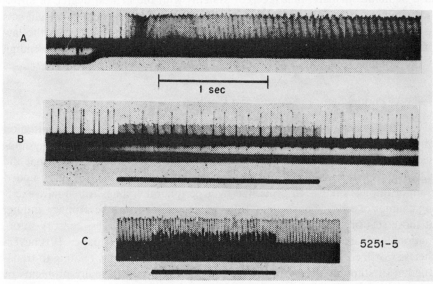

FIGURE 8. Responses from a single afferent fiber from the crayfish caudal photoreceptor, isolated from the ventral nerve cord by fine dissection. A. Response to illumination of the sixth ganglion; lower beam is the record from a monitoring photocell indicating onset of illumination. B. Stimulation in the dark of contralateral uropod nerves, which inhibits spontaneous discharge; C. Same during illumination, producing less evident inhibition.

as primary light receptors and as integrating relay neurons for tactile stimuli. Confusion may be avoided by the fact that one modality (light) yields tonic discharges, whereas the other is phasic and therefore superimposable upon the first.

The fact that a central neuron is here acting in the special capacity of a sensory receptor leads naturally into speculations about the extent to which unspecialized neurons may show the potentiality for activation by sensory stimuli. Uchizono (1961) has demonstrated by electron microscopy the presence of lamellar organelles in crayfish ganglia which resemble to an astonishing degree the rhabdomeres of arthropod eyes, and these structures may be responsible for mediating the light responses just described. Other neurons, too, show light-sensitivity: that of molluscan ganglion cells has been elegantly analyzed by Arvanitaki and Chalazonitis (1960), and there are several other cases. The sensitivity of a variety of neurons and muscle cells to amino acids (e.g., Robbins, 1959; Curtis et al., 1959) is being actively pursued. Low-threshold temperature effects are associated with a number of endings serving other functions (see above), and deformation sensitivity may exist in some sensory neurons primarily associated with other functions. In short, evidence is accumulating that the basic mechanisms underlying various sensory responses may be rather widely distributed among excitable cells, and that the evolution of receptor specificity may involve selective emphasis upon one or two of these properties. A completely speculative addition to this picture might also be made: namely, that receptor systems with the highest degree of specificity and sensitivity are those in which a secondary cell of epithelial origin acts as the primary transducing site. At the moment the departures from the law of stimulus specificity all seem to occur in sense organs in which a nerve ending is the primary receptor.

Ascending Sensory Systems and Coding

This review has dealt primarily with problems related to the initiation of impulses by peripheral receptor endings. While to many sensory physiologists this is the major area of concern, it is important to point out that the significant operations of sensory systems do not end once the frequency-coded train of impulses has been generated by a peripheral ending. An equally exciting chapter of sensory physiology is being written far from the primary ending, at those sets of synaptic junctions which integrate and process sensory information. Such analyses are obviously beyond the scope of this paper. It is nevertheless worth concluding with the note that once the problems relating to transduction of stimulus energy in the nerve ending are solved, many problems of an even more complex nature remain in achieving the final link-up between sensory discharge and the process of perception.

References

Adrian, E. D. 1928. *The basis of sensation.* Christopher's, London.
Arvanitaki, A., and N. Chalazonitis. 1960. Photopotentials d'excitation et d'inhibi-

tion de differents somata identifiables (*Aplysia*). Activation monochromatiques. *Bull. Inst. Oceanogr. Monaco* **1164:**1–83.

Autrum, H. 1950. Die Belichtungspotentiale und das Sehen der Insekten. *Z. vergl. Physiol.* **32:**176–227.

Autrum, H., and D. Burkhardt. 1961. Spectral sensitivity of single visual cells. *Nature* **190:**639.

Autrum, H., and U. Gallwitz. 1951. Zur Analalyse der Belichtungspotentiale des Insektenauges. *Z. vergl. Physiol.* **33:**407–425.

Barber, S. 1960. Structure and properties of *Limulus* articular proprioceptors. *J. Exp. Zool.* **143:**283–322.

Békésy, G. von. 1956. Current status of theories of hearing. *Science* **123:**779–783.

Boyd, I. A., and T. D. M. Roberts. 1953. Proprioceptive discharges from stretch-receptors in the knee joint of the cat. *J. Physiol.* **122:**38–58.

Brown, K. T., and T. Wiesel. 1958. Intraretinal recording in the unopened cat eye. *Amer. J. Ophthalmol.* **46:**91–98.

Brown, P. K., and P. S. Brown. 1958. Visual pigments of the octopus and cuttlefish. *Nature* **182:**1288–1290.

Bullock, T. H. 1953. Comparative aspects of some biological transducers. *Fed. Proc.* **12:**666–672.

———. 1959. Initiation of impulses in receptor and central neurons. *Rev. Mod. Physics* **31:**504–514.

Bullock, T. H., and F. P. J. Diecke. 1956. Properties of an infra-red receptor. *J. Physiol.* **134:**47–87.

Burke, W. 1954. An organ for proprioception and vibration-sense in *Carcinus maenas*. *J. Exp. Biol.* **31:**127–138.

Cohen, M. G. 1960. The response patterns of single receptors in the crustacean statocyst. *Proc. Roy. Soc. (London), B,* **152:**30–49.

Curtis, D. R., J. W. Phillips, and J. C. Watkins. 1959. The depression of spinal neurons by γ-amino n-butyric acid and β-alanine. *J. Physiol.* **146:**185–203.

Davis, H. 1957. Biophysics and physiology of the inner ear. *Physiol. Revs.* **37:**1–49.

———. 1961. Some principles of sensory receptor action. *Physiol. Revs.* **41:**391–416.

Denton, E. J. 1959. The contributions of the orientated photosensitive and other molecules to the absorption of the whole retina. *Proc. Roy. Soc. (London), B,* **150:**78–94.

Denton, E. J., and F. S. Warren. 1957. The photosensitive pigments in the retinae of deep-sea fish. *J. Mar. Biol. Ass. U. K.* **36:**651–662.

Eckert, R. O. 1961. Reflex relationships of the abdominal stretch receptors of the crayfish. I. Feedback inhibition of the receptors. *J. Cell. Comp. Physiol.* **57:**149–162.

Edwards, C., and D. Ottoson. 1958. The site of impulse initiation in a nerve cell of a crustacean stretch receptor. *J. Physiol.* **143:**138–148.

Engström, H., and J. Wersäll. 1958. The ultrastructural organization of the organ of Corti and of the vestibular sensory epithelia. *Exp. Cell. Res. Supp.* **5:**463–492.

Eyzaguirre, C., and S. W. Kuffler. 1955. Processes of excitation in the dendrites and in the soma of single isolated sensory nerve cells of the lobster and crayfish. *J. Gen. Physiol.* **39:**87–119.

Fuortes, M. G. F. 1959. Initiation of impulses in visual cells of *Limulus*. *J. Physiol.* **148:**14–28.

Goldsmith, T. 1958. On the visual system of the bee (*Apis mellifera*). *Ann. N. Y. Acad. Sci.* **74:**223–229.

Granit, R. 1947. *Sensory mechanisms of the retina*. Oxford, London.

Gray, J. A. B. 1959. Initiation of impulses at receptors, pp. 123–145. In *Handbook of physiology*, I, Amer. Physiol. Soc.

Gray, J. A. B., and M. Sato. 1953. Properties of the receptor potential in Pacinian corpuscles. *J. Physiol.* **122:**610–636.

———. 1955. The movement of sodium and other ions in Pacinian corpuscles. *J. Physiol.* **129:**594–607.

Grundfest, H. 1957. Electrical inexcitability of synapses and some consequences for the central nervous system. *Physiol. Revs.* **37:**337–361.

Hartline, H. K., H. G. Wagner, and E. F. MacNichol, Jr. 1952. The peripheral origin of nervous activity in the visual system. *Cold Spr. Harb. Sympos. Quant. Biol.* **17:**125–141.

Hensel, H., and I. Witt. 1959. Spatial temperature gradient and thermoreceptor stimulation. *J. Physiol.* **148:**180–187.

Hodgkin, A. L. 1948. The local electric changes associated with repetitive action in a non-medullated axon. *J. Physiol.* **107:**165–181.

Hodgson, E. S., and K. D. Roeder. 1956. Electrophysiological studies of arthropod chemoreception. *J. Cell. Comp. Physiol.* **48:**51–75.

Hubbard, R., P. K. Broan, and A. Kropf. 1959. Action of light on visual pigments: Vertebrate lumi- and meta-rhodopsins. *Nature* **183:**442–450.

Hubbard, S. J. 1958. A study of mechanical events in a mechanoreceptor. *J. Physiol.* **141:**198–218.

Hunt, C. C. 1952. Muscle stretch receptors; peripheral mechanisms and reflex function. *Cold Spr. Harb. Sympos. Quant. Biol.* **17:**113–123.

Hunt, C. C., and S. W. Kuffler. 1951. Stretch receptor discharges during muscle contraction. *J. Physiol.* **113:**298–315.

Hunt, C. C., and A. K. McIntyre. 1960a. Properties of cutaneous touch receptors in cat. *J. Physiol.* **153:**88–98.

———. 1960b. An analysis of fiber diameter and receptor characteristics of myelinated cutaneous afferent fibers in cat. *J. Physiol.* **153:**99–112.

Hunt, C. C., and E. R. Perl. 1960. Spinal reflex mechanisms concerned with skeletal muscle. *Physiol. Revs.* **40:**538–579.

Jielof, R., A. Spoor, and H. de Vries. 1952. The microphonic activity of the lateral line. *J. Physiol.* **116:**137–157.

Katz, B. 1950a. Action potentials from a sensory nerve ending. *J. Physiol.* **111:**248–260.

———. 1950b. Depolarization of sensory terminals and the initiation of impulses in the muscle spindle. *J. Physiol.* **111:**261–282.

Kennedy, D. 1958. Responses from the crayfish caudal photoreceptor. *Amer. J. Ophthalmol.* **46,** II:19–26.

———. 1960. Neural photoreception in a lamellibranch mollusc. *J. Gen. Physiol.* **44:**277–299.

Kennedy, D., and M. S. Bruno. 1961. The spectral sensitivity of crayfish and lobster vision. *J. Gen. Physiol.* **44:**1091–1104.

Kennedy, D., and R. D. Milkman. 1956. Selective light absorption by the lenses of lower vertebrates, and its influence on spectral sensitivity. *Biol. Bull.* **111:**375–386.

Kuffler, S. W. 1953. Discharge patterns and functional organization of mammalian retina. *J. Neurophysiol.* **16:**37–68.

Kuffler, S. W., and C. Eyzaquirre. 1955. Synaptic inhibition in an isolated nerve cell. *J. Gen. Physiol.* **39:**155–184.

Lippold, O. C. J., J. G. Nicholls, and J. W. T. Redfearn. 1960a. Electrical and mechanical factors in the adaptation of mammalian muscle spindle. *J. Physiol.* **153:**209–217.

————. 1960b. A study of the afferent discharge produced by cooling a mammalian muscle spindle. *J. Physiol.* **153**:218–231.

Löwenstein, O., and T. D. M. Roberts. 1949. The equilibrium function of the otolith organs of the thornback ray (*Raja clavata*). *J. Physiol.* **110**:392–415.

————. 1951. The localization and analysis of the responses to vibration from the isolated elasmobranch labyrinth. A contribution to the problem of the evolution of hearing in vertebrates. *J. Physiol.* **114**:471–489.

Löwenstein, O., and A. Sand. 1940. The mechanism of the semicircular canal. A study of the responses of single-fibre preparations to angular accelerations and to rotation at constant speed. *Proc. Roy. Soc. (London)*, B, **129**:256–275.

Lowenstein, W. 1956a. Modulation of cutaneous mechanoreceptors by sympathetic stimulation. *J. Physiol.* **132**:40–60.

————. 1956b. Excitation and changes in adaptation by stretch of mechanoreceptors. *J. Physiol.* **133**:588–602.

Matthews, B. H. C. 1933. Nerve endings in mammalian muscle. *J. Physiol.* **78**: 1–53.

Miller, W. H. 1957. Morphology of the ommatidia of the compound eye of *Limulus*. *J. Biophys. Biochem. Cytol.* **3**:421–428.

Moncrieff, R. W. 1955. The sorptive properties of the olfactory membrane. *J. Physiol.* **130**:543–558.

Murray, R. W. 1956. The thermal sensitivity of the lateralis organs of *Xenopus*. *J. Exp. Biol.* **33**:798–805.

————. 1959. The response of the ampullae of Lorenzini to combined stimulation by temperature change and weak direct currents. *J. Physiol.* **145**:1–13.

Ottoson, D. 1954. Sustained potentials evoked by olfactory stimulation. *Acta Physiol. Scand.* **32**:384–385.

Pringle, J. W. S. 1956. Proprioception in *Limulus*. *J. Exp. Biol.* **33**:658–667.

Prosser, C. L. 1934. Action potentials in the nervous system of the crayfish. II. Responses to illumination of the eye and caudal ganglion. *J. Cell. Comp. Physiol.* **4**:363–377.

Quillam, T. A., and M. Sato. 1955. The distribution of myelin on nerve fibers from Pacinian corpuscles. *J. Physiol.* **129**:167–176.

Robbins, J. 1959. The excitation and inhibition of crustacean muscle by amino acids. *J. Physiol.* **148**:39–50.

Rose, J. E., and V. B. Mountcastle. 1959. Touch and kinesthesis, pp. 387–429. In *Handbook of physiology* I, Amer. Physiol. Soc.

Ruck, P. 1961. Electrophysiology of the insect dorsal ocellus. II. Mechanisms of generation and inhibition of impulses in the ocellar nerve of dragonflies. *J. Gen. Physiol.* **44**:629–639.

Rushton, W. A. H. 1958. Kinetics of cone pigments measured objectively on the living human fovea. *Ann. N. Y. Acad. Sci.* **74**:291–304.

Sand, A. 1938. The function of the ampullae of Lorenzini with some observations on the effect of temperature on sensory rhythms. *Proc. Roy. Soc. (London)*, B, **125**:524–553.

Schneider, D. 1957. Electrophysiologische Untersuchungen von Chemo- und Mechanorezeptoren der Antenne des Seidenspinners *Bombyx mori*. L. *Zeits. f. vergl. Physiol.* **40**:8–41.

Steinhausen, W. 1931. Über den Nachweis der Bewegung der Cupula in der intakten Bogengangs ampulla des Labyrinthes bei der Natürlichen rotatorischen und calorischen Reizung. *Pflüg. Arch. ges. Physiol.* **228**:322–328.

Uchizono, K. 1961. Possible photoreceptors in the sixth ganglion of crayfish. *Fed. Proc.* **20**(1):325.

Walcott, C., and W. G. Van der Kloot. 1959. Physiology of the spider vibration receptor. *J. Exp. Zool.* **141:**191–244.

Wald, G. 1959. The photoreceptor process in vision, pp. 671–692. In *Handbook of physiology, Neurophysiology* I, Amer. Physiol. Soc.

Wiersma, C. A. G., and E. G. Boettiger. 1957. Unidirectional movement fibers from a proprioceptive organ of the crab, *Carcinus maenas. J. Exp. Biol.* **36:**102–112.

Witt, I., and H. Hensel. 1959. Afferente Impulse aus der Extremitätenhaut der Katze bei thermischer und mechanischer Reizung. *Pflüg. Arch. ges. Physiol.* **286:**582–596.

Wolbarsht, M. L. 1960. Electrical characteristics of insect mechanoreceptors. *J. Gen. Physiol.* **44:**105–122.

Wolbarsht, M. L., and V. G. Dethier. 1958. Electrical activity in the chemoreceptors of the blowfly. *J. Gen. Physiol.* **42:**393–412.

Zotterman, Y. 1936. Specific action potentials in the lingual nerve of cat. *Scand. Arch. Physiol.* **75:**106–119.

Sensory Neural Patterns and Gustation

ROBERT P. ERICKSON

Reprinted from *First International Symposium on Olfaction and Taste.* New York: Pergamon Press, 1963, pp. 205–213.

At present there is no thorough understanding of the nature of the afferent neural message for taste quality.* This is due in large part to our lack of knowledge about the significant aspects of the taste stimulus. However, it is possible to come to a partial analysis of the neural message *without* this knowledge about the stimulus. The nature of this analysis will be made clear by reference to those sensory systems where the neural message has been worked out in some detail.

Method to Determine Number of Sensory Fiber Types

In color vision there are probably very few receptor types, these being represented in the optic nerve by a corresponding number of fiber types.† Assume that there are only three such receptor-fiber types, and let the three

---

* "Taste quality" refers to the "salt-sour-sweet-etc." aspect of taste as distinct from intensity.

† Although perhaps inexact, the assumption is made in this paper that the stimulus sensitivity functions of receptors are reflected without change in their lower-order afferent neurons, and that arguments referring to one apply also to the other.

curves in Figure 1*A* represent the responsiveness of these three types to the various wavelengths of light. Since in taste the significant parameters of the stimulus are not understood fully (as pH, etc.), let us suppose that in vision also the nature of the stimulus for color is not understood. Assume that four colors are available as stimuli and recordings are obtained from a series of

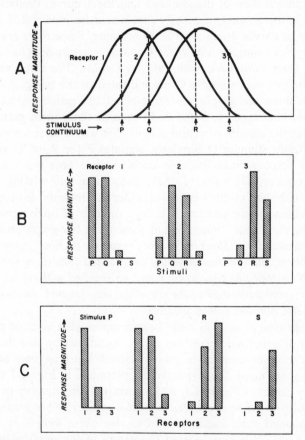

FIGURE 1. Afferent fiber types and patterns of neural activity.

A. Afferent fiber-types (or receptor types). Curves 1, 2, and 3 represent the responsiveness of three hypothetical afferent fiber types (or receptor types) along a hypothetical stimulus continuum. P, Q, R, and S represent four stimuli along this stimulus continuum. The responsiveness of a fiber type to one of these stimuli is indicated by the intersection of the response curve and the ordinate erected at the stimulus.

B. Responsiveness of the three fiber types to the four stimuli in A. In each of the bar graphs is shown the responsiveness of one of the fiber types to each of the stimuli in A. If recordings were obtained from one of the fiber types shown in A using these stimuli, one of these three "response profiles" would be obtained, depending upon which fiber type was being sampled. There would be as many "response profiles" as fiber types.

C. Across-fiber patterns. In these bar graphs are shown the patterns of activity across the three fiber types produced by the four stimuli in A. Each stimulus produces a characteristic pattern across the three fiber types. There would be as many across-fiber patterns as stimuli.

single optic nerve fibers using first the stimulus indicated as Q in the figure. What kind of recordings will result? It is seen from the ordinate erected at Q that the amount of neural activity that would be recorded may take only three values depending on which type of optic nerve fiber was being sampled. If the recording was from fiber type 1, the value that would be obtained is indicated by the intersection of this ordinate and the 1 curve; similarly, for fiber types 2 and 3, the amount of activity that would be obtained is represented by the values of curves 2 and 3 at the Q ordinate. *Since there are only three fiber types in this example, only three response magnitudes (including zero) could result from stimulation with any given color.* The three values which would be obtained with stimulus Q are indicated in the bar graphs in Figure 1*B*. In these three bar graphs are represented the activity which would be recorded from fiber types 1, 2 and 3. In each of these three graphs, the bar for Q indicates the amount of neural activity that would be recorded from that fiber type with the stimulus Q. Similarly, stimulus P (or R, or S) would evoke characteristic response magnitudes in each of these fiber types as indicated. Whenever we record from fiber 1, then, using these four stimuli, we will get a bar graph with the "profile" indicated under 1. Similarly, fiber types 2 and 3 will yield characteristic profiles. If a large number of optic nerve fibers are sampled using these four stimuli, one of these three bar graph profiles will be obtained from each fiber. *Since only three "response profiles" could be derived from these fibers, the conclusion would be reached that there are only three fiber types. Note that this conclusion could be reached without having knowledge of the relevant parameter of the stimulus (wavelength), and without being able to vary the stimulus systematically.*

The same kind of analysis could be accomplished in audition demonstrating the effect of a multiplicity of fiber types. Again assume that the significant aspect of the stimulus for pitch is not understood, but four tones are available as stimuli. If these many fiber types were represented in Figure 1 there would be very many curves in Figure 1*A,* and a corresponding number of bar graphs in Figure 1*B. It would be concluded from the number of bar graph profiles of responses obtained from auditory neurons that there were very many fiber types, even if we did not understand the nature of the stimulus, and did not vary it systematically.*

Determination of the Number of Gustatory Fiber Types

The above considerations give us some clues concerning the sensory neural message for taste quality. Many investigators have collected the type of bar graph for taste shown in Figure 1*B.* Some examples are shown in Figures 2 and 3. Those in Figure 2 were obtained from single second-order neurons in the nucleus of the solitary tract of rats anesthetized with pentobarbital sodium. KCl-filled glass micropipettes were used. Similar bar graphs

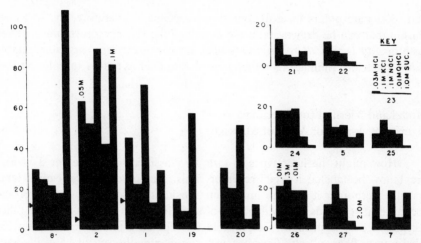

FIGURE 2. Receptor profiles analogous to those shown in Figure 1B. Recordings obtained from single neurons in the nucleus of the solitary tract of the rat. Bar heights indicate number of impulses recorded in the first second of evoked activity. Small triangles indicate spontaneous level of activity.

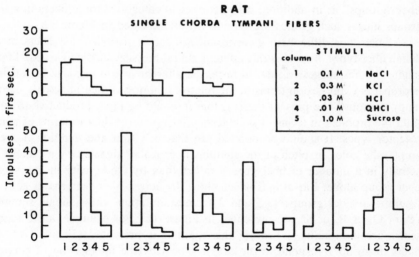

FIGURE 3. As Figure 2 except recordings obtained from single chorda tympani fibers.

describing the responsiveness of first-order neurons in the chorda tympani nerve of the rat are shown in Figure 3. With reference to Figure 1B, it would not be easy to place these graphs into a few groups on the basis of the profiles they present, but rather there would be very many groups. (It is, of course, not necessary that these groups be represented by smooth, uninterrupted curves on uninterrupted continua; e.g., it would be impossible to devise a strictly continuous baseline out of a series of diverse anions. These could, at best, designate points on a discontinuous baseline.) Therefore, the first conclusion that can be drawn about the nature of the sensory neural message for taste quality is that *there are many fiber types representing gustatory quality* as for pitch discrimination, rather than a few fiber types as in color vision.

Model and Method to Determine
Significant Aspect of Afferent Message

How might the fiber types in taste be classified? Let receptor 3 in Figure 1 now be labeled a "red" receptor. This is a somewhat misleading label because, although it has its maximum sensitivity in the red region of the spectrum, it responds to a wide range of stimuli, and in concert with the other receptor types, is probably responsible for signaling many wavelengths. To label a taste fiber a "salt" fiber because it is maximally sensitive to salts likewise may be misleading because it, as the red receptor, is probably responsible for signaling a number of stimuli. Actually, until the stimulus dimensions for taste quality are established, a fiber's point of maximum sensitivity cannot readily be established. Because of the possibility of a very large number of fiber "groups" as in audition, it is incorrect to categorize these fibers in a few groups unless such groups are established as indicated in Figure 1*B*.

Since it is difficult to give meaningful labels to individual fibers or to define fiber types, how may this afferent neural message best be viewed? Pfaffmann (1) has suggested that, in taste, the afferent neural message for quality is probably expressed in terms of the relative amounts of neural activity across many neurons. The present thesis is that it would be more productive to consider the problem in terms of such across-fiber patterns than in terms of many receptor types. It should be pointed out that in vision and audition, for example, the color or pitch of the stimulus is probably signaled by a pattern of activity in a number of fiber groups rather than by the activity in any single fiber group alone. Bar graphs which show the across-fiber patterns of activity resulting in fiber groups 1, 2 and 3 from stimulation with a single stimulus (P, or Q, or R, or S) are presented in Figure 1*C*. For example, let Q represent a green stimulus. Whenever this stimulus is presented (Figure 1*A*), all fibers in group 1 respond to the extent shown by the intersection of curve 1 with the ordinate at Q, all fibers in group 2 respond to the extent shown by the intersection of curve 2 and this ordinate, and similarly for all fibers in group 3. The resulting across-fiber patterning is given in Figure 1*C,* stimulus Q. These three levels of activity in these fiber groups would form a pattern to signal the stimulus Q, or green. Presumably this kind of pattern signals the quality of the stimulus in vision and audition.

Can evidence be obtained that in gustation too, the significant aspect of the neural message is actually the pattern of activity across many taste neurons? There are two steps to the resolution of this question, one physiological and the other behavioral. First, the across-fiber patterns of response for a number of taste solutions must be observed. Second, it must be determined if these patterns are actually significant for the interpretation of the qualities of the taste stimuli. In the experiments which follow, neural patterns were determined for several taste substances; predictions concerning the discriminability of these taste solutions were then made from their neural patterns and tested in behavioral experiments.

Determination of Significant Aspect of Afferent Message; Physiological and Behavioral

First, the responsiveness of a number of chorda tympani fibers to several taste solutions was determined in the rat anesthetized with pentobarbital sodium. Some of these data are presented in Figure 4 in a way which shows the across-fiber pattern. Here the fibers are arranged along the baseline in order of their responsiveness to NH_4Cl. Any other arrangement would be satisfactory for the present purposes. The degree of their responsiveness to this solution is indicated by the black dots connected with the solid lines. In this way is shown a pattern of the amount of neural activity across many neural units, and is the across-fiber NH_4Cl pattern.* According to the present hypothesis this pattern is what signals the quality of NH_4Cl at least as far as these 13 fibers are concerned.

A very important test of the pattern theory of taste quality sensitivity is that if the quality of a stimulus is actually signaled by this kind of patterning, then stimuli which give similar patterns should taste somewhat alike. Conversely, stimuli producing highly dissimilar patterns should taste considerably different. In Figure 4 we see that KCl produces a pattern quite similar to that produced by NH_4Cl, at least as contrasted with the NaCl pattern. A measure of the similarity of these patterns is given by the correlation between the amplitudes of the responses produced by these solutions in these fibers. The product-moment correlation coefficient between the amplitudes of responses to NH_4Cl and KCl for these 13 fibers is $+0.83$, indicating a close similarity between these patterns. The pattern produced by NaCl, as indicated by the unconnected open circles in Figure 4, is not very similar to either the KCl or NH_4Cl patterns. In Table 1 are shown correlation coefficients based on a larger number of fibers. Thus, the neural patterns predict that for the rat, KCl and NH_4Cl should have similar tastes, but neither of them should taste very much like NaCl.

(It is clear from Table 1, in which are presented correlations between the amount of response of the fibers tested to a number of taste solutions, that

---

* Some other aspect of the across-fiber pattern of neural activity more subtle than number of impulses in the first second of evoked activity may prove more predictive of behavior.

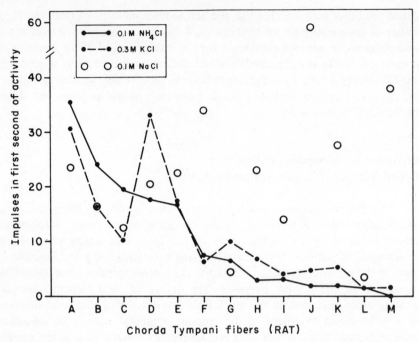

FIGURE 4. Across-fiber patterns analogous to those shown in Figure 1C, except that connected points are used instead of bars, and 13 fibers are shown instead of three. Single rat chorda tympani fibers. Fibers arranged along baseline in order of responsiveness to NH₄Cl. KCl pattern similar to NH₄Cl pattern. Neither of these patterns similar to the NaCl pattern.

NH_4Cl, KCl *and* $CaCl_2$ all produce similar neural patterns, and that LiCl produces a neural pattern very similar to that produced by NaCl. High correlations also suggest that these stimuli are relatively adjacent on the stimulus continua. However, it can be demonstrated that low correlations indicate little more than that the neural patterns produced are dissimilar; the relative placement of these pairs of stimuli on the stimulus continua are indicated more by the *form* of the correlation scattergram than by the degree of correlation.)

Now let us turn to the behavior predicted from the neural data. Two stimuli may be defined as perceptually similar to the extent that a response learned to one of them will generalize to the other. Thus, if these neural patterns are the basis for taste quality sensitivity, a response learned to one stimulus should generalize to another stimulus producing a similar neural pattern, but not as much to one giving a different pattern. If such predictions are borne out, it would be indicated that such neural patterns actually are the basis of taste quality sensitivity.

Two behavioral tests were employed, both based on the generalization of shock-based avoidance of drinking from one salt to others. In the first test, three rats each learned to avoid drinking one of three salts, KCl, NH₄Cl or

Table 1.

Correlations between single chorda tympani fiber responses to a number of taste solutions. Only one concentration of each solution used. In each cell is given first the product-moment correlation coefficient, then the number of fibers upon which this correlation is based, and finally, for the larger correlations, the probability that a correlation of this magnitude would occur by chance if the correlation were actually zero.

LiCl	CaCl₂	NH₄Cl	KCl	HCl	QHCl	1.0 M Sucrose	
+0.94	−0.30	−0.11	−0.09	+0.39	+0.20	+0.17	
12	11	25	25	17	18	10	0.1 M NaCl
<0.01							
	−0.32	−0.30	−0.21	+0.31	+0.15	+0.46	
	11	14	14	12	13	11	0.1 M LiCl
		+0.77	+0.74	+0.45	−0.22	−0.25	
		12	12	12	11	10	0.3 M CaCl₂
		<0.01	<0.01				
			+0.88	+0.58	+0.11	−0.19	
			28	18	21	14	0.1 M NH₄Cl
			<0.01	<0.05			
				+0.59	−0.09	−0.18	
				18	21	14	0.3 M KCl
				0.01			
					+0.39	−0.12	
					17	11	0.03 M HCl
						+0.13	
						14	0.01 M QHCl

NaCl in a single tube test (total of nine rats). Shocks (1 mA for 0.3 sec were delivered through the feet whenever the rat drank for about 2 sec. On several days following the avoidance training, recovery of drinking, the training stimulus or another salt was noted. Being shocked for drinking KCl resulted in a depression of drinking rates for both KCl and NH₄Cl, but not so much depression of NaCl drinking. Similarly, being shocked for drinking NH₄Cl resulted in a depression of drinking rates for both NH₄Cl and KCl, but not so much for NaCl. The depression of drinking from being shocked for NaCl generalized somewhat to both the other salts, but not selectively more to one than the other.

In the second behavioral test, two rats each learned to avoid drinking one of the three salt solutions used in the first behavioral test in a three-tube test (total of six rats). Shocks (3 mA) were applied between the metal drinking tube and the floor whenever the rat drank for about 2 sec. Each rat was first trained to avoid one of the three salts, and then tested for degree of avoidance of all three. In both tests, the following concentrations were used in a random fashion to insure that the discriminations were not developed on the basis of intensity differences: KCl and NH₄Cl—0.01, 0.03, and 0.1 M; NaCl—

0.003, 0.01, 0.03 and 0.1 м. The results are similar to those obtained in the first behavioral test. Depression of drinking generalized between KCl and NH₄Cl, but not so much between either of these and NaCl.

To summarize the results of the behavioral tests, responses learned to KCl generalized to NH₄Cl and vice versa. Responses learned to either KCl or NH₄Cl generalized much less to NaCl and vice versa. It appears that, for the rat, KCl and NH₄Cl taste more nearly alike than either do to NaCl. Therefore, in addition to concluding that there are many fiber types in gustation, one may conclude that *the neural message for gustatory quality is a pattern made up of the amount of neural activity across many neural elements.*

These data support an across-fiber pattern theory for taste quality sensitivity. These patterns which signal the quality of the taste stimulus are developed across a great number of fibers. The various fibers involved show considerable diversity in their sensitivity to taste stimulation; this diversity in sensitivity prevents easy fiber classification, but provides the basis for the across-fiber patterns.

Acknowledgements

The able technical assistance of David A. Marshall and John A. Pooler, and the advice of C. Alan Boncau and Irving I. Diamond were very much appreciated.

Reference

Pfaffmann, C. 1955. Gustatory nerve impulses in rat, cat and rabbit. *J. Neurophysiol.* **18,** 429–440.

Coding in the Auditory Nervous System

I. C. WHITFIELD

Reprinted from *Nature*, Feb. 25, 1967, Vol. 213.

The idea of auditory analysis by resonant structures is one of some antiquity. The earliest theories were framed in terms of cavity resonances, for the inner ear was then thought to be filled with air. Quite explicit theories of this type are to be found at the beginning of the seventeenth century. From the time of du Verney [1] onwards, however, the solid structures to which the auditory nerve is distributed came to be regarded as the resonators, and the only changes between 1700 and 1850 resulted from a continuing search for the precise location of the resonators, the field of search being progressively opened up by improvements in microscopic and histological technique. The postulated resonance seems to have been regarded mainly as a means of magnifying the weak sound stimulus rather than as an analytic mechanism, although du Verney did consider that as a result of differential vibration the auditory nerve would "receive different impressions which represent in the brain the various characteristics of tones." Haller [2] appears to have been the first to speculate on the possibility of distinguishing sound frequencies by the frequency of the "tremors" in the auditory nerve fibres and thus to have foreshadowed the other great group of auditory coding theories—the frequency or "telephone" theories first formalized by Rutherford in 1886.

In 1857 Helmholtz [3] produced his famous theory, which can probably be regarded as the first attempt to formulate a detailed system of auditory coding. He did this by combining three previously enunciated principles. The first of these was Ohm's law of auditory analysis. It is a matter of common experience that, in notes sounded by most musical instruments, it is possible with practice to distinguish both the fundamental and one or two overtones. Ohm extended this observation in his hypothesis, and stated that any complex periodic sound wave behaved—as far as the ear was concerned—as if it consisted of a series of suitably related sine waves corresponding to its Fourier components.

Helmholtz was quick to recognize that a system of tuned resonators is precisely the kind of structure to realize Ohm's proposal physically, and he therefore emphasized the analytic rather than the magnifying properties of the resonance hypothesis of cochlear function already established.

The third principle was that which is now commonly known under the name of Müller's doctrine of specific nerve energies. Müller proposed, in effect, that there are five different kinds of sensory nerves—one for each of the five senses—and that stimulation of one particular kind of nerve, by whatever means, evokes specifically the sensory quality to which it is related. Other people carried the subdivision further and the idea reached its fullest extension with Helmholtz's proposal of a specific fibre or group of fibres for each distinguishable pitch. The Helmholtz theory, in its original form, was a pure place theory. Each subjectively distinguishable tone had a corresponding resonator in the cochlea and each resonator was supplied by an individual nerve fibre or group of fibres distinct from all others. Frequency was thus coded in terms of activity or inactivity in particular fibres, and intensity in terms of the degree of that activity.

There are a great many problems raised by the Helmholtz hypothesis, of most of which Helmholtz was himself aware. It is not possible to discuss them in detail here; they have been well treated by Weaver.[4] It is sufficient to point out the two general headings: the identity of the resonators, and their selectivity. In spite of the greatly increased detail which the compound microscope had revealed by the mid-nineteenth century—in particular the structure of the organ of Corti—it never proved possible to identify any component which would account in number and range of physical properties for the number and range of the known discriminable frequencies. Likewise, it proved impossible to reconcile the high degree of selectivity called for in the resonators with the experimentally determined decay time of the system.

These two difficulties caused Helmholtz later to abandon the idea of highly selective resonators and to suggest only that one particular resonator was most highly excited by a tone while those for some distance on each side would be excited to lesser extents. He thus implicitly abandoned the specific nerve energy "one tone, one fibre" code in favour of a code in which there was a non-unique array of fibres subjected to a unique pattern of activation.

Although both the general principle and the details of resonance in the cochlea continued to be matters of argument, the theory was quite widely accepted and taught in elementary textbooks for some seventy years. Perhaps its very elegance and simplicity made people feel it ought to be true and encouraged its acceptance.

Behaviour of the Cochlear System

The essence of the Helmholtz theory was a series of transverse mechanical resonators, distributed along the length of a tapering basilar membrane. Tones of different pitch would set into vibration different but highly localized regions along the length of this membrane. Until the early 1940s no one had actually looked at the basilar membrane during activation of the ear by a sound stimulus. Then Békésy,[5] who had been working for some time on cochlear models, published several papers on the mechanics of real ears. The essence of his method was to examine the vibrating membrane through an artificial window in the cochlea with the aid of stroboscopic illumination. He found indeed that there was a region of maximum vibration of the membrane for a given frequency of stimulus, and that this maximum moved from the apex towards the base of the cochlea as the sound frequency was increased. The maxima were not very sharp, however, and considerable overlap of the vibration envelopes was evident between frequencies an octave or more apart. The method also made it possible to determine the relative phase of the vibration, and the result proved crucial against a resonance theory. The phase lag of displacement of the basilar membrane relative to the driving force increases progressively from the base to the apex of the cochlea, reaching values as large as 5π at the apical end; the lag at the position of maximum displacement may be 2π or more. These values are not compatible with a true resonant system. The disturbance can best be thought of as a travelling wave originating at the basal end of the membrane and travelling towards the apex of the cochlea. As it travels it gradually increases in amplitude and then dies away rather abruptly. With high frequency driving forces the peak amplitude is reached close to the basal end, and the wave does not travel very far before dying out. With lower driving frequencies the wave travels farther and farther along the cochlea, and the maximum is progressively displaced towards the apical end (Fig. 1).

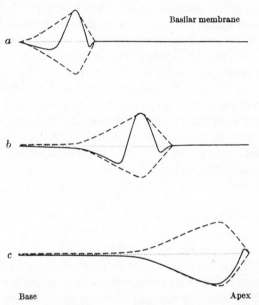

FIGURE 1. "Instantaneous" pictures of the travelling wave on the basilar membrane for a high frequency, *a*; a middle frequency, *b*; and a low frequency stimulus, *c*. The dashed envelopes show how the disturbance travels farther along the membrane from base to apex before reaching a peak and dying out.

The basilar membrane carries on its surface a rather complex structure known collectively as the organ of Corti. This structure contains the hair bearing cells which form the mechano-neural transducers. Vibration of the basilar membrane results in deflexion of the hairs attached to these cells and this, in turn, by a process not fully understood, results in a discharge of impulses in the sensory nerve fibres associated with these cells. The greater the amplitude of vibration of the membrane, the faster are impulses discharged by the nerve.

Although the innervation of the cochlea is quite complex, in general terms we can say that the 30,000 to 40,000 fibres of the auditory nerve are evenly distributed to hair cells along the whole length of the basilar membrane. Because the vibration envelope of one tone can overlap that of other tones an octave or more away, and because the extent of the envelope varies with intensity, we might expect that a single auditory nerve fibre could be activated by many different tones, and this proves to be the case. Near its threshold a fibre responds to only a small range of frequency, but as the sound intensity is increased it responds over a greater and greater range until at high intensities it may be responding to any frequency within a band several octaves wide.[6] Each fibre thus has a triangular frequency/intensity response area which roughly mirrors the shape of the vibration envelope.

Because any one fibre responds to a wide band of frequencies, it would be expected, conversely, that a large number of auditory nerve fibers will be discharging at any given stimulus frequency. Schuknecht [7] has shown that at the quite moderate sound pressure level of 40 dB, between 15 and 25 per cent of the whole system is activated by any one single frequency. But 25 per cent of 40,000 fibres is 10,000 fibres. It follows that if the frequency is changed by 1 per cent—an easily detectable change—something like 200 fibres will be added to one end and a similar number subtracted from the other. In other words, 98 per cent of the active fibres are activated by both tones. When we remember that the total number of fibres activated depends on intensity as well as frequency along the array, it is clear that there is no question of there being specific groups of fibres for specific discriminable frequencies. How then does the system function?

Possible Pulse Interval Codes

An alternative to the resonance hypothesis was put forward by Rutherford [8] in the 1890s and has become known as the "telephone theory." Rutherford suggested that, rather than peripheral analysis taking place, the auditory nerve transmitted a frequency replica of the sound. Little was known in those days about the properties of the nerve impulse, but subsequent work has shown that it is not possible for a nerve to carry trains of impulses at frequencies greater than at most 1,000 per sec, and it usually cannot sustain rates greater than 500/sec for more than a very short time. This leaves a large proportion of the audible spectrum without representation. To deal with the frequencies above 500 c/s, it has been suggested that some form of alternation takes place.[4] According to this idea, a frequency of 10,000 c/s would be dealt with by twenty fibres each firing 500 pulses/sec and firing in rotation. Of course, this would only signal the frequency element of the sound, and considerably more fibres would be required to deal with the intensity parameter, but there are some 40,000 fibres available so that the hypothesis does not immediately fail on this score.

The primary question, however, is the experimental one: do the pulses in auditory nerve fibres bear any relation in time to the stimulus frequency? At low stimulus frequencies (say, 200 c/s) there is undoubtedly a very strong relationship. However, there is a good deal of "jitter" in the system which causes this relationship to become progressively less and less obvious as the stimulus frequency is increased. In the auditory nerve this relationship fails somewhere between 2,000 and 4,000 c/s, according to the time and space over which one chooses to integrate the measurements. The situation gets progressively worse as one ascends the neural pathway, owing to the variable nature of synaptic delays (the variation may be as much as 300 μsec). This means, in effect, that for anything but the very lowest frequencies, a frequency code would have to be converted to some other form at a very early stage in the neural path. There is no evidence that any such conversion takes place. We do not, for example, find that single neurones at the higher levels of the nervous pathway respond only to narrow frequency bands; the band of frequencies to which a given fibre responds at, say, the collicular level is just as great as that of an auditory nerve fibre. We must conclude that although frequency representation is a possible mechanism for low frequencies, it is not a valid one for high frequencies.

Even at low frequencies there is a further problem to be considered. It is very easy when recording nerve impulses on an oscilloscope, or using them to prepare a pulse interval histogram, to distinguish a frequency of 990 from a frequency of 1,000. However, for the nervous system to do this, it too must have a suitable clock and there is no evidence that a neural clock of this degree of accuracy exists.

We have considered two types of coding—individual channel activity and mean pulse frequency. Let us now consider another. The pulse trains in a nerve fibre are not, in detail, evenly spaced in time. This is especially true at higher levels in the system. It is clearly possible that a pulse interval code could exist, and such a code has a potentially high information capacity. In the past ten years or so, the possibility of such a code in the nervous system has attracted a lot of attention and a great deal of work has been done on analyses. So far, little encouragement has been forthcoming. Examination of such "patterns" in the auditory system has served only to support the conclusion that the distributions of pulse intervals are random.

In the early stages of the system, if we discount the relative deficiency of short intervals imposed by the refractory properties of the excitable elements, and any residual first order patterning of the type referred to here, there remains only an interval distribution which could adequately be accounted for by a random process. At higher neural levels the distributions are complicated by multiple delay paths, but there still appears nothing obviously specific to the stimulus. The objection raised here would also seem to apply even more cogently to the use of a pulse interval code: is there in the nervous system any mechanism for decoding such a pattern? Again we know of none.

Coding of Stimulus Frequency and Intensity

Before going further, it may be worth while to consider what the auditory system actually has to do in hearing, say, a steady tone or a vowel sound. If we make measurements of the frequency and intensity difference limina

(DLs) over the whole range of hearing, we can construct a two-dimensional diagram consisting of a number of cells or compartments which show at a glance the size of the DLs in any particular region.[9] If we count up the total number of these cells we find there are about 340,000. However, although many people have greater or lesser degrees of absolute pitch it would be absurd to suggest that anyone when presented with a tone at random can say "That is 6,130 c/s at 30 dB above threshold," and the auditory system is not called on to transmit data for any such choice. Intensity difference limina are normally determined by comparing adjacent stimuli. Again, although speech has a highly complex waveform of potentially very high information content, little of this is used at any one time. Even highly degraded waveforms such as differentiated clipped speech yield 92 per cent intelligibility scores.[10] It seems that a very few frequencies, usually called the formant frequencies, or perhaps even the second formant alone, are sufficient to characterize the speech sounds as far as intelligibility is concerned.[11]

Let us see, therefore, how far we can get with a rather simple code. We have already seen that the pattern of activity in the array of auditory nerve fibres for a tonal stimulus is like that of Figure 2 with fibres firing at various

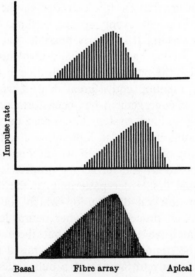

Basal   **Fibre array**   **Apical**

FIGURE 2. Diagram to show the distribution of activity in the array of fibres originating from the basilar membrane. The height of each line represents the mean rate of nerve impulses in the corresponding fibre. The upper and middle diagrams represent two different stimulus frequencies, while the lowest diagram represents an increased stimulus intensity. In actuality there would be several hundred times as many fibres activated as are shown here.

rates according to the degree of excitation of the part of the membrane from which they arise. In this array we could, for example, assess intensity in terms of the discharge rate of the most highly excited fibre, or by the total number of fibres carrying any activity. Likewise, we could assess the stimulus frequency by the position of the most active fibre (the position of the "peak") or by the relative position of the two ends of the array of active fibres. Neither of these two latter criteria is very good, however, as a small percentage of "noise" pulses added at successive synaptic junctions could easily blur their locations.

If we examine the behaviour of a single auditory fibre at a higher level beyond the first cell station (cochlear nucleus) we observe two differences from an auditory nerve fibre.[12,13] First, the discharge rate is no longer a monotonic function of stimulus intensity, so that intensity cannot be signalled purely in terms of discharge rate. Secondly, over a rather wide range of stimulus intensity there is little change in firing rate. The curve tends to increase rather rapidly near threshold as the intensity is raised, and then to flatten off, falling again somewhat at very high intensities. Allanson and Whitfield [14] have pointed out that this effect leads to a transformation in which the noise-sensitive auditory pattern is transformed into one in which all the fibres are substantially either "hard on" or "hard off" (Fig. 3). In other words, if we

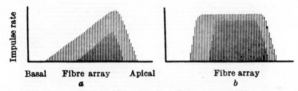

FIGURE 3. Transformation of pulse rate distribution in the fibre array effected by the cochlear nucleus, *a*, input pattern; *b*, output pattern. Thick lines represent a low stimulus intensity, thinner lines a high intensity. Other conventions as in Figure 2 (after Whitfield, 29).

consider only whether there is activity or no-activity in a given fibre, then the frequency is signalled by the relative position of the two edges, and the intensity by the number of active fibres between those edges. Such an arrangement is not only very resistant to degradation, but presents the information in a form which should be eminently detectable by the nervous system which is well adapted to locating regions of abrupt change in activity.

An immediate difficulty arises. Suppose we have not one single tone as stimulus, but two or more simultaneously as will certainly occur very often in real life. Because of the considerable overlap of activity, the auditory nerve pattern might look something like Figure 4*A*, and this, after transformation, might be expected to give rise to a single block of active output fibres indistinguishable from that produced by a single, much louder tone, the frequency of which is located somewhere between the two tones we are considering. If we actually try the experiment, we find that although the fibres in the "overlap" region are activated by either of the two tones sounded alone, if we sound them simultaneously these fibres are actually inhibited and fail to

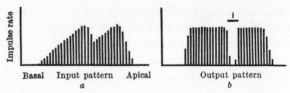

FIGURE 4. Input/output relations for a stimulus involving two frequencies. Note the inhibition (*i*) in the "overlap" region. Conventions as in Figure 2 (after Whitfield, 29).

respond (Fig. 4*B*). This type of inhibition is a common feature of sensory pathways.[15,16] The effect of its existence is clearly to preserve the identity of separate stimuli—in this case the blocks of active fibres corresponding to the two tones.

It is also found experimentally that the fibre array preserves an orderly anatomical arrangement at least as far up as the inferior colliculus.[13] This means that channels which are adjacent frequency-wise are also spatially adjacent. The activity in the total array in response to a complex sound signal will therefore appear rather like that shown diagrammatically in Figure 5*A*.

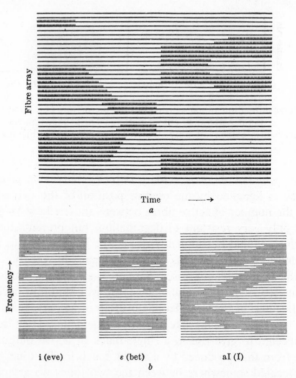

FIGURE 5. *a*. Distribution of pulse activity in the array of fibres in the central auditory pathway, and the way this may vary with time as the components of the stimulus vary in frequency and intensity. *b*. Distribution of speech energy in different frequency bands for two vowels and a diphthong (after Potter, Kopp and Green, 30).

It is instructive to compare this with the time course of the formant frequencies of speech sounds (Fig. 5*B*). The evidence of Figure 5*A* also suggests why discrimination between two successively presented tones, which would only require detection of the fact that the edge has moved, is so much more readily carried out than the absolute identification of frequency which would require memory identification of specific channels.

So far, we have considered only steady states and the relations between them. Identifications of frequency changes, however, are also important. For example, the feature which appears to distinguish between the consonants b, d, and g is whether the second formant frequency rises towards its final value, remains constant, or falls towards the final value respectively.[17] If we examine neurones in the auditory part of the cerebral cortex, we find that there are such units which are specifically responsive to frequency changes.[18] A given neurone will fire only when presented with a falling frequency, while another will fire only when the frequency is rising (Fig. 6). The precise value of the frequency is largely unimportant provided there is a sufficient excursion in the correct direction. Provided the change is not too slow, the rate of change is not very critical.

FIGURE 6. *a*. Response of a neurone in the auditory cortex to a rising frequency. The signal bar represents a steady tone of 12 kc/s which then rose linearly at the point shown to a new steady value of 13·2 kc/s. The rise time was 50 msec. In *b* the frequency returned from 13·2 k/cs to 12 kc/s in the same way; this failed to stimulate the neurone (after Whitfield and Evans, 18).

It seems likely that the qualities of pitch and intensity are distinguished by levels below the cortex, as discriminations of this type can be made, for example, by cats in the absence of the relevant cortical areas. Temporal patterns of sound, in which the only differences are those of the sequence of the tones and not their identity, cannot, however, be distinguished in these circumstances. There is some evidence of a similar situation in man.

Transient Phenomena and Sound Localization

So far we have been considering either steady state phenomena, or signals involving only fairly slow and limited changes of a single frequency. However, the ear has also to operate on a wide range of transient signals. One of the defects of the resonance theory was its failure to deal with this aspect of cochlear behaviour and its concentration on steady state frequency analysis. It is possible theoretically to produce for any waveform a pure frequency analysis, a pure time analysis, or any intermediate compromise. The mechanics of the cochlea do indeed represent such a compromise between the needs of frequency identification and the necessity for the temporal location of wave fronts. The latter are, of course, of particular importance to the organism in the location of sound sources.

If a short impulse is applied to the ear, a "travelling bulge" is produced on the basilar membrane which propagates from the base to the apex of the cochlea. This wave has a velocity of the order of hundreds of metres per second near the base and slows to only three or four metres per second near the apex. Experiment shows that as a result of the passage of this bulge a given auditory nerve fibre discharges one or more impulses with a pulse interval corresponding to the steady-state frequency for which that fibre would be maximally excited.[19] There is thus a close link between the temporal pulse pattern produced by an impulse and that produced by a low frequency tone, and it would appear that the same mechanism could well process both. The "click" has a marked superiority over the tone, however, in that it excites temporarily identifiable pulses in fibres at the basal end of the cochlea, and the steep wave front means that these initial pulses will be especially accurately timed.

For localization of a sound source, the relative time of arrival of the sound at the two ears and the relative timing of the corresponding nerve impulses could provide some of the necessary data. In criticizing the telephone and related theories of frequency analysis, we noted the way in which the relation between nerve impulse position and stimulus envelope, fairly good in the auditory nerve, became progressively degraded as more and more synapses were introduced along the pathway. We argued that this potential source of information could only be used if it were transformed at an early stage into some other code. In the process of sound localization such a transformation does take place. There appears to be a special structure for this purpose—the medial (or accessory) olivary nucleus, which is situated in the brainstem at about the level at which the auditory nerves enter it. The nucleus is a plate like structure which has a sheet of nerve cells each innervated on one face by fibres of the auditory nerve of its own side, and on the opposite face by corresponding fibres of the auditory nerve of the opposite side. Hall,[20] using click stimuli, has shown that the probability that one of these cells will fire depends on the relative time of arrival of the stimulus at the two ears. Thus, if the stimulus to the ipsilateral ear precedes that to the contralateral ear by 500 μsec the probability of the neurone firing might be, say, 0·75. If the ipsilateral stimulus lags by 500 μsec the corresponding probability would be only 0·45. Relative intensity of the stimuli has a similar effect; if the ipsilateral click is more intense than the contralateral one, then the probability of firing is increased and vice versa. Artificial manipulation of the timing and intensity of dichotic clicks enables us to demonstrate the phenomenon of time intensity trading [21] in the apparent position of a source, but for a real single source the two effects reinforce one another, as the signal will be both earlier and louder at the nearer ear. Because this situation involves a higher probability of a particular cell firing, it will mean that more fibres leaving this nucleus will be activated; the code has been transformed from one in which the information is contained in the relative timing of impulses to one in terms of the number of active fibres. The end result of the transformation thus has the same form, and the same resistance to degradation, as the frequency code discussed earlier. Of course, the number of active fibres on a given side will be a function of the absolute intensity of the signal, as well as of its relative intensity, and to this extent there is an ambiguity. The relative number of active fibres, however, on the two sides is to a first approximation independent of the absolute intensity and thus could give a measure of lateralization. Although such a model has been proposed,[22] the anatomical site of a comparator has not yet been located. Nevertheless, at the cortex there are cells which, while they are readily activated by quite weak sounds anywhere in the quadrant from dead ahead to a position opposite one ear, are quite unaffected by much stronger signals originating in the corresponding quadrant on the opposite side of the head.

Centrifugal Control

Finally, let me turn to the question of the control of the auditory input. Everyone is familiar with the phenomenon of "not hearing the sitting room clock tick until it stops." Continuously present or irrelevant signals tend to be suppressed at the expense of more immediately important ones. This control takes place quite early in the system. Thus the electrical response in the cochlear nucleus to a sound signal has been shown to disappear if the signal is repeatedly presented over a long period.[23] Distraction of attention by the presentation of an "interesting" visual stimulus may have a similar effect.[24]

These "gating" operations, which selectively control the input, appear to be mediated by centrifugal pathways which parallel the ascending auditory system all the way from the cortex to the periphery. Even right out at the cochlea it is possible to inhibit activity in individual groups of auditory nerve fibres by stimulation of the centrifugal olivo-cochlear bundle.[25] Farther up the system, within the brainstem, the possibilities become more varied. Stimulation of one set of descending fibres will shut off the response to sound of a particular neurone in the cochlear nucleus;[26] on the other hand, stimulation of a different set of these fibres increases the sensitivity of cochlear nucleus cells, and may lower the sound threshold of a particular cell by as much as 15 dB.[27] It is clear that these fibres control the sensory throughput at all stages. It is less clear if they simply control whether or not information gets through at all, or if they actually determine the route it takes.

Until quite recently, views on auditory localization tended towards the view that somewhere in the system there should be an area or set of structures uniquely activated by a discriminable stimulus. From this locus activity would presumably "fan out" to produce a complex widespread response on the motor side. A diagrammatic representation might be made from two pyramids with a common apex. As we have seen, experiment simply does not support this concept of sensory organization. Just why such an arrangement should have been thought necessary is unclear. Among spinal reflexes, the classical "scratch reflex" involves interconnection of a complex sensory pattern with a complex motor pattern, yet no one has ever postulated a "scratch" unit or claimed that there were unique pathways leading to it. The "pyramid" theory, if it were true, would of course have simplified our concept of the discrimination mechanism, as we should only require a gate to operate at a single point. However, the existence of widespread centrifugal connexions means that not only is diffuse gating a practical means of controlling a "learned" discrimination, but that this gating could take place at almost any neural level. It is well established, for instance, that direct connexions exist between auditory nuclei and motor pathways at the upper medullary level.[28] These are generally described as "auditory reflex" pathways, but there seems no reason why they should not be "conditional" pathways whose activity or quiescence is controlled by the centrifugal system.

In summary, then, let me reiterate two points. There is no evidence anywhere in the auditory system for groups of neurones responding uniquely to particular discriminable stimuli, and multi-channel correspondences probably exist between the sensory system and effector systems, equivalent to those at the spinal level. The elaborateness of the sensory pathway seems to lie in its connectivity; there is no evidence to date for the existence of elaborate code patterns in individual fibres.

References

1. du Verney, J. G. *Traité de l'Organe de l'Ouie* (Paris, 1683).
2. Haller, V. von, *Primae Lineae Physiologiae* (Gottingen, 1751).
3. Helmholtz, H., *Gesellsch. Deutsch. Naturf. Aerzte. Amtl. Ber.*, **34**, 157 (1859).
4. Wever, E. G., *Theory of Hearing* (Wiley, New York, 1949).
5. Békésy, G. von, in *Experiments in Hearing* (McGraw-Hill, New York, 1960).
6. Tasaki, I., *J. Neurophysiol.*, **17**, 97 (1954).
7. Schuknecht, H. F., *Neural Mechanisms of the Auditory and Vestibular Systems*, ch. 6 (Thomas, Springfield, 1960).
8. Rutherford, W., *J. Anat. Physiol.*, **21**, 166 (1886).
9. Stevens, S. S., and Davis, H., *Hearing, Its Psychology and Physiology* (Wiley, New York, 1938).
10. Licklider, J. C. R., and Pollack, I., *J. Acoust. Soc. Amer.*, **20**, 42 (1948).
11. Thomas, I. B., *Tech. Rept. 10, Biol. Computer Lab.* (Univ. Illinois, 1966).
12. Hilalai, S., and Whitfield, I. C., *J. Physiol.*, **122**, 158 (1953).
13. Rose, J. E., Greenwood, D. D., Goldberg, J. M., and Hind, J. E., *J. Neurophysiol.*, **26**, 294 (1963).

14. Allanson, J. T., and Whitfield, I. C., *Third London Symposium on Information Theory*, 269 (Butterworth, London).
15. Whitfield, I. C., *J. Physiol.*, **128**, 15P (1955).
16. Hartline, H. K., *Rev. Mod. Physics*, **31**, 515 (1959).
17. Delattre, P. C., Liberman, A. M., and Cooper, F. S., *J. Acoust. Soc. Amer.*, **27**, 769 (1955).
18. Whitfield, I. C., and Evans, E. F., *J. Neurophysiol.*, **28**, 655 (1965).
19. Kiang, N. S., *M.I.T. Research Monograph No. 35* (M.I.T. Press, Cambridge, 1965).
20. Hall, J. L., *J. Acoust. Soc. Amer.*, **37**, 814 (1965).
21. Shaxby, J. H., and Gage, F. H., *Med. Res. Council Spec. Rept.*, **166**, 1 (1932). David, E. E., Guttman, N., and van Bergeijk, W. A., *J. Acoust. Soc. Amer.*, **31**, 774 (1959).
22. van Bergeijk, W. A., *J. Acoust. Soc. Amer.*, **34**, 1431 (1962).
23. Hernández-Péon, R., and Scherrer, H., *Fed. Proc.*, **14**, 71 (1955).
24. Hernández-Péon, R., Scherrer, H., and Jouvet, M., *Science*, **123**, 331 (1956).
25. Fex, J., *Acta Physiol. Scand.*, **55**, suppl. 189 (1962).
26. Comis, S. D., and Whitfield, I. C., *J. Physiol.*, **188**, 34P (1967).
27. Whitfield, I. C., *Bionics Symposium* (in the press) (1967).
28. Rasmussen, G. L., *J. Comp. Neurol.*, **84**, 141 (1946).
29. Whitfield, I. C., *Brit. Med. Bull.*, **12**, 105 (1956).
30. Potter, R. K., Kopp, G. A., and Green, H. C., *Visible Speech* (van Nostrand, New York, 1947).

Integrative Processes in Central Visual Pathways of the Cat

DAVID H. HUBEL

Reprinted from *Journal of the Optical Society of America*, Jan., 1963, Vol. 53, No. 1, pp. 58–66.

An image falling upon the retina exerts an influence on millions of receptors. It is the task of the central nervous system to make sense of the spatial and temporal patterns of excitation in this retinal mosaic. Unless we know something of how the nervous system handles the messages it receives, we cannot easily come to grips with the problems of perception of form, movement, color, or depth.

For a study of integrative sensory mechanisms the visual system of mammals offers the advantage of a comparatively direct anatomical pathway. At each stage, from bipolar cells to the striate cortex, we can compare activity of cells with that of the incoming fibers, and so attempt to learn what each structure contributes to the visual process. In this paper I summarize a series of studies on the cat visual system made by Torsten Wiesel and myself. I concentrate mainly on experiments related to form and movement.

It is often contended that in studying a sensory system we should first learn to understand thoroughly the physiology of receptors, and only then proceed to examine more central processes. In the visual system one should presumably have a firm grasp of rod and cone physiology before looking at bipolar and retinal ganglion cells; one should thoroughly understand retinal mechanisms before taking up studies of the brain. Unfortunately it is not always possible to be so systematic. In the case of the visual system, orderly progress is impeded by the great technical difficulties in recording from single retinal elements, especially from the rods and cones and from bipolar cells. At the single-cell level, knowledge of the electrophysiology of these structures is consequently almost entirely lacking. If we wish to learn how the brain interprets information it receives from the retina we must either struggle with retinal problems of formidable difficulty or else skip over the first two stages and begin at a point where the appropriate single-unit techniques have been worked out, i.e., the retinal ganglion cell.

The subject of retinal ganglion-cell physiology is complicated by the fact that studies have been made in a wide variety of vertebrates and under a number of different experimental conditions. Here I only describe the receptive field organization of retinal ganglion cells in the cat. This is necessary for an understanding of the integrative function of the lateral geniculate body since the geniculate receives its main visual input directly from the retina.

Because there is convergence of a number of afferent fibers onto each cell, both for bipolar cells and for retinal ganglion cells, we are not surprised to learn that a single ganglion cell may receive its input ultimately from a large number of rods and cones, and hence from a retinal surface of considerable extent. At first glance it might seem that a progressive increase in the size of receptive fields as we follow the visual pathway centrally must lead to a wasteful and pointless blurring of detailed information acquired by the exquisitely fine receptor mosaic. To understand why fineness of discrimination is not necessarily blunted we must realize that all retinal connections are not necessarily excitatory. The existence of inhibitory connections means that when we shine a spot of light on the receptive field of a given cell we may decrease, rather than increase, the cell's rate of firing. The effect of the stimulus will depend on the part of the receptive field we illuminate. The fineness of discrimination of a cell is determined not by the over-all receptive field size, but by the arrangement of excitatory and inhibitory regions within the receptive field.

With the experiments of Kuffler (1953) it became apparent that in the light-adapted cat, retinal ganglion cells did not necessarily respond uniformly throughout their receptive fields: their discharges might be activated or suppressed by a spot of light, depending upon where on the retina the spot fell. The receptive field of a ganglion cell could thus be mapped into distinct excitatory and inhibitory regions. Two types of cells were distinguished by Kuffler: those with fields having a more or less circular excitatory center with an annular inhibitory surround, and those having the reverse arrangement. These two concentrically arranged field types were called "on"-center and "off"-center fields. The terms "off" center and "off" response refer to the empirical finding that when a spot of light suppresses a cell's firing, turning the spot off almost always evokes a discharge, termed the "off" response. Conversely when we see an "off" discharge we usually find that during the stimulus the maintained firing of a cell is suppressed.

Within the excitatory or inhibitory region of a receptive field one can demonstrate summation, i.e., for a given intensity of stimulus the response increases (number of spikes and frequency of firing increase, latency and threshold decrease) as the area stimulated is increased. On the other hand, when both types of region are included in a stimulus their separate effects tend to cancel. If the entire receptive field is illuminated, for example by diffuse light, a relatively weak response of the center type is usually obtained: an "on"-center cell thus gives a weak "on" response, and an "off"-center cell a weak "off" response. I shall use the term "peripheral suppression" to refer to this antagonistic interaction between center and periphery.

Retinal ganglion cells differ from one another in several ways besides those related to field-center type. Obviously they vary in the location of their receptive fields on the retina. In the cat (Wiesel 1960) and the monkey (Hubel and Wiesel 1960) there are considerable differences in the sizes of receptive-field centers, receptive fields near the area contralis or fovea showing a marked tendency to have smaller centers than fields in the peripheral retina. Even for a given region of the retina there is a large variation in the size of field centers. In the monkey the smallest field center so far measured had a diameter of 4 minutes arc; this was situated 4° from the fovea. It is likely that the centers of foveal fields are much smaller than this. The total extent of a field is more difficult to determine, since the effect of a spot of light upon a cell decreases gradually with increasing distance from the field center. Measurements made by constructing area-threshold curves (Wiesel 1960) suggest that receptive fields may not greatly differ in their total size despite wide variations in center sizes.

Retinal ganglion cells differ also in the effectiveness with which the receptive-field periphery antagonizes the center response. This may be measured by determining the difference between the threshold intensity of a spot covering the receptive-field center and that of a large spot covering the entire field. The difference tends to be greater for cells with small field centers (and hence large peripheral zones) than for cells with large field centers. Since cells with small field centers are especially common in the area centralis, this ability to discriminate against diffuse light is particularly pronounced in that part of the retina.

In the cat we know of no functional retinal ganglion cell types besides the "on"-center and "off"-center cells described by Kuffler. Occasionally diffuse light evokes a discharge both at "on" and at "off." This may occur in either "on"-center cells or "off"-center cells. It depends to some extent on the state of light adaptation, stimulus intensity, and other variables. The receptive fields of cells showing "on-off" responses to large spots do not seem to differ in any fundamental way from ordinary "on"-center or "off"-center cells. There thus seems to be no reason for regarding "on-off" retinal ganglion cells of cat as a distinct type.

In the cat the arrangement of excitatory and inhibitory regions within a given receptive field remains the same for all effective stimulus wavelengths. The fields thus seem to be very different from the more complex opponent-color fields described by Wolbarsht, Wagner, and MacNichol (1961) for goldfish retinal ganglion cells (see discussion of Barlow, in Wolbarsht *et al.,* 1961, p. 176). In the monkey optic nerve and lateral geniculate body there are two types of neurons, one resembling cells of the cat in having receptive-field characteristics that are independent of wavelength, the other showing color-specific responses in many ways similar to those seen in the goldfish (Hubel and Wiesel 1960; DeValois 1960).

In the frog, Maturana, Lettvin, McCulloch, and Pitts (1960) have described retinal ganglion cells with highly complex response properties. Their records were made from unmyelinated axons or their terminal arborizations. If such axons exist in the optic nerves of cats, they have probably escaped detection in physiological studies. Unfortunately cat optic nerves have not yet been examined with the electron microscope, and it is not known whether or not they contain unmyelinated fibers.

Lateral Geniculate Body

Anatomically, the dorsal lateral geniculate body differs from most other structures in the central nervous system, and certainly from the retina and cortex, in its relative simplicity. In a sense it is a one-synapse way station, since its cells receive their major input directly from the optic tract, and since most of them send their axons directly to the visual cortex. It has often been asked whether the lateral geniculate body serves any integrative purpose besides that of relaying incoming messages to the cortex for further elaboration. Although in some ways the lateral geniculate body is a simple structure, an anatomist would hardly contend that it is nothing but a one-to-one relay station. The existence of convergence and divergence, complex dendritic arborizations, and, in the cat at least, cells with short axons terminating within the nucleus itself, all seem to be against such a supposition.

A strong case was made for the presence of one-to-one-synapses in the geniculate by the microelectrode studies of Bishop, Burke, and Davis (1958). By electrically stimulating the severed proximal stump of the optic nerve and recording extracellularly from lateral geniculate cells they were able to record excitatory postsynaptic potentials (or the associated extracellular currents) and show that they were not continuously graded, but, at least for two of the cells they studied, were all-or-nothing. Most excitatory postsynaptic potentials were followed by geniculate spikes. The authors concluded that some lateral geniculate cells can be excited by one impulse in a single optic-nerve fiber. They were inclined to attribute the fact that the lateral geniculate cell occasionally failed to fire to the effects of anaesthesia, rather than to variation in possible additional inputs not detected by their electrode. Since both Bishop, Burke, and Davis (1958) and Freygang (1958) observed lateral geniculate cells for which the excitatory postsynaptic potentials were graded in several discrete steps, it is clear that not all geniculate synapses are of a simple one-to-one type. At least some must have several excitatory inputs.

If there is a "straight through" connection between some optic-nerve fibers and lateral geniculate cells, as Bishop's findings suggest, there should be no differences in receptive fields at the two levels. A study of lateral geniculate cells in the cat (Hubel and Wiesel 1961) showed that lateral geniculate fields indeed have the same concentric center-periphery organization, and like retinal ganglion cells, are of two types, excitatory center and inhibitory center. It is clear enough, then, that in the lateral geniculate body there is no very profound reorganization of the incoming messages. Nevertheless, there was a suggestion that the ability of a receptive-field periphery to antagonize the center response was more marked in geniculate cells than in optic-nerve fibers. This was true even when variations in peripheral suppression with position of receptive fields on the retina (referred to above) were taken into account.

The fact that one can record geniculate spikes together with excitatory synaptic potentials of an all-or-none type suggested the possibility of making a more delicate test of geniculate function, namely, a comparison of the responses and receptive fields of a particular geniculate cell with those of its own excitatory postsynaptic potential (Hubel and Wiesel 1961). When this was done for cells with all-or-none synaptic potentials, it was found that while almost all lateral geniculate spikes were triggered by an optic-nerve impulse, the converse was not true; each synaptic potential did not necessarily trigger a postsynaptic spike. The success rate of the optic-nerve impulse varied widely, depending on how the retina was stimulated. The receptive field centers of the optic nerve fiber and the lateral geniculate cell were, as far as one could judge, precisely superimposed. If one shone a restricted spot of light over the common receptive-field center, the likelihood that an impulse would trigger a postsynaptic spike was very high. If, on the other hand, the entire receptive field including the periphery was illuminated, very few of the synaptic potentials were followed by geniculate-cell spikes. For small spots in the center portion of the field the thresholds of the two units were apparently identical, but for large spots, including diffuse light, they were often several log units apart. Sometimes the geniculate cell would not respond to diffuse light at any intensity.

It was thus possible not only to confirm the impression that peripheral suppression is enhanced by lateral geniculate cells, but to obtain some notion of how the change is brought about.

This result shows clearly that even when we record a single all-or-none excitatory synaptic potential along with a geniculate cell spike, the synaptic potential we observe does not represent the only input to the cell. There must be other inputs which are influenced by illuminating the periphery of the common receptive field. Illuminating the periphery might activate retinal ganglion cells whose "on" centers were distributed over this annular region; if these neurons made inhibitory synaptic connections with the geniculate cell we could explain the cell's failure to be triggered when diffuse light was used. We might equally well suppose that lighting the periphery suppressed the firing of a set of "off"-center retinal ganglion cells making *excitatory* connections with the geniculate cell. Now inclusion of the receptive-field periphery would suppress these cells, removing the tonic asynchronous activation needed to enable the geniculate cell to follow the triggering impulses. The important point is that the geniculate cell must be receiving input from not one, but a large number of optic-nerve fibers. In a cell bound to an optic nerve fiber by a synapse having a "straight through" property, the property is a conditional one, depending on activity of other optic nerve fibers.

I have mentioned the possibility of suppressing a cell's firing by withdrawal of tonic excitation rather than by direct synaptic inhibition. The synapse that we are discussing gives us a vivid example of just that, for in illuminating the field center of an "off"-center geniculate cell we suppress firing by suppressing activity in the main optic-nerve fiber feeding into it. Of course the cell may at the same time be actively inhibited by other optic-nerve fibers (we have no evidence for or against this), but this inhibition would not be the main reason for the cessation of firing. To suppress the firing of any cell in the visual system there need only be one inhibitory link in the entire chain beginning with and including the receptor. In the case of the center of an "off"-center cell in the lateral geniculate we do not know at what stage this inhibitory link occurs. It is apparently not in the geniculate, and there is no evidence for or against its being at the retinal ganglion-cell level.

We may sum up the implications of these experiments as follows: (1) all cat geniculate cells apparently have multiple visual inputs; (2) there is often a particular relationship between a cell and one optic-nerve fiber with which it makes a powerful excitatory synapse; (3) when such a relationship exists, the receptive-field centers of the incoming fiber and the geniculate cell are of the same type, i.e., both are "on"-center or both are "off"-center; (4) the lateral geniculate body has the function of increasing the disparity, already present in the retinal ganglion cell, between responses to a small centered spot and to diffuse light.

The lateral geniculate body may have other functions besides that of increasing the effects of the receptive-field periphery. Cells in which the synaptic potential is graded in several steps must have more than one excitatory afferent. This kind of convergence might produce a geniculate receptive-field center larger than any of the field centers of the afferents. So far this has not been tested experimentally.

Some electrophysiological studies have suggested that the lateral geniculate body receives afferent fibers besides those of the optic tract (Hubel 1960; Widén and Ajmone-Marsan 1960; Arden and Söderberg 1961). Nauta and Bucher (1954) have observed a corticogeniculate projection in the rat, and recently Nauta (personal communication) and Beresford (1961) have found in the cat a topographically precise reciprocal pathway from the striate cortex to the lateral geniculate body of the same side. So far we have found no geniculate cells with the complex properties typical of cortical cells, but fibers with these properties are frequently recorded just dorsal to the lateral geniculate body. A knowledge of the presence of a reciprocal pathway is important if we are to avoid including these units in a study of geniculate cells, particularly if there is any chance that the recording electrode is not in the geniculate but just above it.

A problem that has attracted considerable attention concerns the amount of binocular interaction in the lateral geniculate body (Bishop, Burke, and Davis 1959; Erulkar and Fillenz 1960; Grüsser and Sauer 1960; Hubel and Wiesel 1961). While there is evidence that some geniculate cells can be influenced from the two eyes, it seems to be agreed that the proportion of binocularly influenced cells in the lateral geniculate body is small. This is certainly in keeping with the anatomical findings (Silva 1956; Hayhow 1958). We have so far not succeeded in mapping out, for any geniculate cell, two receptive fields, one in each eye. The marked contrast between the scarcity of binocular interaction in the cat's geniculate and its preponderance in the visual cortex does not argue for any major role of the geniculate in binocular vision.

On anatomical grounds it is well established that alternate layers of the lateral geniculate body receive their input from alternate eyes. This has been confirmed in the cat by physiological methods (Cohn, 1956); cells in a given layer can be driven from one of the two eyes, but not from the other. A precise topographical representation of the contralateral half-fields of vision on each geniculate layer, the maps in the different layers being in register, has been established anatomically for the rhesus monkey (Polyak 1957) by noting trans-synaptic atrophy following small retinal lesions. Although a similar anatomical study in the cat has not been made, the physiological evidence for a precise topographical representation in this animal is clear (Hubel and Wiesel 1961). The receptive fields of simultaneously recorded cells are near to one another and often overlap almost completely. The receptive fields of cells recorded in sequence by an electrode passing normal to the layers are close together or almost superimposed, whereas in an oblique or tangential penetration, fields of successively recorded cells move systematically along the retina. Finally, the maps in successive layers are in register.

From what I have said about the lateral geniculate body it will be apparent that the physiological properties of even that simple structure are far from simple. The fact that a number of incoming optic-tract fibers converge upon one cell presents us with a number of possibilities. Any particular geniculate cell will have its own receptive field with center and surround. Each fiber converging upon the cell will have its own center located in the center or surround of the geniculate cell's field: the incoming fiber may have an "on" center or an "off" center; the synapse it makes may be excitatory or inhibitory. If excitatory, the synapse may be powerful, capable of setting up a spike in the geniculate cell; or it may be weak, contributing to the summed effects of a large number of other incoming fibers. Somehow these and perhaps other possibilities are made use of, to produce a mechanism in which individual incoming impulses may trigger individual postsynaptic impulses, but in which the coupling between the incoming and outgoing signals is varied. Such an ingenious piece of machinery would surely have great appeal to a mechanical or an electrical engineer. It may be worth stressing how different this synapse seems to be from that of the anterior horn cell of the spinal cord, which, because it has been so extensively studied by modern electrophysiological methods, is apt to be taken as a prototype of synapses in the central nervous system.

Visual Cortex

If the lateral geniculate body is anatomically a structure of relative histological simplicity, the primary visual cortex is in contrast one of very great complexity. There is considerable order to the architectural plan of the cortex, yet our knowledge of the connections between cells gives us very little notion of how this structure functions. Of course, it has been known for years that the striate cortex is concerned with vision, and that in most mammals it is indispensable for form vision. What we have not known is how cortical cells handle the messages they receive from the lateral geniculate body. We have had insufficient evidence even to decide whether the messages are modified at all, or just handed on to some still higher centers for further elaboration (cf. Brindley 1960, p. 122).

As long as methods for single-cell recording were not available to neurophysiologists, this question of integrative cortical mechanisms could only be approached in a limited way. Since gross electrodes record only synchronous activity one could only examine attributes shared by all or most cells in a relatively large volume of tissue (the order of 1 mm^3). We know now that the one important physiological quality shared by cells over such a large area of striate cortex has to do with the regions of visual field from which cells receive their projections. It is therefore not surprising that topography was one aspect of visual cortical function to be extensively explored with gross electrodes.

In a series of studies by Talbot and Marshall (1941), Talbot (1942), and Thompson, Woolsey, and Talbot (1950) the cortex was mapped in the cat, rabbit, and monkey according to the retinal areas projecting to it. These authors were able to go well beyond what was known from anatomical studies by showing that in the cat and rabbit there is a double representation of the visual half-field on the cortex of the contralateral hemisphere. The two maps lie adjacent to each other, bounded by a line which Talbot and Marshall termed the "line of decussation." This line receives projections from the vertical meridian. Any retinal region (besides the vertical meridian) projects to two regions on the cortex, one medial to the line of decussation and the other lateral to it. There has been some tendency to assume that the medial representation, called Visual Area I, is the classical striate cortex, whereas Area II is non-striate. There is nothing in the literature to support the latter assumption, though to my knowledge it has never been questioned except by Bard (1956).

The mapping experiments of Talbot and Marshall and of Thompson, Woolsey, and Talbot have since been confirmed for the cat by single-unit techniques. We have confirmed the topographical projection scheme in the cat (Hubel and Wiesel 1962), including the presence of a second visual representation lateral to the first. Daniel and Whitteridge (1961) have repeated the experiments in the monkey and have extended the map to buried parts of the cortex. Although Talbot and Marshall did not describe a second visual area in the monkey, Wiesel and I have recently found electrophysiological evidence for a precise retinotopic projection to nonstriate visual cortex.

The introduction of microelectrodes supplies us with a powerful means of studying properties of individual cortical cells, especially those properties that are not common to cells in a large volume of nervous tissue. To learn what kinds of transformations the visual cortex makes on the incoming visual signals we may compare responses of single cortical cells with those of afferent fibers from the lateral geniculate body. If we were to find no differences in receptive fields of cells in these two structures we would indeed be disappointed, for it would mean either that in spite of its anatomical complexity the striate cortex did virtually nothing, or else that our present microelectrode techniques were not equal to the problem. The second alternative is a possible one, since the elaborative functions of the cortex might be discernible only by examining simultaneously large numbers of cells and comparing their firing patterns, perhaps with the help of computers. As it turns out, there *are* differences in receptive fields, differences which give us a fair idea of some of the functions of the cortex. Here I only attempt to summarize some of our own work (see Hubel and Wiesel 1959, 1962); for other microelectrode investigations of the visual cortex the reader may refer to several recent symposia (Rosenblith 1961; Jung and Kornhuber 1961).

In the striate cortex we have found no cells with concentric "on"- or "off"-center fields. Instead there has been an astonishing variety of new response types. These differ one from another in the details of distribution of excitatory and inhibitory regions, but they have one thing in common: that areas giving excitation and inhibition are not separated by circles, as in the retina and geniculate, but by straight lines. Some cells, for example, have receptive fields with a long narrow excitatory area flanked on either side by inhibitory areas, whereas others have the reverse arrangement, an inhibitory area flanked on the two sides by excitatory areas (Hubel and Wiesel 1962, Text-Fig. 2). Some fields have only two regions of opposite type separated by a single straight line. Summation occurs just as in the retina and geniculate, and the most effective stationary retinal stimulus for a cortical cell is one falling on either the excitatory parts of a receptive field or the inhibitory parts, but not on both simultaneously. Consequently stimuli such as long narrow dark or light rectangles, or boundaries with light to one side and darkness to the other ("edges"), are likely to be the most potent for cortical cells. Each cell will have its own optimal stimulus. Moreover the stimulus that works best in influencing a cell, exciting or inhibiting it, will do so only when shone on the appropriate part of the retina and in the correct orientation. Some cells prefer one inclination, vertical, horizontal, or oblique, others prefer another; and all inclinations seem to be about equally well represented. We have termed the inclination of the most effective stimulus the "receptive-field axis orientation" and have come to realize that this is one of a cell's most important properties. For example, if a stimulus such as a long narrow rectangle of light is shone at right angles to the optimum orientation it has little or no effect. Here the light covers portions of both the excitatory and inhibitory regions, and the two effects oppose each other.

We have already seen that turning on or off a diffuse light is not an ideal stimulus for a retinal ganglion cell. It evokes a response, but a much weaker one than that produced by a centered circular spot of just the right size. I have described how cells in the lateral geniculate body are influenced even less than retinal ganglion cells by diffuse light. In the cortex the process is apparently carried a step further. Here many cells give no response at all when one shines light on the entire receptive field. How the cat detects diffuse light and distinguishes different levels of diffuse illumination is something we do not know. Perhaps the mechanism is subcortical; it is known that the cat can make discriminations of intensity of diffuse light even when it lacks a visual cortex (Smith 1937). The information that a large patch of retina is evenly illuminated may be supplied only by cells that are activated by the boundaries of the patch; the fact that cells with fields entirely within the illuminated area are uninfluenced presumably signals the absence of contours within the patch of light—in other words, that the region is diffusely lit.

One may ask why a diffuse flash of light evokes such a large cortical slow wave, if only a small proportion of cells respond to the stimulus, and these only relatively weakly. Too little is known about slow waves to permit an entirely satisfactory answer. It is possible that a large slow wave may be produced by a small proportion of cells firing weakly but synchronously. It is interesting, however, that the visual evoked response is maximal *outside* the cortical area commonly accepted as striate (Doty 1958), and that within the primary visual area it is maximal well in front of the area centralis representation. Indeed, the area representing central vision gives only a relatively feeble response to a diffuse flash (Doty 1958). We have not thoroughly explored cortical areas representing the far periphery of the retinas: it may be that compared with cells receiving projections from centralis, those with receptive fields in the far periphery respond more actively to diffuse light. This is, in fact, the case with retinal ganglion cells (Wiesel 1960) and with geniculate cells (Hubel and Wiesel 1961).

The amazing selectivity with which cortical cells respond to a highly specific stimulus and ignore almost anything else is explained by the existence of excitatory and inhibitory receptive-field subdivisions. While these mechanisms clearly make use of inhibition, it must be stressed that we have no direct evidence that the cortex contains inhibitory synapses, just as we have none in the case of geniculate or retinal ganglion cells (see discussion of Bremer, in Jung 1960, p. 233). Whenever we suppress firing by turning on a stimulus, the effect may be produced by withdrawing tonic excitation as easily as by directly inhibiting, and so far the appropriate methods of distinguishing the two possibilities have not been used in the visual system.

In their behavior cells whose receptive fields can be divided into excitatory and inhibitory regions are probably the simplest of the striate cortex. It is therefore reasonable to suppose that at least some cells with simple fields receive their projections directly from the geniculate (Hubel and Wiesel 1962; Text-Fig. 19). In the striate cortex we find cells of a second type whose properties we have called "complex." Cells with complex receptive fields do not respond well to small spots of light, and it has not been possible to map their fields into separate excitatory and inhibitory regions. They behave as though they received their afferents from a large number of cortical cells with simple fields, all of these fields having the same axis orientation, but varying slightly from one to the next in their exact retinal positions. A complex cell thus responds to an appropriately oriented slit, edge, or dark bar, not just when it is shone in one highly critical retinal position, as we find with simple cells, but over considerable regions of retina, sometimes up to 5°–10° or more. Presumably whenever the properly oriented stimulus is applied within this area, it activates some cells with simple fields (different ones for different positions of the stimulus) and these in turn activate the complex cell. For example, a typical complex cell might be activated by a horizontal slit of light regardless of its exact position within a region several degrees in diameter. For such a cell changing the orientation by more than 5°–10° renders the stimulus ineffective, as does making it wider than some optimum width (e.g., more than ¼°). It is as though such a cell had the function of responding to the abstract quality "horizontal," irrespective of the exact retinal position.

The idea that a complex cell receives its input from a large number of simple cells all having the same receptive-field axis orientation has a remarkable parallel in the functional anatomy of the cat striate cortex. Cells that are close neighbors almost always have receptive-field axis orientations that are, as far as one can tell, identical. By making long penetrations in the manner of Mountcastle (Mountcastle 1957; Powell and Mountcastle 1959) one can show that the regions of constant axis orientation extend from surface to white matter, with walls perpendicular to the cortical layers (Hubel and Wiesel 1962). Within one of these regions, or "columns," there occur all functional types of cell, including simple and complex. All the cells in a column have their receptive fields in the same general region of retina, but there is a slight variation in exact receptive-field position from one cell to the next. If we assume that a complex cell receives its input from cells with simple fields in the same column, this constancy of receptive-field axis orientation together with the slight differences in position of fields is sufficient to account for all of the complex cell's properties. A column is thus considered to be a functional unit of cortex, to which geniculate axons project in such a way as to produce simple cortical fields all with the same axis orientation, and within which simple cells converge upon complex ones.

From the standpoint of cortical physiology it is interesting that these visual columns are in many ways analogous to the columns in the cat somatosensory cortex, described in 1957 by Mountcastle, and confirmed for the monkey by Powell and Mountcastle (1959). A columnar organization may be a feature of many cortical areas. It seems surprising that this type of organization, which must depend primarily on anatomical connections, should have no known anatomical correlate.

As far as we know all striate cortical cells in the cat can be categorized as simple or complex; there do not seem to be still higher orders of cells in this part of the brain. We are inclined to think of complex cells as representing a stage in the process of form generalization, since we can displace an image by several degrees on the retina, as long as we do not rotate it, and the population of complex cells that is influenced by the borders of the stimulus will not greatly change. The same is true if we distort the image, for instance by making it smaller or larger. As far as we know, this is the first stage in the mammalian visual pathway in which such an abstracting process occurs.

It is important to realize again that the size of a receptive field does not have any necessary bearing on a cell's ability to discriminate fine stimuli. In the cat a typical cortical receptive field in or near the area centralis may have a diameter of $1°-2°$, and complex fields range in size from $2°-3°$ up to $10°$ or more. Nevertheless the optimum stimuli for these cells are likely to be of the order of 10 minutes of arc in width. In a simple field this corresponds to a dimension such as the width of a long narrow receptive-field center. The presence of convergence at each stage of the visual pathway does lead to increased receptive-field size, but not to a loss of detail. This is the result of an interplay between inhibitory and excitatory processes.

So far I have not made any reference to one of the most important aspects of vision, namely movement. A moving stimulus commands attention more than a stationary one; clinically, movement is generally one of the first types of visual perception to return after a cortical injury (for references, see Teuber,

Battersby, and Bender 1960, p. 19); even for the perception of stationary objects, eye movements are probably necessary (Ditchburn and Ginsburg 1952; Riggs, Ratliff, Cornsweet, and Cornsweet, 1953). It is not surprising, then, to find that a moving spot or pattern is in general a powerful stimulus for cortical cells. To understand why this is so we must return for a moment to a consideration of cells with simple fields. If we bring a spot from a neutral region of retina into a cell's excitatory area we produce an "on" response; if we remove a spot from the "off" region of a cell we evolve an "off" discharge. If we combine the two maneuvers by moving a spot from an "off" area into an "on" area, the two mechanisms work together to produce a greatly enhanced response. Of course, the cortical cell is most efficiently activated by the stimulus if it is a slit, dark bar, or edge, and if it is oriented in the direction appropriate for the cell. If the receptive field of the cell is not symmetrical (if one flank is smaller or produces less powerful effects than the other), the responses to two diametrically opposite directions of movement may be different. For example, a cell may fire when a spot is moved from left to right across the retina, but not when it is moved from right to left.

Now let us consider how a moving stimulus influences a complex cell. According to the scheme proposed above, a cell with complex properties receives its input from a number of cells with simple fields whose positions are staggered. Because of these differences in field position, a moving stimulus will activate first one simple cell and then another. The complex cell will thus be continuously bombarded and will fire steadily as the stimulus moves over a relatively wide expanse of retina. A stationary stimulus shone into the receptive field of a complex cell evokes as a rule only a transient response because of the adaptation which presumably occurs at the receptors and at subsequent synapses. The moving pattern would bypass much of this adaptation by activating many cells in sequence.

The same mechanism may play a part in the perception of stationary objects by making use of the saccadic eye movements which, at least in man, seem necessary for the persistence of a visual impression. A visual image as it passes across the moving retina presumably activates numbers of simple cells briefly and in sequence, leads to a more steady activation of a much smaller number of complex cells.

From what has been said so far it will be apparent that the striate cortex has a rich assortment of functions. It rearranges the input from the lateral geniculate body in such a way as to make lines and contours the most important stimuli. Directionality of stimuli must be accurately specified; the presence of a columnar system based on receptive-field axis orientation testifies to the importance of this variable. What appears to be a first step in the process of perceptual generalization results from a cell's responding to a property of a boundary (its orientation) apart from its exact position. Movement also becomes an important stimulus parameter, whose rate and direction both must be specified if a cell is to be effectively driven.

To this list one more function must be added, that of combining the pathways upon the two eyes. In contrast to the lateral geniculate body, most cells in the cat cortex (probably at least 85%) receive input from the two eyes (Hubel and Wiesel 1962, Part II). By mapping out receptive fields in each eye separately and comparing them we can begin to learn about the mechanisms of binocular vision, and perhaps ultimately something about binocular depth perception and binocular rivalry.

The primary visual, or striate, cortex is probably only an early stage of the visual pathway. Yet, unfortunately, we have very little knowledge of the pathway from this point on. Except in the rat (Nauta and Bucher 1954) and cat (Beresford 1961) the points to which the striate cortex projects are not known. Even less is known about the connections of the neighboring nonstriate visual cortex, called 18 and 19, or parastriate and peristriate; we have no accurate description of what areas project to them, or of where they send their projections. There even seem to be doubts as to the validity of the distinction between the two areas (Lashley and Clark 1946). Clearly, more will have to be learned about the anatomy before neurophysiologists can make much progress in parts of the pathway beyond the striate cortex.

The work I have described may help to show how visual messages are handled by the brain, at least in the early stages of the process. The analysis takes us to what are probably at least sixth-order neurons in the visual pathway. Our understanding of cells with complex fields will be incomplete until we know how these properties are used at the next stage of integration, just as our grasp of the significance of retinal and geniculate receptive-field organization was incomplete without a knowledge of cortical receptive fields. There is no way of foreseeing what the next transformations will be, but to judge from what we have learned so far one would guess that the process of abstraction will go on, and that response specificity will increase. But it is well to remember that central nervous physiology is in a descriptive and exploratory phase. Our ignorance of CNS processes is such that the best predictions stand a good chance of being wrong.

References

G. Arden and U. Söderberg, "The Transfer of Optic Information through the Lateral Geniculate Body of the Rabbit," in *Sensory Communication,* edited by W. A. Rosenblith (MIT Press and John Wiley & Sons, Inc., New York, 1961), pp. 521–544.

P. Bard, *Medical Physiology* (C. V. Mosby Company, St. Louis, Missouri, 1956), p. 1176.

W. A. Beresford, "Fibre Degeneration following Lesions of the Visual Cortex of the Cat," in *Neurophysiologic und Psychophysik des visuellen Systems,* edited by R. Jung and H. Kornhuber (Springer-Verlag, Berlin, 1961).

P. O. Bishop, W. Burke, and R. Davis, "Synapse Discharge by Single Fibre in Mammalian Visual System," *Nature* **182,** 728–730 (1958).

————, "Activation of Single Lateral Geniculate Cells by Stimulation of Either Optic Nerve," *Science* **130**, 506–507 (1959).

G. S. Brindley, *Physiology of the Retina and the Visual Pathway* (Edward Arnold, Ltd., London, 1960).

R. Cohn, "Laminar Electrical Responses in Lateral Geniculate Body of Cat," *J. Neurophysiol.* **19**, 317–324 (1956).

P. M. Daniel and D. Whitteridge, "The Representation of the Visual Field on the Cerebral Cortex in Monkeys," *J. Physiol. (London)* **159**, 203–221 (1961).

R. L. De Valois, "Color Vision Mechanisms in the Monkey," *J. gen. Physiol.* **43**, Pt. 2, 115–128 (1960).

R. W. Ditchburn and B. L. Ginsburg, "Vision with Stabilized Retinal Image," *Nature* **170**, 36–37 (1952).

R. W. Doty, "Potentials Evoked in Cat Cerebral Cortex by Diffuse and by Punctiform Photic Stimuli," *J. Neurophysiol.* **21**, 437–464 (1958).

S. D. Erulkar and M. Fillenz, "Single-Unit Activity in the Lateral Geniculate Body of the Cat," *J. Physiol. (London)* **154**, 206–218 (1960).

W. H. Freygang, Jr., "An Analysis of Extracellular Potentials from Single Neurons in the Lateral Geniculate Nucleus of the Cat," *J. gen. Physiol.* **41**, 543–564 (1958).

O.-J. Grüsser and G. Sauer, "Monoculare und binoculare Lichtreizung einzelner Neurone im Geniculatum laterale der Katze," *Pflüg. Arch. ges. Physiol.* **271**, 595–612 (1960).

W. R. Hayhow, "The Cytoarchitecture of the Lateral Geniculate Body in the Cat in Relation to the Distribution of Crossed and Uncrossed Optic Fibers," *J. comp. Neurol.* **110**, 1–64 (1958).

D. H. Hubel, "Single Unit Activity in Lateral Geniculate Body and Optic Tract of Unrestrained Cats," *J. Physiol. (London)* **150**, 91–104 (1960).

D. H. Hubel and T. N. Wiesel, "Receptive Fields of Single Neurones in the Cat's Striate Cortex," *J. Physiol. (London)* **148**, 574–591 (1959).

————, "Receptive Fields of Optic Nerve Fibres in the Spider Monkey," *J. Physiol. (London)* **154**, 572–580 (1960).

————, "Integrative Action in the Cat's Lateral Geniculate Body," *J. Physiol. (London)* **155**, 385–398 (1961).

————, "Receptive Fields, Binocular Interaction and Functional Architecture in the Cat's Visual Cortex," *J. Physiol.* **160**, 106–154 (1962).

R. Jung, "Microphysiologie corticaler Neurone: Ein Beitrag zur Koordination der Hirnrinde und des visuellen Systems" in *Structure and Function of the Cerebral Cortex*, edited by D. B. Tower and J. P. Schadé (Elsevier Publishing Company, Amsterdam, 1960).

R. Jung and H. Kornhuber, Editors, *Neurophysiologie und Psychophysik des Visuellen Systems* (Springer-Verlag, Berlin, 1961).

S. W. Kuffler, "Discharge Patterns and Functional Organization of Mammalian Retina," *J. Neurophysiol.* **16**, 37–68 (1953).

K. S. Lashley and G. Clark, "The Cytoarchitecture of the Cerebral Cortex of Ateles: a Critical Examination of Architectonic Studies," *J. comp. Neurol.* **85**, 223–305 (1946).

H. R. Maturana, J. V. Lettvin, W. S. McCulloch, and W. H. Pitts, "Anatomy and Physiology of Vision in the Frog (*Rana pipiens*)," *J. Gen. Physiol.* **43**, Pt. 2, 129–176 (1960).

W. B. Mountcastle, "Modality and Topographic Properties of Single Neurons of Cat's Somatic Sensory Cortex," *J. Neurophysiol.* **20**, 408–434 (1957).

J. H. Nauta and V. M. Bucher, "Efferent Connections of the Striate Cortex in the Albino Rat," *J. comp. Neurol.* **100**, 257–286 (1954).

S. Polyak, *The Vertebrate Visual System,* edited by H. Klüver (The University of Chicago Press, Chicago, 1957).

T. P. S. Powell and V. B. Mountcastle, "Some Aspects of the Functional Organization of the Cortex of the Postcentral Gyrus of the Monkey: a Correlation of Findings Obtained in a Single Unit Analysis with Cytoarchitecture," *Johns Hopkins Hospital Bull.* **105**, 133–162 (1959).

H. A. Riggs, F. Ratliff, J. C. Cornsweet, and T. N. Cornsweet, "The Disappearance of Steadily Fixated Visual Test Objects," *J. Opt. Soc. Am.* **43**, 495–501 (1953).

W. A. Rosenblith, Editor, *Sensory Communication* (MIT Press and John Wiley & Sons, Inc., New York, 1961).

P. S. Silva, "Some Anatomical and Physiological Aspects of the Lateral Geniculate Body," *J. comp. Neurol.* **106**, 463–486 (1956).

K. U. Smith, "Visual Discriminations in the Cat: V. The Postoperative Effects of Removal of the Striate Cortex upon Intensity Discrimination," *J. genet. Psychol.* **51**, 329–369 (1937).

S. A. Talbot, "A Lateral Localization in the Cat's Visual Cortex," *Federation Proc.* **1**, 84 (1942).

S. A. Talbot and W. H. Marshall, "Physiological Studies on Neural Mechanisms of Visual Localization and Discrimination," *Am. J. Ophthalmol.* **24**, 1255–1263 (1941).

H.-L. Teuber, W. S. Battersby, and M. B. Bender, *Visual Field Defects after Penetrating Missile Wounds of the Brain* (Harvard University Press, Cambridge, Massachusetts, 1960).

J. M. Thompson, C. N. Woolsey, and S. A. Talbot, "Visual Areas I and II of Cerebral Cortex of Rabbit," *J. Neurophysiol.* **13**, 277–288 (1950).

L. Widén and C. Ajmone-Marsan, "Effects of Corticipetal and Corticifugal Impulses upon Single Elements of the Dorsolateral Geniculate Nucleus," *Exptl. Neurol.* **2**, 468–502 (1960).

T. N. Wiesel, "Receptive Fields of Ganglion Cells in the Cat's Retina," *J. Physiol.* (*London*) **153**, 583–594 (1960).

M. L. Wolbarsht, H. G. Wagner, and E. F. MacNichol, Jr., "Receptive Fields of Retinal Ganglion Cells: Extent and Spectral Sensitivity," in *Neurophysiologie und Psychophysik des visuellen Systems,* edited by R. Jung and H. Kornhuber (Springer-Verlag, Berlin, 1961).

Eye Movement Control in Primates

DAVID A. ROBINSON

Reprinted from *Science,* Sept. 20, 1968, Vol. 161, pp. 1219–1224. Copyright 1968 by the American Association for the Advancement of Science.

The retinas of most animals in which the eyes face forward have a special area, the fovea centralis, which has a high density of photoreceptors. To see an object with good visual acuity, these animals must move their eyes to place its image on each fovea. The eye movement system is especially well developed in primates. The purpose of this system is to acquire a visual target and then track it so that its image remains on the fovea. To do this, the oculomotor system overcomes, with nervous tissue and muscle, the same problems encountered in tracking systems designed by man. Current research in this field is directed not only toward diagnosis of eye movement disorders in man but also toward understanding how the central nervous system processes information and manipulates signals to achieve the regulation and coordination which this control system displays.

Four Oculomotor Subsystems

All tracking systems made by man or nature have at least two requirements: to acquire a given target rapidly, and then to follow it if it moves relative to the environment. The eye movement systems which perform these two functions are called the saccadic and smooth pursuit systems. When the tracking device is mounted on a moving platform (for example, a shipboard-mounted radar system) an additional requirement is that of stabilizing the tracking device automatically against movements of the platform. For eye movements, this function is fulfilled by the vestibular system. Finally, for depth perception (analogous to stereoscopic range-finding in some gunnery systems) the vergence system controls the degree of convergence of the visual axes of the eyes necessary to maintain the target image on each fovea. In short, the saccadic, smooth pursuit, vestibular, and vergence systems perform the four functions of acquiring targets, tracking them if they move in the environment, compensating for movements of the head in the environment, and tracking in depth.

Almost all eye movements in primates are combinations of the movements produced by each of these subsystems. The tasks are different from each other and appear to be performed by separate neurological control systems specializing in individual tasks. They can be excited independently, and their responses can be observed independently, so that each may be studied in isolation. Figure 1 illustrates this subdivision and the types of movements produced by each system. Except for the vestibular system, which obtains information about movement of the head in space from the semicircular canals, all the systems depend on visual information derived from the retina and carried centrally on the optic nerve. The outputs of the four systems converge on the motor nuclei whose motor cells relay the information along the motor nerves to the extraocular muscles. Each eye is equipped with three pairs of antagonist muscles that rotate the globe in three roughly mutually perpendicular planes: horizontal, vertical, and torsional. This arrangement gives full freedom to the oculomotor system in carrying out its various tasks. The behavioral characteristic of the four subsystems is described in the following sections with emphasis on their differences, which support the notion that they are neurologically distinct.

The Saccadic System

This system is specialized in moving both eyes from one position to another very rapidly. Vision is impaired during a saccade so that it is desirable that little time be lost in the movement to maximize the amount of time in seeing. Figure 1*A* is a record of the horizontal position of a subject's eye in "look-

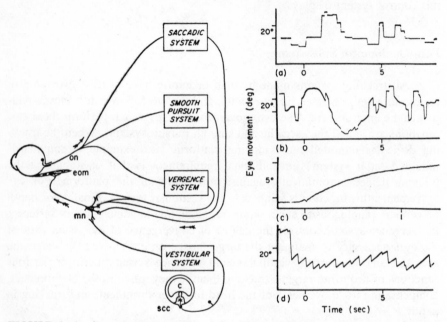

FIGURE 1. A schematic representation of the primate eye movement system emphasizing the four subsystems involved in tracking visual targets. The saccadic system rapidly acquires new targets, the smooth pursuit system tracks the target if it moves in the environment, the vergence system performs binocular tracking in depth, and the vestibular system compensates for head movements. The types of eye movements made by each system are shown in *a, b, c,* and *d,* respectively. Each system converges on the motor nuclei (*mn*) which innervate the extraocular muscles (*eom*) and move the eyeball. Optic nerve, *on;* cupula, *c;* semicircular canal, *scc.*

ing about." Most of the time is spent in periods of steady fixation of different parts of the visual field which are interrupted by quick changes of fixation. Saccades are used for reading or the examination of any object or picture when it and the observer are stationary. The extraocular muscles are among the fastest in the body, and saccades are their fastest product. A 10-degree human saccade lasts 45 milliseconds, and the eye velocity reaches a peak of about 400 degrees per second. During a saccade, the agonist muscle contracts almost maximally, and the antagonist is inhibited completely, so that almost the full reserve of force of the muscles is called upon to make the movement as rapid as possible.

The saccadic system behaves like a sampled-data system. Such systems are unique in that they do not receive information continuously but only at discrete time intervals. When a subject is asked to watch a target that suddenly jumps to one side he will follow it by a saccade after a reaction time of about 200 milliseconds. However if the target jumps back to its starting place after 100 milliseconds the subject will still make a saccade, wholly inappropriate by then, 200 milliseconds after the first target jump to where the target was, and then another 200 milliseconds will pass before he returns his eyes to the starting point (*1*). The system behaves as though, when the target moves, it samples the error and then ceases to take in any new information. After one reaction time it responds with a saccade appropriate to the position error as it existed 200 milliseconds ago. This sampling behavior has been investigated rather thoroughly for the eye movement system (*2*), and is of current interest in other neuromuscular systems involved when man is an operator in a man-machine task (for example, control of jet aircraft and space capsules). The concept of sampled data does appear appropriate to the gross behavior of the saccadic system, although closer scrutiny reveals that during the 200-millisecond period after the initial error sampling takes place, all visual information is not blocked. Subsequent changes in both target velocity and position influence the amplitude of the impending saccade, but the probability that they will do so diminishes with increasing time between the initial sample and the final motor act (*3, 4*).

Saccadic eye movements are, in general, voluntary acts based on visual information, but they can also be made with eyes closed or in total darkness. They also occur during certain periods of sleep (*5*), and are thought to be associated with "watching" the visual imagery of dreams (*6*). There is probably an involuntary side to saccades. When one suddenly perceives movement in the periphery, one's eyes are drawn to it (by a saccade) almost automatically. Thus saccades may be initiated involuntarily by visual stimuli, and voluntarily with or without visual stimuli.

The Smooth Pursuit System

This system, on the other hand, is almost entirely automatic and requires a visual stimulus. Smooth-pursuit eye movements cannot be made in the absence of a moving visual stimulus, and they are involuntary in situations where the entire visual field is in motion. This occurs when looking into a rotating mirror or out the window of a moving train, when the eyes smoothly follow an object until it becomes uncomfortable to continue without a head movement. At that time, the eyes saccade the other way to pick up and track another object. The resulting saw-toothed movement is called optokinetic nystagmus. More commonly the smooth pursuit system tracks only one object moving in a stationary environment. Figure 1*B* shows the eye movements of a subject watching a person walk about. The saccadic system still scans over the person's body, but within each intersaccadic interval the eye velocity matches the velocity of the moving object being observed. Clearly, the value of this pursuit is that it is easier for the visual system to perceive the form and pattern of images if they are stationary on the retina rather than moving. The smooth pursuit system appears to be not concerned with the error itself between target and fovea (which is corrected by the saccadic system), but only with matching the eye velocity to target velocity (7). To do this it apparently extracts from the visual system information concerning the direction and rate of movement of images on the retina and then supplies a signal to the extraocular muscles designed to reduce this rate of movement to zero. Although the smooth pursuit system can produce eye velocities up to 100 degrees per second, it cannot correctly match the velocity of visual stimuli above about 30 degrees per second.

The smooth pursuit system differs from the saccadic system in a number of ways. Two have already been mentioned: its involuntary nature and the fact that target velocity rather than target position is its appropriate stimulus. Experiments in which the target velocity is changed twice in rapid succession indicate that the smooth pursuit system is a continuous rather than a sampled system (3). Its reaction time is only 125 milliseconds. It is slower than the saccadic system and requires 130 milliseconds to effect a step change in eye velocity compared to 20 to 70 milliseconds required by most saccades (8). Barbiturates, alcohol (7), and some disease processes (9) selectively attack the smooth pursuit system before the saccadic system. Another difference appears when the two systems are made to oscillate by external visual feedback. This can be brought about by measuring the subject's eye position and allowing it to change the target position by some electrical or optical scheme. Normally, an eye movement will produce an equal and opposite change in the retinal error between target image and fovea. In the terminology of control theory, the oculomotor system is thus said to have a negative feedback gain of 1.0. External feedback can add or subtract from this value and change the net feedback gain. Almost all control systems oscillate if the negative feedback gain is sufficiently increased, and the oculomotor system is no exception. All three systems—saccadic, smooth pursuit, and vergence—oscillate under increased visual feedback. The vestibular system is not included because it is not a feedback system. The saccadic system oscillates when the net feedback gain is 5.0 at a frequency of about 2 hertz, whereas the smooth pursuit system oscillates at a gain of 8.0 at a frequency of 3.3 hertz (3).

The Vestibular System

This system measures the motion of the head in space and moves the eyes in the head to compensate and maintain the visual axis stable in the environment. Information about head orientation is obtained from the semicircular canals lying in the vestibule of the inner ear. Each is a fluid-filled circular tube with a hinged fluid-tight vane, the cupula (C in Fig. 1), lying across its lumen. Angular acceleration of the head causes the fluid to be "left behind" which deflects the cupula. Nerve cells beneath it sense its deflection, and alter their rate of discharge proportionately. The elements determining the dynamic behavior of the canals (*10*) are the moment of inertia of the ring of fluid, the viscous drag of the fluid as it flows through the canal, and the spring stiffness of the gelatinous cupula which always returns to a neutral position in the absence of applied forces. Because the viscosity is the predominate reacting force, the velocity of the fluid flow is approximately proportional to the angular acceleration of the head. Consequently cupula position (the integral of fluid velocity) is proportional to the angular velocity of the head. Thus, this sense organ behaves like an integrating accelerometer, and in its normal mode of action the neural discharge to the central nervous system is proportional to head velocity (*11*). If the head movements are of too short or too long duration, the viscous reaction force no longer predominates over the inertial or spring forces, and the canal ceases to integrate head acceleration properly. The range of frequencies of head movements over which the semicircular canals behave as integrating accelerometers is approximately 0.017 to 17 hertz.

To stabilize eye position, the incoming vestibular velocity signal must be integrated once more by the nervous system before being translated into eye position by the extraocular muscles. There are three semicircular canals (on each side of the head) lying in three roughly mutually perpendicular planes. They can resolve angular head velocity about any axis in space into three components which are applied in the correct combination to the three pairs of antagonist muscles of each eye to counterrotate them about the same axis. If rotation continues for more than 10 or 15 degrees in the same direction a saccade resets the eyes rapidly in the opposite direction and stabilization then continues to take place for a new visual axis position. If rotation persists it creates the alternating saw-toothed pattern of fast and slow phases (Fig. 1*D*) called vestibular nystagmus. If rotation at a constant velocity is sustained beyond about 10 seconds, nystagmus will cease because such stimulation lies below the physiological bandwith of the system.

Although the smooth pursuit system can compensate for retinal image movement caused by head movement, it cannot do so accurately above 30 degrees per second; yet head movements can easily exceed 300 degrees per second. The vestibular system can compensate for these large velocities and its short direct path through the brain stem insures an almost immediate reaction.

The Vergence System

This is the only system which moves the eyes in opposite directions. It is the slowest of all the systems. In Figure 1*C* a single vergence movement made by a subject looking from a far to a near target is illustrated. The movement lasts for about 800 milliseconds. The reaction time is about 160 milliseconds. It does not appear to be a sampled system (*12*). It oscillates at 2.5 hertz when placed under external negative visual feedback (*12*). The stimulus for this system is the difference between the retinal errors seen by each eye, and it applies to the extraocular muscles a signal that causes the eyes to converge or diverge at 10 degrees per second for each degree of interretinal error *(13)*. When a subject looks from some point A to another, B, which lies at a different angle and depth in his visual field, he first makes a saccade from A to a point in space which allows his two visual axes to just straddle B, and this is followed by a pure vergence movement until both eyes are directed at B *(8)*. This sequence illustrates that the vergence system is a separate neurological system that can only create equal and opposite eye movements that summate with the conjugate movements of the other systems.

The Final Common Path

The motor nerves and muscles form a unit called the final common path because it is shared by all four subsystems. It is useful to know the way nervous activity in the final common path is converted through the tension developed in the muscles to eye position. The scheme describing the mechanics of the globe and one antagonist pair of extraocular muscles is shown in Figure 2. The globe is held in the bony orbit by many passive tissues such as the optic nerve, fat pad, suspensory ligaments, and conjunctiva, whose viscoelastic properties are represented by the springs and dashpots of the passive orbital viscoelastic elements. Each muscle also has its passive elements. Electrical activity in the nerves, which may be thought of as the control signal, is converted to active state tension (F_1 and F_2) in the two muscles. This force is transmitted to the globe through the mechanical elements of the active portion of muscle.

If a subject fixates straight ahead and one eye is drawn aside (by pulling on an opaque suction contact lens firmly seated on the eye), the static spring stiffness of all the elements (Fig. 2) is found to be 1.2 grams per degree *(14, 15)*. The detachment of the two muscles from the globe during corrective surgery reveals that about 20 percent of this figure lies in the passive orbital elastic elements and 30 percent in the two passive muscle elastic elements combined *(16)*. The remaining 50 percent resides in the length-tension relation of muscle and indicates that as the muscles are lengthened they are capable of generating more tension. Such studies *(16)* also indicate that when the eye looks straight ahead both muscles exert a tonic force of about 14 grams. During steady deviations the force increases in the agonist (up to 50 grams) and decreases in the antagonist until the difference just balances the restraining force of the passive tissues. The maximum force of human extraocular muscles is estimated at 150 grams. If the eye, drawn aside by the contact lens, is suddenly released, it returns with a small initial rapid motion followed by a slower motion that lasts over 700 milliseconds and constitutes 75 percent of the total movement. This step response indicates that the system appears to be largely overdamped. The small fast motion has been investigated by applying sinusoidal forces to a contact lens on the eye *(17)* and demonstrating that the inertia J resonates with a stiff spring (thought to be the series elastic component) at 35 hertz with a damping factor of 0.5. Theoretical studies *(18)* suggest that the principal source of viscosity, which constitutes the greatest mechanical impedance to rapid movements, resides in the force-velocity relationship of muscle itself.

From what is now known about the mechanics of the system in Figure 2, it is almost possible to predict the control signals needed to produce saccadic, smooth pursuit, and vergence movements. Even so, it is desirable to observe these signals more directly by fastening the contact lens to a strain gauge which prevents the eye from moving but measures the net force which the isometric muscles exert in their efforts to rotate the globe (3, 14, 19). Figure 2 (A-C)

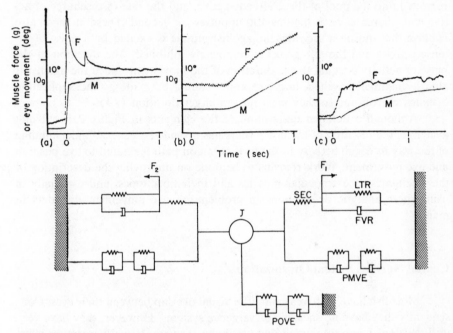

FIGURE 2. A model of the mechanics of the extraocular muscles, globe, and suspensory tissues. The globe, of moment of inertia J, is held in the bony orbit by passive orbital viscoelastic elements (POVE). Each muscle has passive viscoelastic elements (PMVE) and an active portion composed of a series elastic component (SEC) and a contractile component subdivided into an element with a force-velocity relationship (FVR) and an active state tension generator (F_1, F_2) which displays a length-tension relationship (LTR). The recordings represent net isometric muscle force (F) and eye movement (M) for saccadic (a), smooth pursuit (b), and vergence (c) movements.

illustrates the net isometric force measured in one eye and the movement of the other eye during saccadic, smooth pursuit, and vergence movements. The vergence movement is slow because the tension is only a slightly rounded step function. The smooth pursuit movement is more rapid, because the eye is initially accelerated by a rate of rise of force twice as large as that needed to maintain velocity in the steady state. The saccade is the most rapid movement, because a large pulse of force is applied to overcome the viscous impedance of the mechanical system and maintain a high velocity during the movement. At the end of the movement the pulse of force is removed and replaced by a lower holding force. The 150-gram force of which human extraocular muscles are capable is not used to hold the eye in steady deviation but is held in reserve for the pulse of force associated with saccades.

The control signals during eye movements may also be observed by thrusting needle electrodes into the extraocular muscles to observe their electrical activity (*20, 21*), and by placing microelectrodes into the motor nuclei of animals and recording the action potentials of single motor nerve cells. (*22*). Both methods reveal that when a muscle increases its force, more muscle fibers are recruited into the pool of those already active, and the rate of discharge of active units increases to as high as 400 impulses per second. These methods also confirm that during a saccade, the agonist muscle is excited by a pulse of intense activity and the antagonist is completely inhibited. The duration of the pulse of activity is equal to the duration of the movement. Since the agonist is almost maximally excited, larger saccades cannot be made by the application of much more force so they must have a larger duration (*14*).

Although a detailed description of the elements in Figure 2 is still not available, the research of the last 5 years has provided a general understanding of the way in which activity in the final common path is related to eye position and eye movement. Work remains to be done on improving the description of the mechanics of extraocular muscles and their fiber types, and especially in using these analytic descriptions in problems of eye movement disorders in man.

Central Nervous System Organization

Most fish have no foveas and little visual overlap between their eyes. Consequently they have no saccadic or vergence systems. However, they have very well-developed smooth pursuit and vestibular systems. Visual perception takes place in the optic tectum of the fish, which is more simply organized than the visual cortex of primates; therefore it is important for survival that fish have retinal images that are stabilized by these two velocity compensating systems. However, since the activity of these systems can carry the eye to its mechanical limits, a fast resetting mechanism had to develop simultaneously with both systems. This system, responsible for the fast phase of vestibular and optokinetic nystagmus, appears to be the forerunner of the saccadic system. As the central nervous system evolved, the cortex developed, the fovea came into existence, and eye movement came under cortical control. The cortex appears to have used the fast-phase brain-stem system for its own purposes to form the saccadic system. As encephalization progressed, the primary visual area shifted from the optic tectum (the homologue of the mammalian superior colliculi) which subserved smooth pursuit movements to the visual cortex and this function has gone with it. In primates it is not clear what visual or eye movement function remains in the superior colliculi (*23*). Figure 3 presents a simplified picture of those portions of the nervous system involved in eye movements.

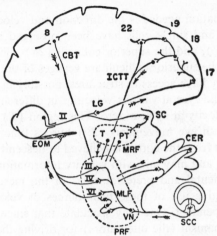

FIGURE 3. A schematic of the major oculomotor pathways in the central nervous system. *CBT*, corticobulbar tract; *CER*, cerebellum; *EOM*, extraocular muscles; *ICTT*, internal corticotectal tract; *LG*, lateral geniculate body; *MLF*, medial longitudinal fasciculus; *MRF*, mesencephalic reticular formation; *PRF*, pontine reticular formation; *PT*, pretectal nuclei; *SC*, superior colliculi; *SCC*, semicircular canals; *T*, tegmentum; *VN*, vestibular nuclei; II, optic nerve; III, IV, VI, oculomotor, trochlear and abducens nuclei and cranial nerves; 17, 18, 19, 22, Brodmann's areas of occipital and parietal visual and association areas; 8, Brodmann's premotor area in the frontal lobes.

The Vestibular System

This is the most localized system. Information concerning head velocity enters the vestibular nuclei and is immediately relayed along the medial longitudinal fasciculus, which distributes the information from the six canals appropriately among the motor nuclei and so to the 12 extraocular muscles. This three-neuron arc (*24*) is inadequate to perform the temporal integration known to take place in the pathway, but multisynaptic pathways exist in the pontine reticular formation and the cerebellum which may perform this function. What generates the fast phase of vestibular nystagmus is unknown, but it depends on the integrity of the brain stem between the vestibular and the oculomotor nuclei (*25*). The pulse of activity that produces the resetting saccade must be distributed in the right proportion to the motor nuclei, so that the direction of the fast-phase movement is opposite to the slow phase. It is likely that the same pulse erases the information stored in the brain-stem integrators so that they may be ready to generate the next slow phase. Since eye and head movements in the same direction are common, the voluntary saccadic system must be capable of completely blocking the action of the vestibular system. These are only a few of the functions executed by this system in ways that are not understood at the nerve cell level.

The Smooth Pursuit System

This system uses information extracted from the visual system, presumably from areas 17, 18, and 19 (Fig. 3) in the cortex and from the superior colliculi. The information needed is the direction and velocity of image movement on the retina and single cells have been observed in the visual cortex (*26*), the retina (*27*), and the superior colliculi (*28*) which seem to provide this information. If the superior colliculi are vestiges of the optic tectum of the fish, they presumably have access to structures, possibly in the tegmental area, organized to move the eyes at various velocities in different directions to keep the retinal image velocity at or near zero. This region (*T*) is known to be intimately involved with eye movements (*29*) but its function is still unclear. Velocity information from the cortex is believed to descend in the internal corticotectal tract (*30*) and may mix with velocity information from the superior colliculi in the tegmental and pretectal areas of the mesencephalic reticular formation. The relative use of these two sources of velocity information is probably species-dependent. One may speculate that since the vestibular system contains a mechanism (the integrators) for driving the eyes at a velocity that is proportional to an input signal and the smooth pursuit system has the same requirement, they may share the same neural networks. Vestibular and optokinetic nystagmus certainly can compete with each other, but it is not known whether they do this at the input to the integrators or at the motor nuclei. Electrical stimulation of areas 18 and 19 (Fig. 3) produces conjugate eye movements to the opposite side (*31*), but most investigations have been carried out in the lightly anesthetized monkey in which all movements are smooth, and no one has yet demonstrated smooth pursuit movements by stimulation of the cortex of the unanesthetized monkey.

The Vergence System

Electrical stimulation of cortical areas 19 and 22 (Fig. 3) produces vergence movements in the lightly anesthetized monkey (*32*). Although this needs verification in the absence of anesthesia, it suggests that here the vergence system extracts visual information of the difference in retinal error between the eyes and sends it, also by the internal corticotectal tract, to the brain stem. This system is not only responsible for movements of convergence and divergence but must also actively maintain fusion of the two retinal images by controlling vertical and torsional muscle balance, so it must have access to all the motor nuclei.

The Saccadic System

Saccades can be evoked by stimulation of cortical area 8 (Fig. 3), known as the frontal eye fields. The movements produced by a brief (30-millisecond) stimulus train in the unanesthetized monkey are conjugate contralateral saccades indistinguishable from the animal's spontaneous saccades (*33*). Stimulation of many sites in the frontal eye fields shows that no other types of eye movement are evoked. At each site, the saccade occurs above a certain stimulus threshold in an all-or-nothing fashion, and the size and direction of the saccade depends not so much on how the cortex is stimulated (above threshold) as on where it is stimulated. Stimulation of different subdivisions of the frontal eye fields produces saccades which range from 2 to 60 degrees in amplitude depending only on stimulus location. These observations support the hypothesis of neurology that the frontal eye fields are the cortical outlet for the voluntary saccadic system. It also suggests that all sizes and directions of saccades required by the animal to look anywhere in his visual field are coded by location in this area of the cortex.

Fibers leave this area and descend in the corticobulbar tract to the pontine reticular formation (the ill-defined region marked *PRF* in Fig. 3) where so much of the oculomotor signal processing takes place and the pulse of activity associated with saccades is generated. It appears that cortical stimulation has access to these pulse generators and sets in motion an irreversible stereotyped chain of neural events in the brain stem that leads to a saccade. If the first stimulus is followed by a second test stimulus it appears that the pulsatile system has a refractory period of about 25 milliseconds during which it cannot be reexcited and a relative refractory period of 40 milliseconds during which it can be reexcited only by an increased stimulus intensity. The combination of threshold, all-or-nothing response, and a refractory period are characteristics which often occur together in pulse generator devices either made by man (for example, the one-shot multivibrator) or nature (for example, the nerve action potential). However, if the second test stimulus is delivered to the opposite cortex, there is no refractoriness and it produces a second saccade in the opposite direction which can occur so soon after the first that it mechanically interferes with it. When this happens the first saccade appears to be canceled in midflight and replaced by the second. This suggests that horizontal saccades are created by two pulse generators, one for left gaze triggered from the right cortex, and the other for right gaze triggered from the left, each of which is post-stimulus refractory and which mutually interact so that only one pulse generator can be on at any one time.

When two cortical points are stimulated simultaneously either on the same or opposite sides, the resulting saccade is a weighted mixture of the two movements evoked by each stimulus separately with the weightings determined by stimulus intensity. For example if the left and right cortices are stimulated together the resulting saccade amplitude can be continuously varied from a right movement through zero to a left movement by varying the ratio of stimulus intensities. Since saccade amplitude is largely determined by the pulse duration of the pulse generators, it appears that some neural network must control this pulse width on the basis of which fibers from the cortex carry the activity rather than the temporal nature of the activity itself. When two sets of fibers are excited at once this network must reach a compromise between them and control the pulse width accordingly.

Summary

The neural organization of the oculomotor system is much more complex than that suggested by Figure 3 and the foregoing descriptions. The final picture of this system must explain a great variety of signal manipulation and coordination. The electrical stimulation of the frontal eye fields just discussed is an example of how functional descriptions of the organization and interaction of elements of the subsystems can be built up. The areas where future research will no doubt concentrate are the mesencephalic and pontine reticular formations into which information flows from many sources. In and through this small volume of neural tissue, a vast amount of information processing and transmission takes place, only a small part of which is concerned with eye movements. However, it is here that the four oculomotor subsystems perform their final transformations on the incoming signals and establish the interactions required between them before passing the total output to the final common path. Stimulation and single nerve cell recording with microelectrodes in animals will probably be the methods used in future research, coupled with techniques to avoid the use of anesthesia and to measure eye movement accurately.

I have tried here to emphasize the importance of function in oculomotor research. A discussion of the evolution of eye movements by Walls (*34*) also puts strong emphasis on function. The oculomotor system is one of the few control systems in physiology where function can be stated with such clarity and the function of each of its subsystems can be stated with equal clarity. With our knowledge about the final common path and an appreciation of the simple task each subsystem must perform it is possible to state what information each system needs, how it must process it, and what form of control signal it must present to the final common path in order to accomplish its goal. This knowledge should help in interpreting the data that will emerge when we seek to discover how all this is accomplished at the nuclear and cellular level.

References and Notes

1. G. Westheimer, *Arch. Ophthalmol.* **52,** 932 (1954).
2. L. R. Young and L. Stark, *IEEE* (*Inst. Elec. Electron. Eng.*) *Trans. Human Factors Electron.* **HFE-4,** 38 (1963).
3. D. A. Robinson, *J. Physiol.* **180,** 569 (1965).
4. L. L. Wheeless, Jr., R. M. Boynton, G. H. Cohen, *J. Opt. Soc. Amer.* **56,** 956 (1966).
5. A. F. Fuchs and S. Ron, *Electroencephalogr. Clin. Neurophysiol.* **23,** 244 (1968).
6. W. Dement, in *The Oculomotor System,* M. B. Bender, Ed. (Harper and Row, New York, 1964), p. 366.
7. C. Rashbass, *J. Physiol.* **159,** 326 (1961).
8. A. L. Yarbus, *Eye Movements and Vision* (Plenum, New York, 1967).

9. G. K. von Noorden and T. J. Preziosi, *Arch. Ophthalmol.* **76**, 167 (1966).
10. A. J. Van Egmond, J. J. Groen, L. B. W. Jongkees, *J. Physiol.* **110**, 1 (1949).
11. G. M. Jones and J. H. Milsum, *IEEE (Inst. Elec. Electron. Eng.) Trans. Bio-Med. Eng.* **BME-12**, 54 (1965).
12. B. L. Zuber and L. Stark, *IEEE (Inst. Elec. Electron. Eng.) Trans. Syst. Sci. Cyb.* **SSC-4**, 72 (1968).
13. C. Rashbass and G. Westheimer, *J. Physiol.* **159**, 339 (1961).
14. D. A. Robinson, *ibid.* **174**, 245 (1964).
15. D. S. Childress and R. W. Jones, *ibid.* **188**, 273 (1967).
16. D. A. Robinson, D. M. O'Meara, A. B. Scott, C. C. Collins, in preparation.
17. J. G. Thomas, *Kybernetik* **3**, 254 (1967).
18. G. Cook and L. Stark, *Commun. Behav. Biol.* **1**, 197 (1968).
19. D. A. Robinson, *J. Pediat. Ophthalmol.* (31 Aug. 1966), p. 31.
20. Å. Björk and E. Kugelberg, *Electroencephalogr. Clin. Neurophysiol.* **5**, 595 (1953).
21. J. E. Miller, *Amer. J. Ophthalmol.* **46**, 183 (1958).
22. K. P. Schaefer, *Pflüger's Arch.* **284**, 31 (1965).
23. P. Pasik and T. Pasik, in *The Oculomotor System*, M. B. Bender, Ed. (Harper and Row, New York, 1964), p. 40.
24. J. Szentágothai, *J. Neurophysiol.* **13**, 395 (1950).
25. R. Lorente de Nó, *Ergeb. Physiol.* **32**, 73 (1931).
26. D. H. Hubel and T. N. Wiesel, *J. Neurophysiol.* **28**, 229 (1965).
27. H. B. Barlow, R. M. Hill, W. R. Levick, *J. Physiol.* **173**, 377 (1964).
28. R. M. Hill, *Nature* **211**, 1407 (1966).
29. J. E. Hyde and R. C. Eason, *J. Neurophysiol.* **22**, 666 (1959).
30. E. C. Crosby and J. W. Henderson, *J. Comp. Neurol.* **88**, 53 (1948).
31. I. H. Wagman, H. P. Krieger, M. B. Bender, *ibid.* **109**, 169 (1958).
32. R. S. Jampel, *Amer. J. Ophthalmol.* **48**, 573 (1959).
33. D. A. Robinson and A. F. Fuchs, in preparation.
34. G. L. Walls, *Vision Res.* **2**, 69 (1962).
35. Supported by PHS research grant AM-05524 from the National Institute of Arthritis and Metabolic Diseases.

Interaction of Cortex and Superior Colliculus in Mediation of Visually Guided Behavior in the Cat

JAMES M. SPRAGUE

Reprinted from *Science*, Sept. 23, 1966, Vol. 153, No. 3743, pp. 1544–1547. Copyright 1966 by the American Association for the Advancement of Science.

Visual fields of the cat can be ascertained and measured rather accurately by means of a simple perimetric test in which animals are trained to fixate and to respond to food stimuli. When tested in this fashion with monocular masks, the horizontal visual field of each eye includes about 130°, that is, the field of the right eye extends from 100° right to 30° left of fixation. The area of binocular overlap so measured (60°) is somewhat reduced from the actual amount by presence of the mask. Field deficits after lesions can be measured with an accuracy of about 10°. After recovery or compensation of a field deficit, bilateral stimulation can demonstrate inattention or neglect of one visual field by preferential response to stimuli in the opposite field. This and other "clinical" behavioral tests for deficits in visually guided behavior (following of moving stimuli, blink to threat, placing, depth perception in jumping and avoidance of obstacles, and choice of food-baited plaques placed on opposite sides of a runway) have been used and are described in detail elsewhere (1).

Deficits in visually guided behavior, measured in these ways, follow unilateral removal of the superior colliculus (1) and of various areas of the occipito-temporal cortex (2). Unilateral colliculectomy which does not invade

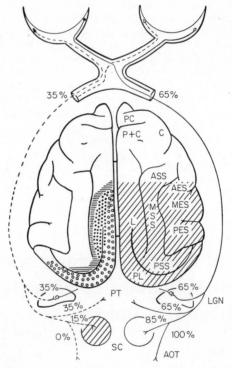

FIGURE 1. Schematic drawing to show the primary visual pathways in the cat. The approximate percentage of crossed and uncrossed fibers, based on estimates from anatomical studies (7), is shown at the level of the optic chiasm, the lateral geniculate nucleus (LGN), pretectum (PT), superior colliculus (SC), and accessory optic system (AOT). Note that the percentages present at the chiasm are maintained at LGN and PT, but not at SC and AOT. Diagonal hatching in the right cortex and left colliculus indicates the crossed lesions described in the text. Symbols plotted on the left cortex show the topography of area 17 (circles), 18 (dots), and 19 (lines), taken from Otsuka and Hassler (8).

the pretectum or the underlying tegmentum results initially in contralateral homonymous hemianopia complete to the vertical meridians, marked ipsiversive circling, and a deficit in contralateral movements of the eyes, although compensation occurs in all of these changes in the succeeding several weeks. Responses to stimuli in the contralateral fields appear gradually, beginning at the middle and extending to about 60° lateral; between 60° and 100° responses are irregular and when present are slow. Simultaneous bilateral stimulation always results in response to the ipsilateral side, even when the contralateral stimulus is larger and has greater movement. Tactile and acoustic deficits also occur in this preparation (*1*).

Alteration in visual behavior after various unilateral cortical lesions in the cat has been thoroughly described (*2*), together with the resulting thalamic degeneration. Removal of the striate cortex (area 17), largely sparing areas 18 and 19 (see Fig. 1), results in only minimal and transient deficits or in no deficit at all. Progressively larger occipito-temporal ablations, which in addition to the striate cortex include areas 18 and 19 and the middle and posterior suprasylvian gyri (with severe atrophy of the dorsal lateral geniculate nucleus), result in deficits which when compensated are similar to those that occur after colliculectomy. Only when the lesion includes all of these areas plus the auditory cortex and temporal fields (that is, extends from the splenial sulcus to or near the rhinal fissure, Fig. 2) is the deficit one of contralateral hemianopia

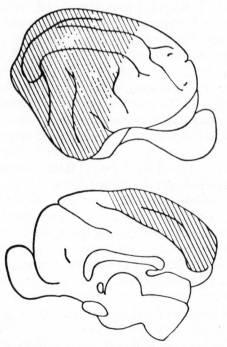

FIGURE 2. Drawings of the lateral and medial aspects of the cat's brain to show the extent of removal of occipito-temporal cortex that results in total hemianopia.

complete to, or within a few degrees ($< 10°$) of, the vertical meridians (*3*). Except for this evidence of macular sparing, the half-field blindness was total and showed no compensation during survival periods up to 1 year in six cats. The importance of completeness of the lesions is shown by other animals, in which sparing of only part of the striate cortex or the middle suprasylvian gyrus resulted in considerable recovery. In contrast, unilateral removal of the frontal cortex resulted in no visual deficits (*2*). Thus, cortex lying outside of the classically defined first (area 17) and second (areas 18 and 19) visual fields make a significant contribution to the mediation of visually guided behavior. This conclusion is in agreement with the conclusions of others who used pattern and intensity discrimination tests (*4*).

From these results it is apparent that visually directed behavior is mediated at both cortical and midbrain sites, and it is the purpose of this report to describe the interaction between these two levels of the brain which can be seen after sequential chronic lesions. Thus, after full compensation and stabilization of deficits following subtotal occipito-temporal cortical lesion, the ipsilateral colliculus was removed, while in other animals the sequence was reversed. When the two lesions were placed on the *same side* of the brain, partial contralateral field deficits, residual after the first lesion, were converted into total hemianopia as a result of the second lesion, regardless of the sequence. This marked potentiation was found when the cortical lesion involved areas 17, 18, and 19 and the middle and posterior suprasylvian gyri, or area 17 alone, and the ensuing total hemianopia showed no further compensation, provided area 17 was completely removed and the colliculus largely destroyed in each case. No potentiation of the collicular deficit was found after removal of the frontal cortex. Thus, despite the obvious contribution of extrastriate cortex in the mediation of visually guided behavior, this cortex is not capable of functional compensation in the absence of area 17 and the superior colliculus.

When cortical and tectal lesions are placed sequentially on *opposite sides* of the brain, the resultant effects do not summate but instead are opposed. This process is dramatically shown by first removing the entire right occipito-temporal cortex from splenial sulcus to rhinal fissure, a lesion that results in total hemianopia of the left fields (Figs. 1 and 2). Despite vigorous training of these animals for extended postoperative periods up to 1 year, no compensation of this deficit was discernible. This deficit represents the end-point in the severity of visual loss caused by a unilateral lesion. After subsequent removal of the left colliculus contralateral to the cortical lesion, marked changes were apparent as soon as animals recovered from anesthesia. Table 1 shows the nature of these changes in one animal (cat 73) with almost complete collicular removal (Fig. 3). Thus visual responses returned to the previously hemianopic left fields (*5*). The initial deficit induced in previously normal right fields by the tectal lesion was expected from previous studies (see *1*) but was less marked than that seen in animals with only tectal lesions.

After compensation the responses to the peripheral fields of both sides

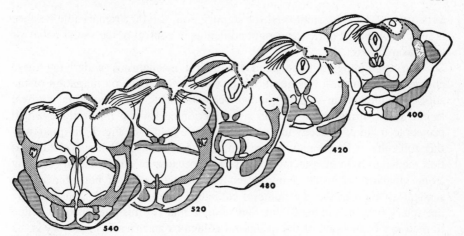

FIGURE 3. Drawings of selected sections to show extent of the lesion in the superior colliculus in cat 73. Area of total destruction enclosed by dashed lines; partial cell and fiber loss indicated by dots.

were similar; they were slower than in the normal cat and were evoked only by moving stimuli. Only those stimuli near the midline evoked brisk responses and only here were responses obtained to stationary objects. This field of maximal acuity lay within the area of binocular overlap and extended somewhat more lateral on the right side (30°) than on the left (10°). Two other cats gave similar results but showed recovery of responses to stimuli in the left visual fields only to 60°; in one of these (cat V8), with histology available, the lesion was limited to the caudal two-thirds of the colliculus with sparing of the lateral part in much of the lesion area (Fig. 4). The neural state of these animals can be understood by reference to Figure 1, in which these two lesions are indicated by diagonal hatching. It will be seen that responses to stimuli in the right visual fields are mediated by the intact left hemisphere, while responses to the left side are mediated by the intact right superior colliculus and possibly other midbrain

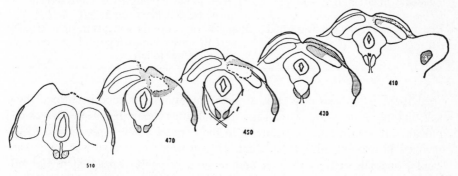

FIGURE 4. Drawings of selected sections to show the extent of the lesion in the superior colliculus in cat V8.

structures. After time is allowed for stabilization, a rather remarkable balance is seen between left cortex and right colliculus in control of the visual behavior as measured here.

In attempting to understand the neural mechanisms underlying these changes, one must ask this question: In view of the active participation of the superior colliculus in visually guided behavior, why, after the initial cortical lesion, is the ipsilateral colliculus not functioning for the hemiretinae which project to it "look" directly into the hemianopic field (see Fig. 1)? Apparently this colliculus is functionally depressed, either because of removal of facilitation mediated by corticotectal fibers (6) or because of an inhibition resulting from imbalance of visual centers after the cortical lesion, or both. Since subsequent ablation of the contralateral colliculus returns visual responses to the previously hemianopic fields, one may assume that (i) this phenomenon is due to recovery of function of the ipsilateral colliculus and (ii) this recovery is the result of removal of an inhibition that emanates from the tectum of the opposite side.

Table 1.

Summary of visual deficits that follow cortical lesion and the changes that occur after subsequent removal of the contralateral superior colliculus.

Deficits after right cortical lesion	*Deficits after subsequent lesion in left superior colliculus*
Total hemianopia left fields	Response to stimuli in left fields (0° to 100°)
Normal right fields (0° to 100°)	Response to stimuli in right fields 0° to 45° initially, improving slowly to 70°, then to 100°
Following only to right	Following only to left initially, slowly appearing on right, but left favored
Blink to lateral threat only on right	Blink to threat initially only on left, slowly appearing on right
Lateral visual placing only on right	Placing initially on left, slowly appearing on right
Tendency to circle right	Marked initial circling to the left, slowly reduced to tendency to circle left
Eye movements and pupils normal	Pupils normal; eye movements to right initially absent, slowly improving to almost normal, slightly better to left

If the hypothesis of a crossed tectal inhibitory influence is correct, then splitting the commissure of the superior colliculus should be as effective as removal of the colliculus contralateral to the cortical lesion. This proved to be the case in two animals. In one (cat V3), in which the lesion was limited to caudal one-half of the collicular commissure, responses appeared to the left visual fields 3 weeks after commissurotomy. Recovery began at the midline (vertical meridian) and by 10 weeks included the full field of 100°; apart from mild pupillary dilatation and sluggishness of response to light, other signs which follow colliculectomy (Table 1) were absent. In the other cat, which was not killed but which had more extensive tectal split that apparently extended into the pretectum (evidenced by maximal pupillary dilatation), recovery of responses to the left were first observed at 6 weeks, again beginning at the vertical meridian, and by 16 weeks had extended to 60°. Delay in the return of vision to the previously hemianopic fields after tectal commissurotomy, in contrast to the immediate recovery after collicular ablation, should be pointed out, although I have no immediate explanation.

The hemianopia that follows unilateral removal of the cortex that mediates visual behavior cannot be explained simply in classical terms of interruption of the visual radiations that serve cortical function. Explanation of this deficit requires a broader point of view, namely, that visual attention and perception are mediated at both forebrain and midbrain levels, which interact in their control of visually guided behavior. Hemianopia caused by cortical lesion is due to an imbalance of these neural centers that subserve vision, resulting in an alteration of function at the midbrain level. Imbalance can be redressed and vision restored to the previously hemianopic field by subsequent lesion in the superior colliculus.

References and Notes

1. J. M. Sprague and T. H. Meikle, Jr., *Exp. Neurol.* **11**, 115 (1965).
2. J. M. Sprague, in *The Thalamus,* D. P. Purpura and M. D. Yahr, Eds. (Columbia Univ. Press, New York, 1966).
3. These observations are probably related to the fact that in the cat the lateral geniculate nucleus projects to cortical fields outside of area 17 [see 2, T. H. Meikle, Jr., and J. M. Sprague, *Int. Rev. Neurobiol.* **6**, 149 (1964), and L. J. Garey, *Nature* **207**, 1410 (1965)].
4. R. E. Myers and R. W. Sperry, *Arch. Neurol. Psychiat.* **80**, 298 (1958); R. W. Sperry, R. E. Myers, A. M. Schrier, *Quart. J. Exp. Psychol.* **12**, 65 (1960); T. Gualtierotti, *Amer. J. Physiol.* **200**, 1215 (1961); P. M. Meyer, *J. Comp. Physiol. Psychol.* **56**, 397 (1963); J. P. Baden, J. C. Urbaitis, T. H. Meikle, Jr., *Exp. Neurol.* **13**, 233 (1965).
5. One animal was prepared with unilateral removal of all cortex, rhinencephalon, and basal ganglia; visual deficits were similar to those shown on the left side of Table 1. After 1 year the contralateral colliculus was completely removed and there followed a delayed (6 weeks) and partial (30°) recovery of responses to the previously hemianopic fields. The cat was killed soon after so that further extension of this field cannot be ruled out.
6. D. Jassik-Gerschenfeld, P. Ascher, J. A. Guevara, *Arch. Ital. Biol.* **104**, 30 (1966).
7. A. M. Laties and J. M. Sprague, *J. Comp. Neurol.,* in press.
8. R. Otsuka and R. Hassler, *Arch. Psychiat. Ztschr. Neurol.* **203**, 212 (1962).
9. Supported in part by research grant NG-05506 from NIH.

Study Questions for Part II

1. Although it can be said that "we are immersed in a sea of stimulation," only a small part of the total stimulus influx ever activates appropriate receiving areas of the brain. Starting at the level of the sensory cell (for example, a group of rods or cones in the eye), see if you can draw a diagram of how stimuli are transduced into a pattern of excitation organized to convey meaning. In drawing this model, be sure to consider the organization of "receptive fields" existing at different levels of the CNS, for example, between the eye and the visual cortex of the brain.

2. Suppose we were able to keep stimulus energy impinging upon a sense organ very constant. How do you think it would be possible to alter the perception of the stimulus without changing any of its physical characteristics (for example, consider the phenomenon of lateral inhibition at the receptor, on-off receptive fields, and so forth)?

Part III

Arousal and Attention

We began this text by studying the cellular and synaptic mechanisms responsible for the generation and conduction of neural information. Next, you read how the organization of excitatory and inhibitory cells into "receptive fields" elaborated the neural code into a more complex, yet more coherent, message. The resulting patterns of neural firing became part of the substrate of activity necessary for organized behavior; but even though the code as initiated at the level of the receptor, and subsequently modified at different levels of the CNS, is critical, this transduction and transmission is not sufficient for conscious experience.

One principle that physiological psychologists agree upon is that the organism must be awake for most forms of organized behavior to take place. For example, contrary to public opinion, experiments have demonstrated that learning while asleep does not occur, thus suggesting that at least a minimum level of arousal is necessary. However, we do not want to imply that conscious experience is a required condition for all forms of information processing in the CNS. To illustrate, it has been shown that people in deep coma have a highly synchronized, slow-wave EEG record, characteristic of dream-free, deep sleep. These people also show almost no EEG or behavioral response to intense physical stimuli. Yet, if the patient's name is whispered into his ear, a desynchronization of the EEG characteristic of arousal can be observed. Another example might be that of a mother who sleeps through the passage of noisy trucks directly beneath her window, yet awakens to the whimpering of her child across the hall.

In the present section we will explore the phenomenon of selective attention and arousal. We know that organisms of all sorts can actively control their response to various stimuli present in the environment. For instance, at a loud cocktail party you can focus in on a particular conversation, phase

127

out of that and in on another, and perhaps even switch in on a third at some other time. You can do this without taking a step in any direction and while even appearing to "pay attention" to the conversation directly in front of you.

Scientists have long been interested in the CNS mechanisms that permit this highly adaptive form of behavior: that of filtering out redundant or uninteresting input or conversely amplifying important or novel sensory stimulation. The brain mechanisms that permit this behavior are also intimately involved in controlling sleep and wakefulness as well as shaping the character of our perceptual world.

As we began to learn more about how the brain works, it soon became evident that any model of brain function based upon the notion of simple input-output relationships would be unable to account for the complexity of CNS organization underlying selective response. Areas of the brain were found to do more than serve as passive receptacles of sensory input. Instead, specialized aggregates of nerves were shown to exert significant efferent or *centrifugal* control over incoming messages. Thus, the "message" is more than just the sum of activity in sensory receptors. The final message or "code" that eventually reaches the classical sensory receiving areas of the cortex (e.g., visual, auditory) is very different from the activity generated by stimuli impinging upon the sensory receptor. Indeed, these so-called "centrifugal systems" can actually modify activity in the receptor cells as well as at higher levels of the sensory pathways. Another way of stating it is that the brain can control its own level of arousal and activity and *select* which aspect of the total stimulus environment it will respond to at any given moment.

In order for the organism to selectively attend to certain information, the CNS must be capable of monitoring all incoming messages prior to their registration in consciousness. A model for this activity is detailed in the article by Deutsch and Deutsch. Briefly, the authors assume that a level of excitation or arousal is established by the sensory cortex. The level of arousal serves to "tune" the brainstem and thalamic reticular formation, which then filters out subsequent input whose "excitation value" is lower than the level established by the system. In this manner, the state of the organism at a particular moment, as reflected in the ongoing activity of the CNS, provides a context against which neuronal information is compared and assessed.

An important component of attention is the process of habituation. Habituation often refers to the selective degradation of incoming information by the CNS. As such, the mechanism involved in this process may play a crucial role in the organism's ability to shift his attention from one source of stimulation to another. The next three papers investigate several different, but interrelated, components of habituation. The article by Scheibel and Scheibel is of particular interest (for two reasons). First, the authors provide evidence that suggests that habituation *cannot* be accounted for simply in terms of inhibitory mechanisms. Instead, they suggest that we must look at the interplay of both facilitatory and inhibitory units within the reticular formation. Second, they maintain that this interplay is dependent upon the integrated activity of several different levels within the CNS (e.g., cortical, thalamic, and brainstem activity).

The next article, by Hernández-Peón, details another role of the brainstem reticular formation (RF) in the process of habituation. In this paper, the author argues that not only is the RF capable of attenuating information at the level of the brainstem, but through a system of centrifugal nerve fibers, it can inhibit input at the peripheral sensory synapses as well. Such a system is important to our understanding of how "higher-order" structures modify activity in peripheral, "lower-order" components of the brain.

The article by Glaser and Griffin rounds out our presentation of the structural mechanisms involved in habituation by demonstrating that the role of the frontal cortex is to maintain selective suppression of input rather than to initiate the process of habituation.

The counterpart of habituation is information amplification. The article by Hubel et al. describes the activity of some highly specialized cells in the auditory cortex. These cells respond only when the organism appears to be "paying attention" to a particular sound. It has been argued (see article by Deutsch and Deutsch) that this selective amplification of discrete input may be, in part, responsible for the animal's ability to make an appropriate motor response to incoming information.

The articles on arousal, attention, and habituation deal primarily with the integration and elaboration of information during states of consciousness and provide us with an understanding of the minimum conditions necessary for organizing conscious activity. If we consider attention and its concomitants as a higher form of CNS activity, how then can we characterize sleep? For many years, sleep was considered to be a passive process resulting from a diminution or decrease in sensory inputs to the brain. More recent research, however, has demonstrated that, in fact, sleep may very well involve active excitation and/or inhibition in specific areas of the CNS. The work of Jouvet provides us with an excellent example of research and theory on the physiological substrates of sleep.

In his experiments, Jouvet combines neurophysiology, neuroanatomy, and neurochemistry in an attempt to specify the mechanisms and areas of the brain controlling sleeping and waking. He discusses the specific interaction between serotonin and noradrenaline in brainstem areas and shows that alternations in the levels of these transmitters by lesioning or drug manipulation markedly affect the sleep-wake cycle.

The preceding articles in this section emphasized the critical role of the RF in the maintenance of arousal and attention. However, as you shall see, the results reported in the paper by Adametz cast considerable doubt on the validity of this assumption. The article speaks for itself, and no more need be said about it here.

Thus far, we have considered only anatomically defined constituents of the attentional system. However, it has long been recognized that arousal mechanisms must be susceptible to the influence of hormones such as adrenalin and other biochemical agents. The last article, by Purpura, presents a strong argument for a detailed analysis of the problem of attention at a biochemical level. By joining the circulatory systems of two animals, Purpura demonstrated that stimulation of one animal leads to the elicitation of appropriate physiological components of arousal in the recipient.

Some Monoaminergic Mechanisms Controlling Sleep and Waking

M. JOUVET

Reprinted from *Brain and Human Behavior*. Ed. by A. G. Karczmar and J. C. Eccles.
© by Springer-Verlag, Berlin, Heidelberg, 1972. Printed in Germany.

The nervous system is a super-organization comprising many sub-systems. This truism should be kept in mind when studying sleep mechanisms. The fact that rather limited, specific brain stem lesions are able to suppress either sleep or waking is a good reason to believe that certain systems are specialized to control the sleep-waking rhythm. This is a more promising approach to the problem of sleep-waking mechanisms than that which presupposes that every neuron possess a "built in" waking-sleep rhythm similar to the mysterious periodical firing shown by isolated neurons of Aplysia (Strumwasser, 1965).

The approach to the mechanisms of sleep and waking has recently been helped by the development of new techniques. Indeed, it is rather fortunate that at the time during which lesion and transection experiments were defining the neural structures responsible for sleep and waking within the intricate network of the reticular formation, a new map of the brain, in bright color, became available to neurophysiologists thanks to histochemistry and histofluorescent techniques. This colored map appears to be painted by a modern painter, by a Dufy. The color sometimes overflows the sharp boundaries of classical nuclei of the brain stem as delimitated by Nissl stain. Thanks to this map, the "unspecific" systems of the reticular formation are beginning to acquire some biochemical specificity. It is also fortunate that, at about the same time, progresses in neuropharmacology and biochemistry have permitted us to explore more and more specifically those new systems which are unveiled by histochemistry.

In this paper I will summarize the neurophysiological, neuropharmacological and biochemical evidences which have led to the hypothesis that sleep and waking are controlled by two antagonistic systems: the serotonin-containing neurons of the Raphé system which controls sleep, and the catecholamine-containing neurons of the ponto-mesencephalic reticular formation which controls waking.

I. Serotonin and Sleep

A. Neurophysiological Evidences for the Presence of Hypnogenic Structures in the Lower Brain Stem

It should first be recalled that sleep is no longer considered as a unique phenomenon opposed to waking. On the contrary, in birds and mammals, behavioral sleep is the result of the succession of two different states, slow wave sleep (SWS), and paradoxical sleep (PS) or rapid eye movement or REM sleep, respectively. These two states appear quite regularly and can be quantitatively measured. In brief, a cat spends about 50% of its time sleeping; 75% of this consists of SWS, and 25% of PS occurring in phases of 6 minutes' duration separated by intervals of about 25 minutes (Fig. 1).

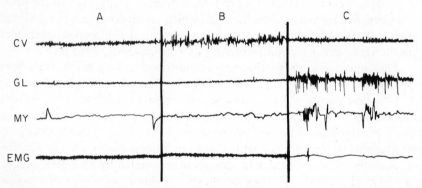

FIGURE 1. Main polygraphic characteristics of waking (A), slow-wave sleep (B), and paradoxical sleep (C) in the cat. The fast cortical activity (occipital cortex, CV) and total abolition of the neck muscle activity (EMG) constitutes the tonic components of PS whereas discharges of ponto geniculo occipital spikes (PGO) which are recorded in the lateral geniculate (GL) and rapid eye movements (MY) compose the phasic components. PGO spikes may be triggered independently of PS by a large variety of drugs (cf. Table 1), whereas the inhibition of muscle tone during PS may be suppressed by a limited lesion of the dorso lateral pontine tegmentum. Calibration: 6 sec and 50 microvolts.

The neural mechanisms which are responsible for the induction of both SWS and PS are mainly, if not exclusively, located in the lower brain stem. This can be illustrated by two experiments (Fig. 2):

1. A total intercollicular transection of the brain stem (cerveau isolé) (Bremer, 1936) is followed by a synchronized cortical activity analogous to SWS. This is explained by the fact that this transection, situated in front of the mesencephalic reticular formation prevents the activating influences from the waking structures to reach the cortex. However, a section situated immediately caudal to the ponto-mesencephalic border (medio pontine pretrigeminal preparation) is followed on the contrary by a significant increase in EEG arousal (Batini et al., 1959). The probable explanation of these facts is that the medio-

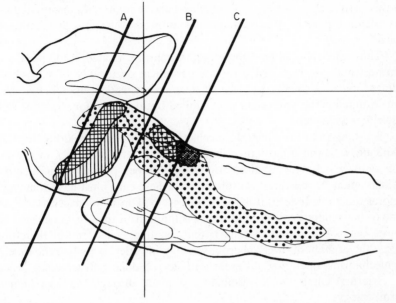

FIGURE 2. Upon a sagittal section of the brain stem (the vertical line represents the frontal plane zero, the horizontal lines represent the horizontal planes HC 0 and HC −10) are projected schematically the serotonin-containing neurons of the Raphé system (in dots) which appeared to be responsible for sleep. The norepinephrine-containing neurons are represented by crossed lines. Those which are responsible for cortical desynchronization (anterior part of group A 6) in the pontine tegmentum and the group of neurons of the mesencephalic tegmentum are represented by lighter crosses than the caudal part of the locus coeruleus, the destruction of which suppresses the muscular inhibition during PS. Vertical hatching indicates the projection of the dopamine-containing neurons of the substantia nigra. Line A represents the intercollicular transection of the brain (cerveau isolé) which totally suppresses cortical activation. Line B represents the most caudal brain stem transection (rostro pontine transection) which increases cortical synchronization. This section is just in front of the group of norepinephrine-containing neurons of the pons. The rostro pontine transection is also the most caudal transection which still permits the periodical appearance of PS (in the pontile cat). Line C represents the medio pontine transection which increases cortical desynchronization. This transection is just caudal to the activating neurons and suppresses serotonergic influences from the caudal Raphé system. The lesion of the Raphé system caudal to transection C induces an insomnia similar to that induced by the medio pontine transection. The lines indicating the transection are idealized. Usually, a transection would destroy the brain on a width of 1–1.5 mm.

pontine transection suppresses ascending deactivating or hypnogenic influences originating in the lower brain stem, caudal to the transection. Thus, somewhere in the lower brain stem (caudal pons and/or medulla) there should be some neurons which are responsible for synchronizing the EEG and possibly for inducing SWS.

2. The existence of structures responsible for PS in the lower brain stem are solidly established: a chronic pontile cat (the entire brain of which in front of the pons has been removed) still shows clearly the periodical behavioral and

central manifestations of PS. On the other hand, a limited lesion situated in the dorso lateral part of the pontile tegmentum may selectively suppress PS (Jouvet, 1962).

Thus, there should be some group of neurons located in the pontine tegmentum which are responsible for the periodical occurrence of PS. All these findings indicate also that the states of sleep are dependent upon *active* mechanisms situated in the brain stem since limited brain stem lesions are able to suppress either SWS or PS.

Thus, in order to explain the mechanisms of both SWS and PS, one should deliminate with the utmost precision the groups of cell bodies in the lower brain stem, which actively and periodically dampen directly or indirectly the waking system. Moreover, it is probable that these cells must have some neurohumoral function. Indeed, it is impossible to explain many aspects of sleep in terms of the synaptic millisecond which is the unit of time of the electrophysiologists but is not a unit of time potentials. It appears fruitful therefore to explore the domain of "wet" neurophysiology in order to analyse the biochemical mechanisms operating at the level of sleep inducing structures.

The first entry into this domain was made through the door of neuropharmacology.

B. Neuropharmacological Analysis of the Role of Serotonin in Sleep: from Possibility to Strong Probability

Many factors have made difficult the study of the role of serotonin in sleep mechanisms.

Serotonin does not cross the blood-brain barrier in mature mammals. On the other hand, it is not sure at all that 5-hydroxytryptophan (5HTP), the immediate precursor of serotonin, which readily crosses the blood-brain barrier, is decarboxylated only in the serotoninergic neurons. Finally, when one desires to affect the metabolism of serotonin, the numerous drugs such as the inhibitors of monoamine oxidase, reserpine, etc. which act upon the catabolism of serotonin or its liberation, also act upon catecholamines.

These three limitations are, however, counterbalanced by a recently arisen opportunity due to the development of a "specific" * inhibitor of the first step of the synthesis of serotonin.

Mandell and Spooner (1968) humorously referred to the experiments which were the first to draw attention to the possible entry of serotonin among the possible candidates for the role of sleep "neuromodulator," as "monoamine game."

Early, this "game" involved "tricks" concerning the blood-brain barrier. In chicks, whose blood-brain barrier is permeable, the injection of serotonin was able to induce sleep-like behavior and cerebral synchronization (Spooner

---

* I define the "specific inhibitor" with regard to the short 2–3 years' period during which it is shown that a drug acts "only" upon a specific enzyme, until new experiments demonstrate that it is not the case.

and Winters, 1967). Koella and his coworkers (1966) have also made numerous attempts to by-pass the blood-brain barrier in mammals: by local applications of serotonin at the level of the area postrema or by means of its intraventricular administration they could induce behavioral and EEG signs of SWS, or augmentation of the recruiting response in the cat.

Another indirect approach was employed subsequently when long-term quantitative recording of sleep became available routinely. This approach made it evident that most of the drugs which act upon brain monoamines also interfere with sleep.

1. Producing a decrease in serotonin and catecholamines, reserpine (0.5 mg/kg in the cat) suppressed SWS for 6–8 hours and PS for one day. A subsequent injection of 5HTP, which is believed to restore a normal level of brain serotonin, resulted in the immediate reappearance of SWS, whereas the injection of DOPA following reserpine led to an earlier reappearance of PS. This indicated that serotonin may be involved in SWS whereas PS may necessitate catecholaminergic mechanisms (Matsumoto and Jouvet, 1964).

2. Monoamine oxidase (MAO) inhibitors which act upon both brain monoamines by inhibiting their catabolism and by thus increasing their level in the brain were shown to act dramatically upon sleep states. Most of MAO inhibitors utilized (nialamid, pheniprazine) have a very selective and long-lasting suppressive effect upon PS in the cat without interfering with SWS. This suppressive effect is so intense that it is even obtained when the "need" for PS is greatly enhanced following the deprivation of the latter (Jouvet, 1967). This result suggested that MAO could be involved in the transition from SWS to PS. However, these facts had only a limited significance in view of the complexity of the biochemical mechanisms of the brain; indeed, most of these drugs could act upon both indolamines and catecholamines.

3. More recently, some drugs decreasing selectively brain serotonin levels have been discovered. P-Chloromethamphetamine (PSMA) was the first drug known to deplete brain serotonin and its metabolite 5-hydroxyindol acetic acid (5HIAA) without altering catecholamines level. Its mechanisms of action are still unknown but it is probable that it does not act through inhibition of serotonin synthesis (Pletscher et. al., 1963). This drug (20 mg/kg) induced in the cat a very marked arousal which resembled that induced by amphetamine and included agitation and mydriasis. This arousal lasted 16–20 hours and was followed by a gradual recovery of both SWS and PS and by an almost continuous discharge of PGO spikes (Delorme et al., 1966). We have not been able to counteract the arousal due to PCMA by either high 50 mg/kg or low dose of 5-HTP (10 mg/kg). In fact, this precursor of serotonin has caused, under these circumstances, the death in four cats through a still unknown mechanism.

Fortunately, another drug has recently made possible the study of serotonin metabolism in the brain in a manner compatible with the physiological condition of the animal. It has been shown that p-chlorophenylalanine (PCPA) decreases the level of serotonin in the rat's brain without altering the level of catecholamines (Koe and Weismann, 1966). The following experiment demonstrates that PCPA inhibits the synthesis of brain serotonin by interfering with anabolism of the latter at the level of tryptophan-hydroxylase in the cat (Pujol et al., 1969). As shown in Figure 3, slices of cat cerebral cortex or brain

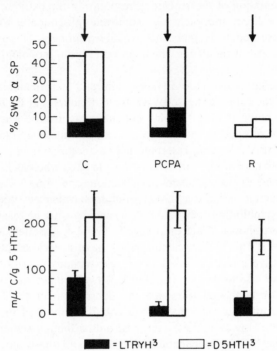

FIGURE 3. In the upper part of the figure, the effect of the injection, i.p., of 5 mg/kg of 5HTP upon sleep. The left hand column represents the percentage of SWS (white) and of PS (black) during the six hours which precede the injection of 5 mg/kg of 5HTP. The right hand column indicates the percentage of SWS and PS during the 6 hours which follow the injection, in normal control (C) cats (mean of 4 experiments), in cats having received 400–500 mg/kg of PCPA 30 to 50 hours previously (mean of 5 experiments), and in cats, the Raphé system of which has been subtotally destroyed (R mean of 16 experiments). It is evident that 5HTP has a significant hypnogenic effect only in PCPA-treated cats. In the lower part of the figure, biosynthesis of $5HT^{H3}$ in slices of cerebral cortex incubated either in $TRYH^3$ (black) or in $DL5HTP^{H3}$ in Krebs Ringer solution. Abscissae: amount of $5HT^{H3}$ (mean and SEM) expressed in mμ curie/g in the 6 normal control cats (C), in four cats pretreated 40 hours previously with 400–500 mg/kg of PCPA or in four cats the Raphé system of which was destroyed subtotally 7 to 9 days before. See text for further explanation. (*From Pujol et al., 1969.*)

stem were incubated for 30 minutes in vitro in Krebs-Ringer solution containing ^{3}H-tryptophan and D L ^{3}H-5HTP, and the amount of ^{3}H-5HT was measured subsequently. There was an 80% decrease of ^{3}H-5HT synthetized from ^{3}H-tryptophan (as compared with control animal) in cats pretreated with 500 mg/kg of PCPA forty hours before. On the other hand, the synthesis of ^{3}H-5HT from ^{3}H-5HTP was normal.

The action of PCPA upon the sleep states of the cat, rat and monkey has been extensively studied (Delorme et al., 1966; Mouret et al., 1968; Koella et al., 1968; Weitzman et al., 1968). After a single injection of 400 mg/kg of PCPA in the cat, no apparent effect on behaviour or on the EEG was observed during the first 24 hours. This fact demonstrates that the drug in itself has no direct pharmacological action upon the brain. Following this period, an abrupt decrease of both states of sleep occurred and after about 30–40 hours an almost total insomnia appeared as shown by a stable, unexcited waking behaviour, mild mydriasis, and an almost continuous low-voltage, fast cortical activity. The recovery of sleep began after the 40th hour and was accompanied by the appearance of permanent phasic waves in the lateral geniculate body and occipital cortex (similar to the phasic PGO activity which is observed in the lateral geniculate during SWS immediately preceding PS, or during PS). Very discrete episodes of PS may appear, either following short episodes of SWS or even directly following waking. SWS episodes of longer duration gradually reappeared at shorter intervals. Normal qualitative and quantitative patterns of sleep were resumed after about 200 hours.

With the administration of PCPA, a significant correlation has been found to exist between the diminution of the frequency of SWS (Fig. 4) and the

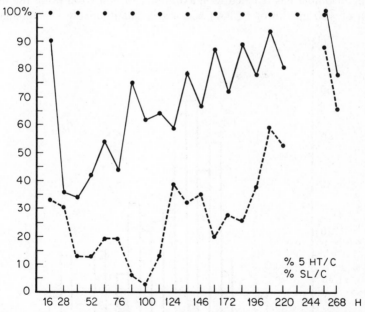

FIGURE 4. Effects of p-chlorophenylalanine on sleep and telen-diencephalon concentrations of serotonin in the rat. After intraperitoneal injection of PCPA (500 mg/kg), there is a decrease in the amount of slow-wave sleep (SWS) and in serotonin (5HT) concentration, followed by a slow return to normal values after 268 hours. *Solid line*: Percentage of slow-wave relative to the amount for a control rat; each point represents the mean percentage per 12-hour period (black dots at top indicate night hours, 7 P.M. to 7 A.M.). *Dashed line*: Percentage of serotonin (relative to the concentration for a control rat); for the purpose of this analysis, two animals were killed every 12 hours. There was no significant alteration of either noradrenaline or dopamine. (*From Mouret et al., 1968.*)

decrease of cerebral serotonin in the rat whereas there was no significant alteration of catecholamine level. Koella et al. (1968) have also observed the same
correlation in the cat brain.

It is evident, by looking carefully at the two curves obtained in the rat
or in the cat that this correlation is not absolute; return to normal sleep levels
usually occurred before endogenous serotonin levels approached control values,
and there was no explanation for the small transient relative increase of brain
serotonin on the 4th or 5th days without concomitant temporary increase of
sleep. It is probable that the determination of 5HIAA and of the turnover of
serotonin after injection of PCPA should give much more fruitful data since
very little is known at the present time about possible storage and functional
pool of serotonin at the level of terminals of serotonin-containing neurons.

Since PCPA inhibits only the first step of the synthesis of serotonin at the
level of tryptophan hydroxylase, it is possible to by-pass its blocking action and
thus reestablish higher levels of serotonin by injecting 5HTP (which readily
crosses the blood-brain barrier); this procedure was employed to manipulate
the state of sleep of the animal following the administration of PCPA. A single
injection (I.V. or I.P.) of a very small dose of 5HTP (2–5 mg/kg) performed
when the insomnia has reached its maximum (30 hours following the administration of 400 mg/kg of PCPA) restored a quantitatively and qualitatively

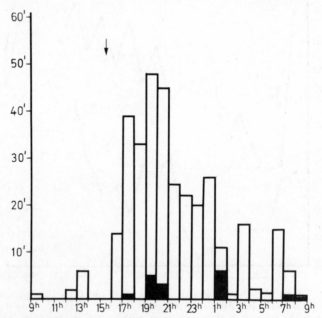

FIGURE 5. Hypogenic effect of 5HTP in PCPA-treated cats. Ordinates: time (in
minutes) spent either in SWS (white) or PS (black) every hour. Abscissae: time in hours.
On the left, insomnia 36 hours after the injection of 400 mg/kg of PCPA. The arrow
signals the injection (IV) of 5 mg/kg of DL5HTP. There is a return to normal amount
of SWS and PS for 7 hours.

normal pattern of both states of sleep during 6–8 hours (Fig. 5). Interestingly enough, when a larger dose of 5HTP (30–50 mg/kg) was injected, only SWS reappeared during the first hours and PS was delayed for 4–5 hours. This suggests that after the inhibition of tryptophan hydroxylase, in the absence of endogenous substrate, the serotonin-containing neurons are able to synthetize very quickly serotonin from a small amount of exogenous 5HTP, whereas it appears that larger quantities of exogenous 5HTP interfere at some other site with the normal process of PS.

Other experiments have shown that whereas a cat receiving multiple dose of 150–200 mg/kg PCPA each day for one week exhibits a severe and long-lasting insomnia, an animal receiving balanced daily doses of 5HTP with the same amount of PCPA may show normal or even increased states of sleep during several days. These experiments show rather conclusively that sleep mechanisms can be manipulated at will by interfering "only" with the synthesis of serotonin at least for one week (Jouvet, 1969).

These results which are in agreement with the previous finding that 5HTP is able to restore SWS when injected after reserpine led to the hypothesis that SWS requires the presence of serotonin at the terminals of serotonin-containing neurons. In view of the pharmacological data demonstrating that PS is selectively eliminated for a long period of time by MAO inhibitors, it is suggested that a deaminated metabolite of serotonin may be responsible for the triggering of PS. Among those deaminated metabolites, 5-hydroxy-indolacetaldehyde could possibly be involved since it has been shown that this product may have some central hypnogenic effect in the chick (Sabelli et al., 1969).

However, these neuropharmacological results, alone, cannot be accepted as a conclusive evidence for the decisive role of serotonin in the triggering of sleep. It must be admitted that PCPA alters not only brain serotonin but also the serotonin level in the total body. It is therefore very difficult to eliminate a possible peripheral factor in the very significant decrease of sleep which follows PCPA.

Thus, only a method permitting the selective decrease of brain serotonin should give unequivocal results. In the absence of such a method it is fortunate that it is now possible, with the help of histochemical and histofluorescence techniques to map out monoaminergic neurons and thus to reconcile the neurophysiological results which show that the neurons located in the lower brain stem are responsible for sleep with biochemical and neuropharmacological data which demonstrate that serotonin is involved in sleep.

C. Histochemical Anatomy of the Brain Stem
Monoamines-Containing Neurons in the Cat

1. MONOAMINE OXIDASE.   With the histochemical method of Glenner, MAO could be localized in some restricted regions of the cat's brain stem, particularly in the dorso lateral part of the pontine tegmentum (nucleus locus

coeruleus and subcoeruleus, and nuclei parabrachialis medialis and lateralis (Figure 8).

2. MONOAMINE-CONTAINING NEURONS.   The existence of regional brain differences in the distribution of catecholamines and serotonin suggested the relation of this distribution to some neuroanatomical organization. This hypothesis was confirmed later when it was demonstrated that limited lesion of the medial forebrain bundle could decrease serotonin in the telencephalon (Heller et al., 1962). However, the great advance in our knowledge of the topography of monoamine-containing neurons comes from the work of Hillarp

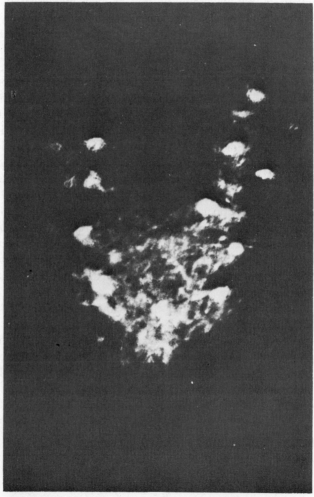

FIGURE 6. Nucleus Raphé obscurus in the cat, Histofluorescent technique of Falk. (*From Jones, 1969.*)

and Falk (cf. Falk et al., 1962) and Dahlstrom and Fuxe (1964). By using histofluorescent techniques, these authors could map out precisely the location of nerve cells containing monoamines in the rat. The serotonin-containing cell bodies, which showing bright yellow fluorescence, were located mostly in the Raphé system, from the nucleus Raphé abscurus in the caudal part of the medulla (Fig. 6) to the nucleus Raphé linearis at the junction between the pons and the mesencephalon. These neurons have about the same distribution in the cat (Pin et al., 1968) as shown in Figure 7. However, several discrete yet important differences between the rat and the cat were observed. Not present in the rat, serotonin-containing cells were seen in the case of the cat in the nuclei of the IV and III nerve, in Edinger-Westphal nucleus and in the magno cellularis part of the red nucleus.

In the pons of the cat, the catecholamine-containing neurons were located mostly in the dorso lateral part of the pontine tegmentum regions of the n. locus coeruleus, subcoeruleus, parabrachialis medialis and lateralis and were very closely related with the localization of MAO.

In the cat's mesencephalon, green fluorescent cells containing catecholamines, surrounded by diffuse fibers, were observed in the mesencephalic reticular formation; these cells probably correspond to those of the group A 8 in the rat. The origin of this group of cells was found in the griseum centralis of the mesencephalon; in the cat, these cells could be clearly traced as descending in reticular formation to beneath the red nucleus. Corresponding to the group A 9 cells of the rat, large green fluorescent cells were contained in the zona compacta of the substantia nigra and in the medial lemniscus. Finally, catecholamine type cells were observed in the region dorsal to and surrounding the nucleus interpeduncularis similar to the cells of the group A 10 in the rat. These three groups of cells in the mesencephalon were found to merge with one another in the brain stem of the cat.

The cell bodies of the serotonin- and norepinephrine-containing neurons were shown to send terminals into widespread regions of the brain and spinal cord (Dahlstrom and Fuxe, 1964). Moreover, it was shown that the sectioning of the axon would suppress specific fluorescence of the corresponding terminals after a delay of about 8–10 days. This finding permitted to attack specific groups of monoamine-containing neurons by stereotaxically-oriented coagulation, and to correlate such a destruction with biochemical analysis allowing a certain amount of time between destruction of the nerve cells and the sacrifice of the animal. Fortunately for the neurophysiologist, the localization of serotonin-containing cell bodies as a concentrated group in the Raphé system makes possible their destruction by stereotaxic techniques. Since the biochemical results of this procedure could be analyzed quantitatively, as the topographical methods could give an arbitrary measurement of the extent of the lesion of the nerve cells, and since quantitative determination of sleep states was available through polygraphic recordings, it was possible to investigate a possible correlation between these three variables.

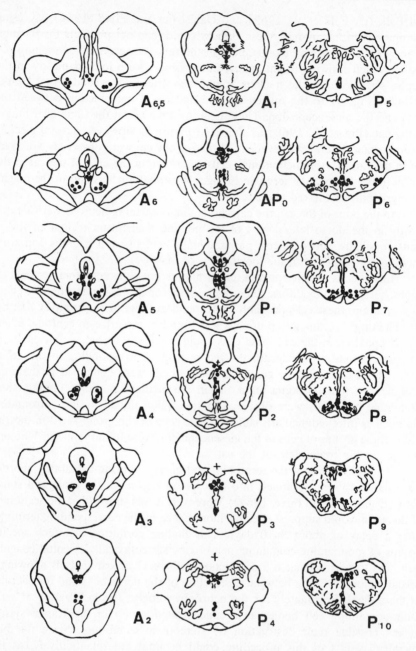

A

FIGURE 7. A. Topography of serotonin-containing cell bodies (dots) in the brain stem of the cat. Frontal section according to Horsley-Clark coordinates. B. Topography of catecholamine-containing cell bodies in the pons and mesencephalon of the cat. The nebular-like formation of the mesencephalic tegmentum is represented in black. (*From Pin et al.*, 1968.)

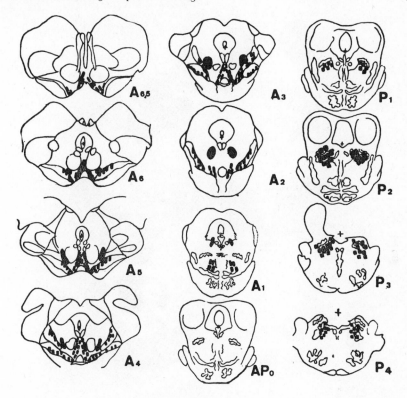

B

D. Selective Decrease of Brain Serotonin
and Insomnia after Destruction of the Raphé System

The destruction of the serotonin-containing neurons of the Raphé system was performed stereotaxically in chronically implanted cats. Following the operation, the animals were continuously (22 hours a day) recorded for a period of 10–13 days, this being the critical duration for the voiding of the serotonergic terminals. On the 13th day, the cats were sacrificed always at the same hour (11 a.m.) in order to avoid possible circadian variation, and the histological evaluation of the lesioned area of the brain stem and the bio-chemical analysis of the intact regions of the brain (telencephalon-diencephalon) were carried out. A valid quantification of the sleep states was obtained in terms of the percentages of SWS and PS in the course of 10–13 days of recording. Moreover, the volume of the lesion was measured by means of the topograph-ical analysis and represented as the percentage of Raphé system destroyed; finally the monoamine levels of the brain were measured and expressed as the percentages of the control levels of serotonin and norepinephrine in normal cats sacrificed under the same conditions (Jouvet, 1968–1969, cf. Fig. 8).

Following a subtotal (80–90%) coagulation of the Raphé system, a state

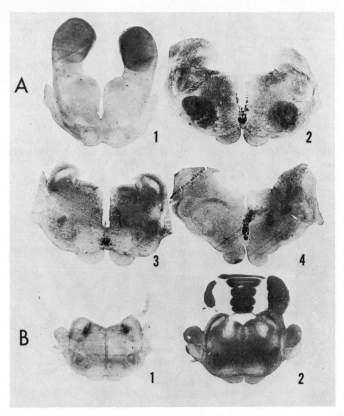

FIGURE 8. A. Subtotal lesion of the Raphé system in the cat. Rostral section at the level of (1) the Raphé centralis superior and dorsalis nuclei, (2) the Raphé pontis, and (3 and 4) the Raphé magnus and pallidus. B. Rostral sections of the pons: (1) Glenner stain shows the monoamine oxidase (dark areas) in the nucleus locus coeruleus, (2) bilateral destruction of the nucleus locus coeruleus which selectively suppresses the muscular inhibition during paradoxical sleep.

of permanent insomnia was observed during the first 3–4 days (Fig. 9): the animals exhibited continuous running movements and a marked mydriasis; they reacted immediately to a moving stimulus with vertical eye movements, as the lateral eye movements are suppressed by the midline lesion. Their cortical activity was permanently fast and exhibited the well-known pattern of the arousal reaction. In the period followed, the percentage of SWS did not exceed 10% of the recording time. In these preparations, PS was never observed. Continuous discharges of pontogeniculate (PGO) spikes in the lateral geniculate or occipital cortex appeared immediately after the destruction of the Raphé, at a rate of 30–40/min. The pattern of discharge was similar to the one which follows injection of reserpine in the normal cat. The rate of discharge of PGO spikes diminished on the 3rd day to 10/min. Partial lesions of the Raphé system (rostral or caudal regions) resulted in an insomnia which was less pronounced particularly due to a gradual recuperation of sleep after

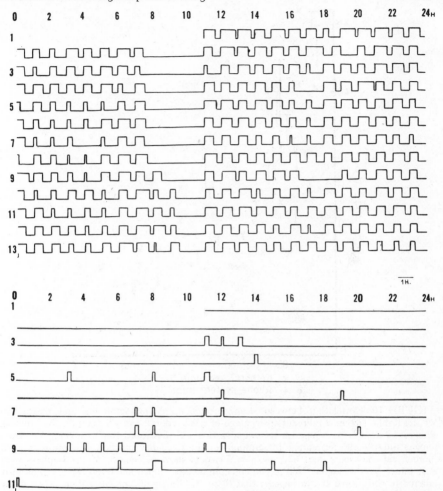

FIGURE 9. Upper part of the figure: sham operated cat recorded during 13 days. The amount of sleep (white rectangular) is 57% of the recording. Lower part of the figure: insomnia following a subtotal destruction of the Raphé system [percentage of total sleep (SWS) during 11 days: 3.5%]. Ordinates: sleep; abscissae: time in hours. Each horizontal line represents one day of recording.

the first two days. In these preparations, PS was found to occur in correlation with the daily percentage of SWS: PS was present only when the SWS frequency surpassed 15%, otherwise the PS was totally absent. Destruction involving less than 15% of the Raphé system at any level did not provoke a significant change in the states of sleep. The biochemical analysis of the insomniac preparations revealed a significant decrease in cerebral serotonin and 5HIAA with no variation in catecholamines in the telencephalon and diencephalon. It was therefore demonstrated that a significant correlation exists between the amount of destruction of the Raphé system, the intensity of the resulting insomnia, and the selective decrease of cerebral serotonin (Fig. 10).

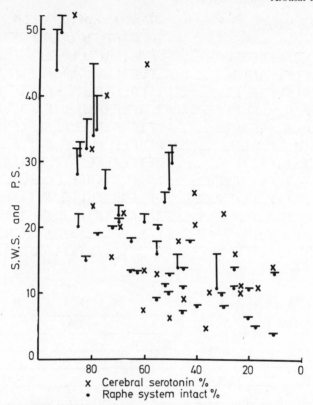

FIGURE 10. Correlation between sleep, telen-diencephalon serotonin, and destruction of the Raphé system. Ordinates: percentage of SWS (dots) and PS (vertical line) during the 10–13 days of postoperative recording in cats with destroyed Raphé system. Abscissae: crosses indicate the percentage of serotonin in the telen-diencephalon (as compared with normal cat—normal value: 622 mg/g $\pm$ 22); dots show percentage of the Raphé system left intact by the lesion. Neither norepinephrine nor dopamine levels were significantly altered in those cats. It can be seen that there exists a significant correlation between the extent of the destruction of the Raphé system, the decrease of telen-diencephalic serotonin, and the decrease of sleep. PS usually does not appear if SWS levels are less than 15% of the recording time.

EFFECTS OF 5HTP AND BIOSYNTHESIS OF SEROTONIN IN CATS FOLLOWING THE DESTRUCTION OF THE RAPHÉ SYSTEM.   In view of the results obtained with PCPA-treated cats, we have investigated both the effects of 5HTP and the biosynthesis of serotonin in Raphé-destroyed cats in which the Raphé system was destroyed (Pujol et al., 1969, see Fig. 3).

The I.P. injection of 5 mg/kg of 5HTP did not significantly alter the continuous arousal which follows subtotal destruction of the Raphé system, whereas it almost immediately restored both SWS and PS when injected during the total insomnia following PCPA. On the contrary, a larger dose of 50 mg/kg of 5HTP induces a synchronized cortical activity which was usually accompanied by a waking behaviour. No PS occurred.

The serotonin synthesis in slices of the cerebral cortex and of the brain stem was studied in vitro in cats, whose Raphé systems were subtotally destroyed ten days before. There was a significant decrease in [H3]serotonin synthetized in vitro from [H3]tryptophan; this may be explained as due to the decrease in tryptophan hydroxylase at the level of terminals ten days after the destruction of the cell bodies. This decrease was well correlated with the decrease in endogenous 5HT.

On the contrary there was no significant decrease in [H3]serotonin synthetized in vitro from [H3]5HTP. This can probably be explained by the fact that 5HTP can be decarboxylated at the level of non-serotoninergic neurons, presumably catecholaminergic, where the nonspecific DOPA decarboxylase is located.

This finding is in accordance with other experiments which show that only tryptophan is the physiological precursor of serotonin in the brain (Moir and Eccleston, 1968). Apparently exogenous 5HTP given at very low doses is able to be decarboxylated preferentially in serotonin-containing neurons only when the endogenous serotonin is lacking (as after PCPA). It is thus possible that high doses of 5HTP (50 mg per kg) (which are usually given in most experiments) do not really induce a specific, physiological state due either to exogenous 5HTP itself or to the presence of serotonin in other, non-serotoninergic monoamine-containing neurons.

Discussion

Although the insomnia obtained by destruction of the Raphé system in the cat or in the rat (Kostowski et al., 1968) resembles closely the insomnia induced by the inhibition of the serotonin synthesis, thus providing a very convincing argument for the role of serotonin in sleep, much work remains to be done in order to understand the mechanisms of action of serotonin and of the organization of the sleep system.

First, it is evident that coagulation is a rather crude technique to bring about the destruction of the serotonin-containing neurons, and it is certain that other adjacent midline neurons are also destroyed together with ascending and descending crossing pathways. The fact that a moderate insomnia (18–20% of SWS and 3% of PS, Michel and Roffwarg, 1967; Mancia, 1969) can be obtained by a sagittal split of the pontine tegmentum (which also inevitably destroys the pontine Raphé system) has recently been taken as an evidence that insomnia could be caused by the interruption of hypothetical crossing ascending pathways coming from bilateral sleep-inducing structures which could be located more laterally in the lower brain stem (Mancia, 1969) although in earlier experiments those hypothetical sleep centers were shown to send ipsilateral uncrossed ascending pathways as indicated by the results of the hemisection of the brain stem (Cordeau and Mancia, 1958). This hypothesis does not seem justified by recent experiments done in our laboratory. Indeed, we have been able to induce total insomnia (less than 2% of

SWS) for 3 or 4 days by slow microinjection (4 to 8 μl) of saline or Ringer solution directly in the Raphé nuclei. With this technique, injection into a site located only 1.5 mm from the midline does not reduce sleep. If the insomnia was caused by the interruption of any crossing ascending pathway, a parasagittal injection should have also induced insomnia.

On the other hand much data concerning the turnover of serotonin neurons are needed. Total sleep deprivation does not significantly alter the concentration of endogenous serotonin (Tsuchiya et al., 1970). However, it has been demonstrated that, in the rat, the brain concentration of serotonin is higher during the day (5 p.m.) at the time when the rat sleeps most of the time than during the night (3 a.m.) (Quay, 1968). The alteration of the circadian rhythm of sleep in the rat, independent of light, has been induced by the change of the feeding schedule (Mouzet and Bobillier, 1970): rats were allowed to have access to food and water only during the day and their night sleep was increased. This alteration of the feeding schedule has been shown to suppress progressively the difference between day and night SWS, whereas the PS was increased during the night, while the biochemical analysis of the brain of the experimental rats carried out at 5 p.m. and 3 a.m. has failed to reveal any difference in brain endogenous serotonin between night and day.

The electrophysiological exploration of the Raphé system is only at its beginning and the data are still contradictory. The stimulation of the Raphé system at low frequency in the rat may induce behavioural and EEG signs of sleep (Kostowski et al., 1969), whereas in other experiments, the stimulation of the Raphé in rats submitted to auditory stimuli has failed to induce sleep (Aghajanian et al., 1967).

Recording from the Raphé system with integrated technique has failed to reveal any significant changes during SWS, whereas there was a very significant tonic and phasic increase in activity during PS (Balzano and Jeannerod, 1970).

Finally, one should remember that serotonin itself is not yet totally accepted as a neurotransmitter since it does not yet totally fulfill the numerous conditions that are necessary before a substance can enter the exclusive club of neurotransmitters.

Nevertheless the numerous data obtained with iontophoretic administration techniques (Roberts and Straughan, 1967) which show that serotonin is able to "inhibit" or to "increase" the firing of brain stem or of thalamic neurons together with the histofluorescent demonstration of serotonin-containing neurons certainly argue for the existence of serotoninergic neurons and place serotonin among the most probable "neuromodulators" involved in SWS.

II. Problem of Paradoxical Sleep

Although we have met PS many times in reviewing the role of serotonin in SWS, it is still impossible to present a global and coherent picture of the intricate mechanisms which trigger PS.

A. Neurophysiological Data

Neurophysiological experiments have shown that PS can be selectively suppressed (both in its tonic and phasic components, including the PGO spikes) by lesion of the pontine tegmentum including nucleus locus coeruleus, subcoeruleus, and the dorsal part of nucleus pontis oralis and caudalis (Jouvet, 1967). Unfortunately, this part of the brain stem appears multicolored in a histochemical map since it contains MAO and catecholamines (mainly norad-renaline)- containing neurons, as well as cells showing cholinesterase and therefore perhaps cholinergic in nature (Shute and Lewis, 1965; cf. however Karczmar, 1969 and 1970).

The lesion of the caudal part of the locus coeruleus is able to selectively suppress the motor inhibition which takes place during PS, but leaves the ascending components of PS, such as the PGO spikes and cortical activation, intact. After such lesions, cats may present a "pseudo hallucinatory" behavior during sleep (Jouvet, 1967; cf. Fig. 8).

Lesions of the rostral part of the locus coeruleus result in a very significant decrease in norepinephrine in the telen-diencephalon, a decrease in waking (see below), but no impairment of or even an increase in the PS.

These results show that the neural structures which trigger PS may be very close to those which are related to waking.

B. Neurochemical Results

Playing the "monoamine game" with PS is difficult since PS appears to be the result of a chain of many events; this complex situation may be summarized as follows:

1. PS appears to depend upon some serotoninergic mechanism which primes its appearance, since after the lesion of the Raphé system or after injection of PCPA, PS appears only if a certain daily level of SWS is reached (15%), and thus requires a certain level of serotonin turnover. Rostral Raphé does not probably contribute to prime PS mechanism since after its destruction, PS may appear directly after waking (narcoleptic attack). However, lesions of the medial and caudal Raphé suppress or strongly decrease PS, which suggests that some serotoninergic terminals originating from the medial and caudal Raphé could trigger its appearance. Another indirect argument in favor of the participation of serotoninergic mechanisms in PS is constituted by the fact that during the PS deprivation, the rat brain 5HIAA is increased (Weiss et al., 1968), whereas there is an increased synthesis and utilization of brain serotonin (Pujol et al., 1968 a).

2. The PGO spikes which usually appear only during or immediately before PS are still a neuropharmacological riddle. The PGO may be so facilitated by drugs that they can appear continuously during waking or SWS while the PS is suppressed. The Table 1 lists the drugs which either facilitate

or inhibit PGO activity and PS. The drugs which act upon PGO belong to three categories:

a) Only eserine and butyrate are able to trigger PGO and PS (in chronic pontile cats, but not in normal cats);

b) Drugs which dissociate PGO from PS such as reserpine: with these drugs, PGO appears continuously even during waking; and, finally,

c) Drugs which suppress selectively PGO and PS without interfering with SWS (Jouvet, 1967).

Although there appears to be a common link (decrease of serotonin) between drugs which facilitate PGO and suppress PS, this does not explain why PS (and PGO) are suppressed by α-methyl DOPA, MAO inhibitors or atropine.

Table 1.

The effect of various drugs on PGO spikes, PS and SWS. Facilitation and suppression indicated by + and −, respectively.

		PGO	PS	SWS
I	Eserine / Physostigmine	+	+	
	Butyrate of sodium	+	+	
II	Reserpine	+	−	−
	Parachloromethamphetamine	+	−	−
	Parachlorophenylalanine	+	−	−
III	MAO inhibitors	−	−	+ (cat)
	5HTP	−	−	+
	αMDOPA	−	−	+
	Atropine	−	−	±

3. The existence of catecholaminergic mechanisms is suggested by the strong inhibitory action of α-methyl DOPA (Dusan-Peyrethon et al., 1968) (which could act as a precursor of α-methyl noradrenaline, "a false transmitter"). The significant increase of the turnover of brain norepinephrine during the rebound of PS which follows its instrumental deprivation in the rat suggests also that changes of activity of central noradrenergic neurons are involved in PS (Pujol et al., 1968 b). However, the significance of these data is lessened by the finding, that, in the cat, the inhibition of the synthesis of catecholamine by α-methyl p-tyrosine (100–300 mg/kg) has no significant effect upon PS (Jouvet, unpublished).

4. Finally, a cholinergic mechanism appears to be involved in PS. This is shown by the potent inhibitory action of atropine (1–2 mg/kg) upon PS in the cat even after its previous deprivation. This is also demonstrated by the very significant increase in PS after the injection of eserine in pontile cats (Matsuzaki, 1969), or by the triggering of very long periods of PS (up to one

hour) by direct injection of carbachol in the region of the n. locus coeruleus (George et al., 1964; Baxter, 1969; cf. also Karczmar et al., 1970 *). Very little is known about the possible interaction between serotonin and acetylcholine (Aprison et al., 1962), and further progress in this field is necessary before we can draw a comprehensive picture of the mechanisms of PS.

Whatever the intimate mechanisms of both SWS and PS may be, one problem remains to be solved. Is another monoaminergic system involved in the continuous arousal which follows the subtotal destruction of the Raphé system? The results which are summarized below strongly suggest, in fact, that catecholamine-containing neurons are involved in waking.

III. Catecholamines and Waking

A. Neurophysiological Evidences for the Existence of a Ponto-Mesencephalic Waking System (See Fig. 2)

Twenty years of brain stem transection or coagulation have delimited with a good accuracy the anatomical structures responsible both for EEG and behavioural arousal. On the basis of the extensive work of Magoun, Moruzzi and others (for references, cf. Rossi and Zanchetti, 1957) the posterior mesencephalic reticular formation and the anterior pontile tegmentum were considered to be the essential structure. The caudal limit of the activating system is well defined by the medio-pontine transection, since a rostro-pontine transection induces a synchronized EEG. The rostral limit of the system is still a matter of discussion since anterior mesencephalic or hypothalamic lesions may induce cortical synchronization not only by lesioning cell bodies, but evidently by interrupting ascending activating pathways.

Those anterior lesions, however, have permitted to dissociate the ascending activating structures from those responsible for behavioural waking. Indeed, posterior hypothalamic lesions may induce a state of coma as well as the occurrence of long cortical activation (Feldman and Waller, 1962), whereas bilateral lesions of the midbrain tegmentum produced the opposite result, that is, behavioural arousal and orientation to stimuli with only fleeting cortical activation. It may be therefore necessary to consider that two mechanisms are involved in waking.

B. Neuropharmacological Analysis of the Role of Catecholamines in Waking: from Contradiction to Probability

Early pharmacological investigations of the role of the catecholamines in central mechanisms employed the systemic injection of the amines (see Rothballer, 1959). In moderate doses, norepinephrine and epinephrine produced

* Cf. also the discussion which followed this presentation.

a cortical activation parallel to an increase in peripheral sympathetic tone. The activating effect of norepinephrine was abolished if the mesencephalic reticular formation was transected or lesioned. It appeared thus possible that the neurons of the reticular formation might be adrenergic.

However, evidence was soon presented that neither norepinephrine nor epinephrine injected directly in the blood stream passed the blood-brain barrier in any significant amount (Weil-Malherbe et al., 1959). This fact led to a total reversal of the situation, and during some time catecholamines were considered as possible "neuromodulators of sleep." Indeed, injected in young chicks in which the blood-brain barrier is absent, noradrenaline produced, EEG-wise and behaviourally, sleep-like states (Key and Marley, 1962). Good examples in favor of the "depressing" or soporific action of catecholamines may be found in a recent paper by Mandell and Spooner (1968) who list 21 instances (from 1914 to 1969, and from chicks to man) of epinephrine or norepinephrine-produced sedation, sleep, deep anesthesia and even unconsciousness. However, it is possible that sedation and EEG slowing induced by norepinephrine could also be due to indirect action of this hormone. In fact, Bonvallet et al. (1954) have shown that the increase of sinoaortic pressure and the excitation of baroreceptors elicit a central shift toward depression and EEG synchronization.

A better knowledge of the biosynthesis of the brain catecholamines, the existence of potent "specific" inhibitors of catecholamines synthesis, the development of techniques allowing the measure of the turnover of central catecholamines have recently again switched the balance in favor of catecholamines as waking "neuromodulator."

Among numerous data which have been accumulated, I will only choose two types of experiments, which appear quite convincing.

1. Inhibition of the synthesis of catecholamines at the level of tyrosine hydroxylase by α-MPT led to a decrease of EEG and behavioural waking in rats, cats and monkeys (Weitzman et al., 1969).

This "depressor" effect of α-MPT may be demonstrated even in a more dramatic way (Fig. 11). α-MPT (150–200 mg/kg) was given I.P. to cats with destroyed Raphé system at the time when behavioural and EEG waking was almost permanent (2 to 6 days after the lesion). Four to six hours after the injection, behavioural sedation became evident: The running movements stopped, miosis appeared, and there was a definite increase of cortical synchronization which lasted for 24 hours; subsequently, there was a rapid return to behavioural and EEG insomnia. The norepinephrine content of the telen- and diencephalon of 3 cats sacrificed at the time of behavioural sedation was decreased by 60% as compared with other cats in which the Raphé system was destroyed, but which did not receive α-MPT. This experiment provides the neuropharmacological evidence that the increase in waking which follows the destruction of serotonin-containing neurons of the Raphé system is caused by the increased activity of central catecholaminergic neurons.

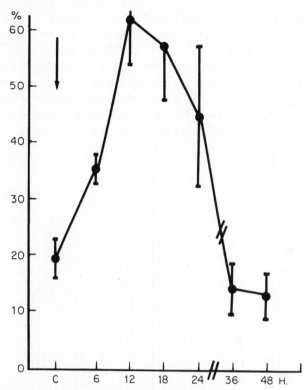

FIGURE 11. Decrease of waking in cats with destroyed Raphé system after α-methyl paratyrosine (α-MPT). Ordinates: percentage of the SWS during the experimental period (6 or 12 hours); abscissae: time in hours. C: percentage of sleep (mean value and SEM) in control conditions in 8 cats, the Raphé system of which was subtotally destroyed 2 to 6 days before. The arrow signals the injection of 150–200 mg/kg of the methyl ester of α-MPT intraperitoneally. There is a very marked increase in cortical synchronization which lasts for about 24 hours after which there is a return to insomnia.

2. The following experiment provides some additional cues about the localization of the central catecholaminergic neurons involved in waking. It is well known that the behavioural and EEG-activating effects of amphetamine depend upon the ponto-mesencephalic reticular formation since destruction of the mesencephalic formation or "cerveau isolé" transection suppresses the amphetamine-induced EEG arousal (Hiebel et al., 1954). On the other hand, in the rabbit, intravertebral injection of amphetamine is not followed by arousal if the basilar artery is tied at the midpontine level (Van Meter and Ayala, 1961). This fact excludes any caudo-ponto-bulbar neurons from being involved in the wakefulness caused by amphetamine. Finally, numerous data tend to demonstrate that the activating effect of amphetamine is due to catecholaminergic neurons such as the increase in the turnover of brain noradrenaline after amphetamine injection (Javoy et al., 1968), or the blockade of behavioural agitation by pretreatment with α-MPT (Hanson, 1967). The

following experiment confirms the probable role of central catecholaminergic neurons in behavioural and EEG waking induced by amphetamine in the cat: whereas a single IM injection of 5 mg/kg of DL amphetamine induces a very marked behavioural (agitation, mydriasis) and EEG waking lasting continually for 11 hours (mean of 5 cats), pretreatment of three animals with a single dose of 200 mg/kg of α-MPT, six hours before the injection of amphetamine considerably shortens both the EEG and behavioural arousal which does not last more than 1 hour and which is followed by SWS (Fig. 12).

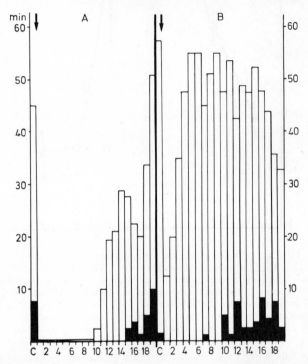

FIGURE 12. Suppression of the waking effect of DL-amphetamine by α-MPT in normal cats. Ordinates: time (in minutes) spent in SWS (white) or PS (black) every hour; abscissae: time in hours. C: control (mean of 6 hours). A. The arrow signals the injection of 5 mg/kg (I.M.) of DL-amphetamine. There is a long-lasting and continuous arousal during 10 hours, followed by a return of sleep (mean of 5 experiments). B. The cats were pretreated by α-MPT (200 mg per kg), 6 hours before. The arrow signals the injection of 5 mg/kg of DL-amphetamine: the waking effect of this drug is almost totally suppressed, although PS is altered during 8–9 hours (mean of 3 experiments).

Although this experiment does not distinguish between the catecholamines which may be involved (norepinephrine or dopamine), it strongly suggests that catecholamine-containing neurons of the rostral pons or caudal mesencephalon are most likely to be involved in behavioural and/or EEG arousal.

For this reason, those groups of neurons (which have been previously mapped out) were the target for destruction, following the same procedure which has been used in the case of the Raphé system.*

C. Alteration of Behavioural and EEG Waking after Destruction of Catecholamines-Containing Neurons of the Ponto-Mesencephalic Reticular Formation

1. DOPAMINE-CONTAINING NEURONS OF THE SUBSTANTIA NIGRA.   Lesions of the catecholamine-containing cell bodies of the substantia nigra (Group A 9) produced a decrease in dopamine in the rostral brain (telencephalon, striatum, diencephalon) and a behavioural state of akinesia and unresponsiveness. Some severely lesioned cats in which dopamine was severely decreased (more than 90%) were almost comatose. Despite such a depressed behaviour, a quantitatively normal EEG record of alternating sleep and waking activity persisted during the comatose state. Long-lasting cortical activation in response to peripheral stimulation was common even in the total absence of behavioural arousal (Jones, 1969; Jones et al., 1969; Fig. 13).

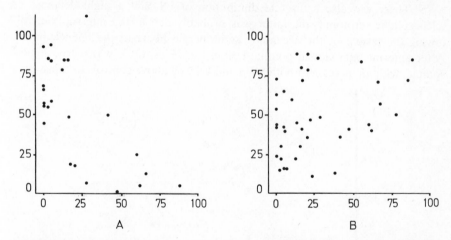

A   B

FIGURE 13. A. Correlation between the amount of destruction of the substantia nigra (abscissae), and the level of dopamine in the telen-diencephalon (in percentages of values obtained in normal cats; ordinates). B. Absence of correlation between the amount of destruction of the substantia nigra (abscissae) and the percentage of cortical synchronization during the 10–13 days of postoperative survival (ordinates). (*From Jones et al., 1969.*)

These results confirm earlier findings (Anden et al., 1966) that the catecholamine-containing cells of the substantia nigra contain dopamine. In view of the numerous anatomical data which suggest the existence of a nigro-striatal ascending system, it appears possible that dopamine could play a role in be-

* Most of this work was performed by B. E. Jones during her stay in my laboratory, cf. Jones, 1969; Jones et al., 1969.

havioural alertness and motor coordination presumably by way of this system. On the other hand, dopamine-containing neurons do not significantly play a role in either cortical synchronization or desynchronization since an almost total disappearance of dopamine from the telen-diencephalon does not induce significant shift in the EEG, sleep-waking alternation.

2. NORADRENALINE-CONTAINING NEURONS OF THE PONTO-MESENCE-PHALIC TEGMENTUM.   The destruction of the green fluorescent cells of the lateral pontine tegmentum (anterior part of locus coeruleus), and of the mesencephalic reticular formation resulted in a slight decrease of dopamine and a significant decrease of norepinephrine, accompanied by a significant decrease of polygraphic waking, i.e., of low voltage, fast activity and of EMG activity; there was no or little impairment of behavioural arousal or motor function. Sensory stimulation produced both behavioural orientation and cortical activation which were, however, contingent upon the presentation and duration of the stimulus. After mesencephalic lesion, the decrease of low voltage fast activity was replaced by a deactivated EEG and to a lesser extent by an increase in SWS. There was also a discrete diminution of PS, and a slight decrease of telencephalic serotonin; the latter was probably due to the interruption, following the lesion, of the ascending serotonergic fibers to the telencephalon. After anterior laterodorsal pontine lesions, however, there was a true hypersomnia, with an increase of both SWS and PS well above control. In those cats,

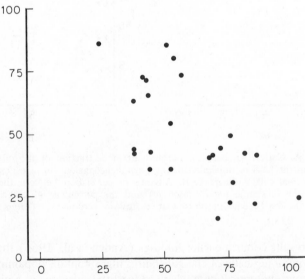

FIGURE 14. Correlation between the level of norepinephrine in the telen-diencephalon (as compared with intact cats) after lesion of noradrenergic neurons of the pons or the mesencephalon (abscissae) and the percentage of cortical synchronization (ordinates) during the 10–13 days of survival. (*From Jones et al., 1969.*) The levels of norepinephrine are expressed as percentages of control values.

an increase of the telencephalic 5HIAA paralleled the decrease of norepinephrine. There was no significant change of telen-diencephalic serotonin.

Finally, in all these cats, there was a significant correlation between the amount of destruction of the norepinephrine-containing neurons, decrease of norepinephrine in the rostral brain, and the decrease of EEG waking (desynchronization) (Fig. 14).

In summary, two mechanisms are implicated in these experiments concerning the maintenance of waking: 1. a dopaminergic mechanism of the nigrostriatal system seems responsible for behavioural arousal and alertness; 2. a noradrenergic system originating in the anterior part of the dorsolateral part of the pontine tegmentum and the mesencephalic reticular formation appears to be responsible for the *tonic* cortical activation which usually accompanies waking. This system, however, does not play a role in the phasic cortical activation which accompanies external stimulation.

Discussion: Some Hypotheses Concerning the Interaction Between the Serotonergic Sleep System and the Catecholaminergic Waking System

The catecholamine-containing neurons of the pons and mesencephalon are much more widespread and diffuse than the serotonergic neurons of the Raphé system. Moreover, many cholinergic neurons are also intermixed with the catecholaminergic neurons (mostly in the locus coeruleus and the substantia nigra) (Shute and Lewis, 1965). It is evident therefore that the coagulation technique is not a specific way to destroy specifically the catecholamine-containing neurons. The fact that direct or intraventricular injections of 6-hydroxydopamine destroy "specifically" and reversibly the catecholaminergic neurons (Ungerstedt, 1968) constitutes a much more powerful method for verifying the above data and for delineating in more detail exact topography and projection of this postulated ascending ponto-mesencephalic, noradrenergic activating system.

Figure 15 summarizes all the biochemical and EEG data obtained since 1966 in 133 cats which were all operated, recorded, sacrificed and biochemically analyzed as already described. They had either lesions of the midline Raphé, or of the bulbar, pontine, or mesencephalic tegmentum, or of substantia nigra. Groups of animals were classified according to the percentage of EEG synchronization during the 10–13 days of the postoperative survival, and to the mean value of the percentage of serotonin and norepinephrine in the telencephalon and diencephalon as compared to controls. It is clear that serotonin and norepinephrine fit two opposite curves: Cats with insomnia (less than 30% of cortical synchronization) have a decreased brain serotonin and a normal brain norepinephrine. Cats with normal or subnormal level of synchronization (30–60%) exhibit normal or subnormal values of both serotonin

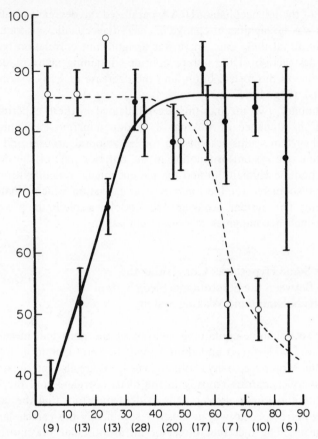

FIGURE 15. Ordinates: mean value and SEM of the percentage of serotonin (black circle) and norepinephrine (white circle) in the telen-diencephalon. Abscissae: percentage of cortical synchronization during 10–13 days of survival after the lesion. The numbers in brackets refer to the number of cats in each group. Other explanations in the text. The normal value (100%) for 50 control cats are respectively 622 $\mu g/g \pm 22$ for serotonin and 399 $\mu g/g \pm 10$ for norepinephrine.

and norepinephrine, whereas cats with increased synchronization show a decreased norepinephrine with normal or subnormal serotonin level in the telen-diencephalon.

Thus, all these results obtained with a combination of histochemical, electrophysiological, neuropharmacological and biochemical techniques suggest that two different and possibly antagonist monoaminergic subcortical ascending systems are responsible for the cortical synchronization and sleep on the one hand, and for the cortical desynchronization and waking on the other.

According to this hypothesis, the ascending sleep system would be composed of most of the cell bodies of the Raphé system, their ascending axons, some of which pass through the medial forebrain bundle, and their terminals.

It is possible (but not yet proven) that some serotonin terminals might have synaptic contacts with the catecholamine-containing cell bodies in the ponto-mesencephalic formation responsible for waking (opening a possibility of a direct interaction between the two antagonist systems):

A. Two Forms of Insomnia

Two different forms of insomnia are thus theoretically possible. 1. One form seems due to the damage to the serotoniergic sleep system: sleep would be impaired by either lesion of the serotonin-containing cell bodies, of their ascending pathways, or even of the terminals. It is possible that the secondary mild insomnia which is observed after a lesion of the preoptic region (McGinty and Sterman, 1968), could be the result of a possible retrograde effect upon the turnover of serotonin-containing cell bodies. Our results also suggest that the decrease of sleep which is observed after a medio pontine transection can be explained by the deconnection of about 2/3 of the Raphé system from the waking system. In fact, lesion localized at the level 2/3 caudal of the Raphé system induced the same amount of insomnia (Jouvet, 1969).

Another characteristic of insomnia created by a lesion is its selectivity. According to the extent of the destruction of the Raphé system, either total sleep or only SWS can be suppressed, PS occurring directly after waking as in narcoleptic attacks. PS can also be selectively suppressed by a lesion of the dorso pontine tegmentum without impairment of SWS.

The total insomnia which is obtained by the inhibition of the synthesis of serotonin with P-chlorophenylalanin obviously involves this system.

Finally, insomnias due to the lesion of serotoninergic neurons or to inhibition of serotonin synthesis have one common characteristic: *the decrease of sleep is not followed by a subsequent rebound of sleep.* This suggests that the common mechanism is a decrease of the turnover of central serotoninergic neurons. 2. Insomnia may also be induced by the activation of the ascending noradrenergic ponto mesencephalic system. This insomnia may be induced either by direct stimulation of the mesencephalon, by nociceptive stimuli, by the instrumental method (the swimming pool technique, Vimont et al., 1966), or by drugs such as amphetamine; it is short lasting unless repeated stimuli or increasing quantities of drugs are employed. It is either a total insomnia, or a selective suppression of PS (by an instrumental method), but never a selective suppression of SWS. This insomnia *is always followed by a rebound SWS and/or PS,* the intensity and duration of which are proportional to the duration of insomnia (Vimont et al., 1966; Dement, 1960). This fact suggests a possible regulation of the biosynthesis and of the turnover of serotinergic neurons by the increased activity of the waking system.

Finally, both forms of insomnia share one common characteristic. They can be suppressed by inhibition of the synthesis of catecholamines by α-methyl-paratyrosine which decreases the turnover of central catecholaminergic neurons.

B. Two Forms of Decreased Wakefulness

Two different forms of decrease in waking are possible. 1. A true hypersomnia consists of an increase of both SWS and PS. This has not yet been obtained for a long duration by any direct stimulation of the Raphé system, but nothing is known about the physiological stimuli which trigger this system at the onset of sleep. Such hypersomnia (above control level) has been obtained with exogenous 5HTP only when endogenous 5HTP has been used up and depleted after the inhibition of tryptophan hydroxylase by PCPA. A true hypersomnia with more than 80% of total sleep (and 20–25% of PS) may also be observed after limited lesion of the anterior part of the noradrenergic neurons of the dorso lateral pontine tegmentum. The fact that this insomnia is accompanied by an increase of telen- and diencephalic 5HIAA suggests that there is an increase of the turnover of central serotinergic neurons and that those pontine noradrenergic neurons might control the synthesis of serotonin in some part of the Raphé system. The existence of projections from the locus coeruleus to the Raphé system, which has been demonstrated in the rat (Loizou, 1969) is in favor of this hypothesis. Theoretically, this form of hypersomnia should be suppressed by PCPA. 2. Decrease of waking (but not true hypersomnia) is observed following the lesion of mesencephalic noradrenergic neurons. After such a lesion, the time originally spent in waking (50%) is occupied by an increase neither of SWS nor of PS, but by a "deactivated EEG" with a pattern different from the stage 1 of sleep (which corresponds to sleep onset). It is possible that the localized lesion of only mesencephalic noradrenergic neurons which leads to a significant decrease of telen- and diencephalic norepinephrine does not suppress the possible control of the Raphé system by the anterior pontine noradrenergic neurons.

Finally, the decrease of waking which is observed after inhibition of synthesis of catecholamines by α-methyl p-tyrosine cannot be considered as a true hypersomnia since the increase of synchronization is not accompanied by a correspondent increase of PS; in fact, usually a slight decrease of PS occurs.

Whatever the organization of these two systems, it appears certain that it is quite difficult to interpret the action of most drugs which act upon both indolamine and catecholamines. According to their prevalent effect upon either serotonin or noradrenaline, inhibitors of MAO may either increase SWS (in the cat; Jouvet, 1967) or have some arousal effect (in the rat; Mouret et al., 1968). Even the effect of a "selective" inhibitor of synthesis of only one monoamine is not without danger. If we admit that only noradrenergic neurons of anterior pons and caudal mesencephalon are responsible for the tonic activation of EEG, it remains possible that other ascending noradrenergic neurons from the caudal pons or medulla may have different functions, the suppression of which might counteract or conceal the effects of the pharmacological inhibition of the noradrenergic systems concerned with the EEG activation.

Finally, it is possible that most of the actions which take place at the terminals of these systems mimic many "trophotropic" and "ergotrophic" effects (Hess, 1944), which are believed to take place in the diencephalon. The existence of the cell bodies of these two antagonistic systems, well below in the lower brain stem, makes this part of the brain stem one of the most important sites for the control of many events which are believed to be of hypothalamic origin.

Even if many effector neurons, responsible for the behavioural and electroencephalographic aspects of sleep and waking are located in the telendiencephalon regions, it is probable that most of the mechanisms which regulate and adapt the activity at the terminal level are located at the place where the enzymes are synthetized, i.e., in the cell bodies of the serotonin-containing neurons of the Raphé system and in the catecholamine-containing cell bodies of the ponto mesencephalic tegmentum.

Acknowledgements

The experiments which are described in this paper have been performed with the help of the Direction des Recherches et Moyens d'Essais, contract 69047, l'Institut National de la Santé et de la Recherche Medicale, and a Grant (EOAR 68-0039) from the European Office of Aerospace Research.

References

Aghajanian, G. K., Rosecrans, J. A., Sheard, M. H.: Serotonin: release in the forebrain by stimulation of midbrain Raphé. *Science* **156,** 402 (1967).

Anden, N. E., Dahlstrom, A., Fuxe, K., Larsson, K., Olson, L., Ungerstedt, U.: Ascending monoamine neurons to the telencephalon and diencephalon. *Acta Physiol. Scand.* **67,** 313–326 (1966).

Aprison, M. H., Kariya, T., Hingtgen, J. N., Toru, M.: Neurochemical correlates of behaviour. *J. of Neurochem.* **15,** 1131–1139 (1962).

Balzano, E., Jeannerod, M.: Activite multi-unitaire de structures sous corticales pendant le cycle veille-sommeil chez le chat. *EEG. Clin. Neurophysiol.* **28,** 136–145 (1970).

Batini, C., Magni, F., Palestini, M., Rossi, G. F., Zanchetti, A.: Effects of complete pontine transections on the sleep-wakefulness rhythm: the midpontine pretrigeminal preparation. *Arch. Ital. Biol.* **97,** 1–12 (1959).

Baxter, B. L.: Induction of both emotional behaviour and a novel form of REM sleep by chemical stimulation applied to cat mesencephalon. *Exper. Neurol.* **23,** 220–229 (1969).

Bonvallet, M., Dell, P., Hiebel, G.: Tonus sympathique et activité électrique cérébrale. *EEG Clin. Neurophysiol.* **6,** 119–144 (1954).

Bremer, F.: Nouvelles recherches sur le mécanisme du sommeil. *Compt. Rend. Soc. Biol.* **122,** 460–463 (1936).

Cordeau, J. P., Mancia, M.: Effect of unilateral chronic lesions of the midbrain on the electrocortical activity of the cat. *Arch. Ital. Biol.* **96,** 374–379 (1958).

Dahlstrom, A., Fuxe, K.: Evidence for the existence of monoamines containing neurons in the central nervous system. *Acta Physiol. Scand.* **62**, suppl. 232 (1964).

Delorme, F., Froment, L., Jouvet, M.: Suppression du sommeil par la P. Chlorometamphétamine et la P. Chlorophénylalanine. *C. R. Soc. Biol.* **160**, 2347–2351 (1966).

Dement, W. C.: The effect of dream deprivation. *Science* **131**, 1705–1707 (1960).

Dusan-Peyrethon, D., Peyrethon, J., Jouvet, M.: Suppression élective du sommeil paradoxal chez le chat par l'alphamethyl DOPA. *C. R. Soc. Biol.* **162**, 116–120 (1968).

Falck, B., Hillarp, N. A., Thieme, G., Torp, A.: Fluorescence of catecholamines and related compounds condensed with formaldehyde. *J. Histochem. Cytochem.* **10**, 348–354 (1962).

Feldman, S. M., Waller, H. J.: Dissociation of electrocortical activation and behavioural arousal. *Nature* **196**, 1320–1322 (1962).

George, R., Haslett, W. L., Jenden, D. J.: A cholinergic mechanism in the brain stem reticular formation: induction of paradoxical sleep. *Intern. J. Neuropharmacol.* **3**, 541–552 (1964).

Hanson, L. C. F.: Evidence that the central action of + amphétamine is mediated via catecholamines. *Psychopharmacologia* **10**, 289–297 (1967).

Heller, A., Harvey, J. A., Moore, R. Y.: A demonstration of a fall in brain serotonin following central nervous system lesions in the rat. *Biochem. Pharmacol.* **11**, 859–866 (1962).

Hess, W. R.: Das Schlafsyndrom als Folge dienzephaler Reizung. *Helv. Physiol. Pharmacol. Acta* **2**, 305–344 (1944).

Hiebel, G., Bonvallet, M., Huve, P., Dell, P.: Analyse neurophysiologique de l'action centrale de la D. Amphetamine. *Sem. Hôp. (Paris)* **30**, 1880–1887 (1954).

Javoy, F., Thierry, A. M., Kety, S. S., Glowinski, J.: The effect of amphetamine on the turnover of brain norepinephrine in normal and stressed rats. *Comm. Behavior. Biol.* **1**, 43–48 (1968).

Jones, B. E.: Catecholamine containing neurons in the brain stem of the cat and their role in waking, M. A. Thesis. 87 p. Tixier Edit. Lyon 1969.

——— Bobillier, P., Jouvet, M.: Effet de la destruction des neurones contenant des catecholamines du mesencephale sur le cycle veille-sommeil du chat. *C. R. Soc. Biol.* **163**, 176–180 (1969).

Jouvet, M.: Insomnia and decrease of cerebral 5 HT after destruction of the Raphé system in the cat. In: *Advances in Pharmacology.* Eds.: S. Garattini and P. A. Shore. New York and London: Academic Press 1968, pp. 265–279.

Jouvet, M.: Biogenic Amines and the States of Sleep. *Science* **163**, 32–41 (1969).

——— Recherches sur les structures nerveuses et les mécanismes responsables des différentes phases du sommeil physiologique. *Arch. Ital. Biol.* **100**, 125–206 (1962).

——— Mechanisms of the states of sleep: A neuropharmacological approach. In: *Sleep and Altered States of Consciousness.* Eds.: S. S. Kety, E. V. Evarts and H. L. Williams. Baltimore: The Williams and Wilkins Co. 1967, p. 86.

Karczmar, A. G.: Is the central cholinergic system overexploited? In: *Symposium on Central Cholinergic Transmission and Its Behavioral Aspects.* Ed.: A. G. Karczmar. *Fed. Proc.* **28**, 147–157 (1969).

——— Central cholinergic pathways and their behavioral implications. In: *Principles of Psychopharmacology.* Eds.: W. G. Clark and J. Del Giudice. New York: Academic Press 1970, pp. 57–86.

——— Longo, V. G., Scotti de Carolis, A.: A pharmacological model of paradoxical sleep: The role of cholinergic and monoamine systems. *Physiology and Behavior* **5**, 175–182 (1970).

Key, B. J., Marley, E.: The effect of the Sympathomimetic amines on behaviour and electrocortical activity of the chicken. *Electroencephalog. Clin. Neuroph.* **14**, 90–105 (1962).

Koe, B. K., Weissman, A.: P-Chlorophenylalanine: A selective depletor of brain serotonin. *J. Pharmacol. Exptl. Therap.* **154**, 499–516 (1966).

Koella, W. P., Czicman, J.: Mechanism of the EEG synchronizing action of serotonin. *Am. J. Physiol.* **211**, 926–934 (1966).

Feldstein, A., Czicman, J. S.: The effect of Para-Chlorophenylalanine on the sleep of cats. *Electroencephalog. Clin. Neurophysiol.* **25**, 481–490 (1968).

Kostowski, W., Giacalonne, E., Garattini, S., Valzelli, L.: Studies on behavioural and biochemical changes in rats after lesion of the midbrain Raphé. *Europ. J. Pharmacol.* **4**, 371–376 (1968).

——— Electrical stimulation of midbrain Raphé: Biochemical behavioural and bioelectrical effects. *Europ. J. Pharmacol.* **7**, 170–175 (1969).

Loizou, L. A.: Projections of the nucleus locus coeruleus in the albino rat. *Brain Research* **15**, 563–566 (1969).

Mancia, M.: Electrophysiological and behavioural changes owing to splitting of the brainstem in cats. *Electroenceph. clin. Neurophysiol.* **27**, 487–502 (1969).

Mandell, A. J., Spooner, C. E.: Psychochemical Research Studies in Man. *Science* **162**, 1442–1453 (1968).

Matsumoto, J., Jouvet, M.: Action de Reserpine, DOPA et 5 HTP sur les deux états de sommeil. *Compt. Rend. Soc. Biol.* **158**, 2135–2140 (1964).

Matsuzaki, M.: Differential effects of sodium butyrate and physostigmine upon activities of para-sleep in acute brain stem preparations. *Brain Research* **13**, 247–265 (1969).

McGinty, J., Sterman, M. B.: Sleep suppression after basal forebrain lesions in the cat. *Science* **160**, 1253–1255 (1968).

Michel, F., Roffwarg, H.: Chronic split brain stem preparation: effect on the sleep-waking cycle. *Experientia* **23**, 126–128 (1967).

Moir, A., Eccleston, D.: The effects of precursor loading in the cerebral metabolism of 5-hydroxy indoles. *J. of Neurochem.* **15**, 1093–1108 (1968).

Mouret, J., Bobillier, P.: *Life Sciences,* in Press.

——— Jouvet, M.: Insomnia following P. Chlorophenylalanin in the rat. *Europ. J. Pharmacol.* **5**, 17–22 (1968).

——— Vilppula, A., Franchon, N., Jouvet, M.: Effets d'un inhibiteur de la monoamine oxydase sur le sommeil du rat. *C. R. Soc. Biol.* **162**, 914–917 (1968).

Pin, C., Jones, B., Jouvet, M.: Topographie des neurones monoaminergiques du tronc cérébral chez le chat. Etude par histofluorescence. *C. R. Soc. Biol.* **162**, 2136–2140 (1968).

Pletscher, A., Burkard, W. P., Bruderer, H., Gey, K. F.: Decrease of cerebral serotonin and 5-HIAA by an arylalkylamine. *Life Sci.* **11**, 828–833 (1963).

Pujol, J. F., Bobillier, P., Buguet, A., Jones, B., Jouvet, M.: Biosynthèse de la sérotonine cérébrale: Etude Neurophysiologique et biochimique après P. Chlorophénylalanine et destruction du système du Raphé. *C. R. Acad. Science* **268**, 100–102 (1969).

Pujol, J. F., Hery, F., Durand, M., Glowinski, J.: Augmentation de la synthèse de la sérotonine dans le tronc cérébral chez le rat après privation sélective du sommeil paradoxal. *C. R. Acad. Sciences.* **267**, 371–372 (1968 a).

——— Mouret, J., Jouvet, M., Glowinski, J.: Increased turnover of cerebral norepinephrine during rebound of paradoxical sleep in the rat. *Science* **159**, 112–114 (1968 b).

Quay, W. B.: Différences in circadian rhythms in 5-Hydroxytryptamine according to brain region. *Amer. J. Physiol.* **215**, 1448–1452 (1968).

Roberts, M. H. T., Straughan, D. W.: Excitation and depression of cortical neurons by 5-hydroxy tryptamine. *J. Physiol. (Lond.)* **193**, 269–294 (1967).

Rossi, G. F., Zanchetti, A.: The brain stem reticular formation anatomy and physiology. *Arch. Ital. Biol.* **95**, 199–435 (1957).

Rothballer, A. B.: The effects of catecholamines on the central nervous system. *Pharmacological Review* **2**, 494–547 (1959).

Sabelli, H. C., Giardina, W. J., Alivisatos, S. G., Seth, P. K., Ungar, F.: Indole-acetaldehydes: Serotonin-like effects on the central nervous system. *Nature (Lond.)* **223**, 73–74 (1969).

Shute, C. C. D., Lewis, P. R.: Cholinergic and monoaminergic systems of the brain. *Nature* **212**, 710–711 (1966).

Spooner, C. E., Winters, W. D.: The influence of centrally active amine induced blood pressure changes on the electroencephalogram and behavior. *Intern. J. Neuropharmacol.* **6**, 109–118 (1967).

Strumwasser, F.: The demonstration and manipulation of a circadian rhythm in a single neuron. In: *Circadian Clocks*. Ed.: J. Aschoff. Amsterdam: North Holland 1965, pp. 442–462.

Tsuchiya, K., Toru, M., Kobayaski, T.: Sleep deprivation: changes of monoamines and acetylcholine in rat brain. *Life Sciences* **8**, 867–873 (1969).

Ungerstedt, U.: 6-Hydroxydopamine-induced degeneration of central monoamine neurons. *Europ. J. Pharmacol.* **5**, 107–110 (1968).

Van Meter, W. G., Ayala, G. F.: EEG effect of intracarotid or intra vertebral arterial administration of d-amphetamine in rabbits with basilar artery ligation. *Electroenceph. clin. Neurophysiol.* **13**, 382–384 (1961).

Vimont, P., Jouvet, M., Delorme, J. F.: Etude de la privation de sommeil paradoxal chez le chat. *Electroenceph. clin. Neurophysiol.* **20**, 439–449 (1966).

Weil-Malherbe, H., Axelrod, J., Tomchick, R.: Blood brain barrier for adrenaline. *Science* **129**, 1226–1227 (1959).

Weiss, E., Bordwell, B., Seeger, M., Lee, J., Dement, W. C., Barchas, J.: Changes in brain 5-HT and 5-HIAA in REM sleep deprived rats. *Psychophysiology* **5**, 209 (1968).

Weitzman, E. D., Rapport, M., McGregor, P., Jacoby, J.: Sleep pattern of the monkey and brain serotonin concentration. Effect of P. Chlorophenylalanin. *Science* **160**, 1361–1363 (1968).

—————— McGregor, P., Moore, C., Jacoby, J.: The effects of alpha-methyl-para-tyrosine on sleep patterns of the monkey. *Life Sciences* **8**, 751–757 (1969).

Discussion of Jouvet's Paper

Alexander H. Friedman, Dept. of Pharmacology, Loyola University Medical Center. I would like to throw in another candidate to the monoamine game for Dr. Jouvet. I refer in particular to the work of Professor Monnier (1969) who reported a waking action for histamine. I refer also to some of our own work (Friedman and Walker, 1968) demonstrating certain circadian rhythms in which histamine levels are peaking during the period when the animal is alert and are 180 degrees out of phase with serotonin levels. And I also refer to the actions of antihistamines as sedatives. And to some of the work of Carl Pfeiffer's group (1969) on histamine levels in individuals suffering from manic or depressive psychoses. So I think perhaps histamine might be incorporated into this monoamine game, and I would like to hear Dr. Jouvet's comments.

Dr. Michel Jouvet. I am sure how I play the game. We play the game only if we have the map. If you give us the map of those histamine-containing neurons, and I think this is possible, the problem will be quickly solved. We will destroy them and then we will agree generally with the sense of your remarks. I am my own critic. The methods of destruction are difficult to accept. But, now we have new techniques which are taking the place of those big bombings. And these are injections of specific drugs which can selectively be taken up by the neurons, and which are poison for those neurons. 6-hydroxy-dopamine is a new tool which we are now using for destroying certain neurons, and I think that now in Sweden, they have one drug, very secret probably, which is able to be selectively taken up by serotonergic neurons and which destroys them; the day when we will know what drug it is, we will use it and try to find further evidence for our data. I don't think the sedative effect of the antihistamines is a sufficient proof of the waking action of histamine, but I agree that histamine and certainly many other amines can be incorporated in the "monoamine game." But at the present time the rules of the game are rather complicated. Concerning histamine, one should be able to map out the histamine-containing neurons and possibly one should destroy them as selectively as possible. It would be important also to inhibit the synthesis of brain histamine as "selectively" as possible.

Alexander H. Friedman: There are some drugs which deplete histamine such as 48/80 but I am not sure whether this is specific for mast cell histamine or histamine in other locations.

References

Friedman, A. H., Walker, C. A.: Circadian rhythms in rat mid-brain and caudate nucleus biogenic amine levels. *J. Physiol.* **197,** 77–85 (1968).

Monnier, M.: Afferent and central activating effects of histamine on the brain. 4th International Congress on Pharmacology, Basel, Switzerland July 14–18, 1969, P168.

Pfeiffer, C. C., Iliev, V., Goldstein, L. Jenney, E. H.: Correlations between histamine, polyamine levels, EEG and psychiatric ratings in schizophrenia, abstracts. 4th International Congress on Pharm., Basel, Switzerland July 14–18, 1969, P170.

Attention:
Some Theoretical Considerations

J. A. DEUTSCH AND D. DEUTSCH

Reprinted from *Psychological Review*, 1963, Vol. 70, No. 1, pp. 80–90. Copyright 1963 by the American Psychological Association, and reproduced by permission.

The selection of wanted from unwanted messages requires discriminatory mechanisms of as great a complexity as those in normal perception, as is indicated by behavioral evidence. The results of neurophysiology experiments on selective attention are compatible with this supposition. This presents a difficulty for Filter theory. Another mechanism is proposed, which assumes the existence of a shifting reference standard, which takes up the level of the most important arriving signal. The way such importance is determined in the system is further described. Neurophysiological evidence relative to this postulation is discussed.

There has, in the last few years, been an increase in the amount of research devoted to the problem of attention, which has been summarized in Broadbent's (1958) important work. Whilst psychologists have been investigating the behavioral aspects of attention, suggestive evidence has also been found by neurophysiologists. We feel that it would be useful at this time to consider the theoretical implications of some of this research.

Our paper is divided into three parts. In the first we consider some of the behavioral findings on attention. In the second a system is proposed to account for various features of this behavior. Although we do not consider it necessary to identify a system of this type with particular neural structures (see Deutsch, 1960) since a machine embodying such a system would also display the behavior we wish to explain, we do, however, venture some tentative hypotheses concerning the neural identification of the proposed system.

Behavioral Considerations

However alert or responsive we may be, there is a limit to the number of things to which we can attend at any one time. We cannot, for instance, listen effectively to the conversation of a friend on the telephone if someone else in the room is simultaneously giving us complex instructions as to what to say to him. And this difficulty in processing information from two different sources at the same time occurs even if no overt response is required. This phenomenon of selective attention has been investigated in a number of experiments. The most important of these deals with the processing of information emitted simultaneously by two separate sound sources (Broadbent, 1954; Cherry, 1953; Spieth, Curtis, and Webster, 1954). Two problems arise from the results of such experiments. The first is how different streams of information are kept distinct by the nervous system, and how a resultant babel is thereby avoided. The second is why only one of the messages (once it has been kept distinct and separate) is dealt with at any one time. A proposed solution to the first problem, based on experiments in which two messages were fed simultaneously one to each ear, was that the messages were kept distinct by proceeding down separate channels (such as different neural pathways). Nor was it difficult for Broadbent (1958) to extend such a notion to other cases. It had been shown in numerous experiments that we are enabled to listen to one of two simultaneous speech sequences while ignoring the other, by selecting items for attention which have some feature or features in common, such as their frequency spectra (Egan, Carterette, and Thwing, 1954; Spieth et al., 1954) and their spatial localization (Hirsch, 1950; Poulton, 1953; Webster and Thomson, 1954). It was supposed that relatively simple mechanisms were responsible for segregation according to these categories, though the principles of their operation were not made clear.

Broadbent's (1958) answer to the second problem, of how one message is admitted to the exclusion of others, followed from the notions we have already considered. It was proposed that there was a filter which would select a message on the basis of characteristics toward which it had been biased and allow this message alone to proceed to the central analyzing mechanisms. In this way, messages with other characteristics would be excluded and so the total amount of discrimination which would have to be performed by the nervous system would be greatly decreased. Whole complex messages could be rejected on the sole basis of possessing some simple quality, and no further analysis of them would occur.

However, it seems that selection of wanted from unwanted speech can be performed on the basis of highly complex characteristics. For instance, Peters (1954) found that if an unwanted message is similar in content to the wanted one, it produces more interference with the adequate reception of the latter than if it is dissimilar to it. This shows that the content of the two messages is analyzed prior to the acceptance of one and rejection of the other. Gray and Wedderburn (1960) have also found that when speech was delivered to subjects in both ears simultaneously, such that a meaningful sequence could be formed by choosing syllables or words alternately from each ear, the subjects reported back the meaningful sequence rather than the series of words or syllables presented to one ear or the other. Treisman (1960) presented two messages, one to each ear, and subjects were asked to repeat what they heard on one ear. The messages were switched from one ear to the other in the middle and it was found that subjects tended to repeat words from the wrong ear just after the switch. "The higher the transition probabilities in the passage the more likely they were to do this" (Treisman, 1960).

Other evidence, indicating that complex discriminations would be required of the filter, has been produced by experiments concerning the selection of novel stimuli, for which function Broadbent (1958) assumes the filter to be responsible. Sharpless and Jasper (1956), studying habituation to auditory stimuli in cats, found that habituation, both behavioral and EEG, was specific not only to the frequency of sound presented, but also to the pattern in which a combination of frequencies was presented. Evidence for human subjects is presented by Sokolov (1960) and Voronin and Sokolov (1960), who report that when habituation has been established to a group of words similar in meaning but different in sound, then arousal occurred to words with a different meaning. Behavioral data on the arousal of curiosity in rats upon the presentation of novel visual patterns are reported by Thomson and Solomon (1954).

Such evidence as the above would require us, on filter theory, to postulate an additional discriminative system below or at the level of the filter, perhaps as complex as that of the central mechanism, to which information was assumed to be filtered.

Howarth and Ellis (1961) have presented an ingenious experimental argument to show that the same discriminatory mechanism functions in normal perception and when, on filter theory, the discrimination would have to be performed at the level of the filter. The case they put forward is as follows. Moray (1959) had shown that if a subject is listening selectively to one channel and ignoring the other, calling his name on the rejected channel will on a certain proportion of instances cause him to switch his attention to this channel. This was explained by assuming that the subject's name had a higher priority for the filter than the message to which he had been attending. Oswald, Taylor, and Treisman (1960) in a well-controlled experiment reported that during sleep a subject tends to respond selectively to his own name. Howarth and Ellis (1961) went on to show that the subject's name has a significantly lower threshold than other names when the subject is required to listen normally and there is masking by noise. After analyzing quantitatively their results and those obtained by Oswald et al. and Moray, they (Howarth and Ellis, 1961) conclude that,

There is, therefore, a very impressive amount of agreement among these three very different experiments concerning the relative intelligibilty of one's own name. It seems an obvious conclusion to suppose that the same pattern-analyzing mechanism is required to account for behavior during dichotic listening or during sleep.

as during ordinary listening under noise. Thus although Broadbent's (1958) filter theory provides an ingenious explanation of the selection of messages by means of simple and few discriminations, such as which ear is being stimulated, it becomes less attractive as an explanation of those cases where complex and many discriminations, discussed above, are needed.

If we may identify levels in filter theory with neural levels, then there is also evidence against a two-level system to account for novelty and habituation on neurological grounds. Sharpless and Jasper (1956) found that specificity of habituation to tonal pattern was destroyed by bilateral regions of cortex concerned with audition. It is known from other work (Goldberg, Diamond, and Neff, 1958) that sound pattern discrimination is a cortical function. On the other hand, frequency specific habituation was maintained with Sharpless and Jasper's lesions and it has been shown that frequency discrimination can be taught to animals without these cortical areas (Goldberg et al., 1958). This shows, first, that the level at which habituation occurs is not the same for both pattern and tone, and second, that the destruction of the level which is essential to normal functioning also destroys an animal's ability to habituate. This renders it plausible to assume that the mechanism responsible for habituation is not on a different level from that responsible for other learning and discrimination.

Theoretical Considerations

This review of the behavioral evidence leads us to the probable conclusion that a message will reach the same perceptual and discriminatory mechanisms whether attention is paid to it or not; and such information is then grouped or segregated by these mechanisms. How such grouping or segregation takes place is a problem for perceptual theory and will not concern us here. We may suppose that each central structure which is excited by the presentation of a specific quality or attribute to the senses, is given a preset weighting of importance. The central structure or classifying mechanism with the highest weighting will transfer this weighting to the other classifying mechanisms with which it has been grouped or segregated.

The main point with which we are concerned is the following. Given that there is activity in a number of structures, each with a preset weighting of importance, how might that group of structures with the greatest weighting be selected? Or, in behavioral terms, how might the most important of a group of signals be selected? Any system which performs such a function must compare all the incoming signals in importance. This could be done by comparing each incoming signal continuously to every other incoming signal and deciding which is the most important by seeing which signal has no other signal which exceeds it in the physical dimension by which "importance" is represented. But a small amount of reflection will suffice to show that such a system is very uneconomical. Each possible incoming signal must have a provision in the shape of numerous comparing mechanisms, through each of which it will be connected to all other possible signals. So that as the number of possible signals increases, the number of mechanisms to compare them all against each other will increase at an enormous rate. If the same comparing mechanisms are to be shared by pairs of signals then the time to reach a decision will increase out of all bounds.

However, there is a simpler and more economical way to decide that one out of a group of entities is the largest. Suppose we collect a group of boys and we wish to decide which is the tallest. We can measure them individually against each other and then select the boy in whom this comparison procedure never yielded the answer "smaller." This is like the system outlined above. The decision smaller will be made in this case when we lower a horizontal plane or ruler down on the heads of two boys. The boy whose head is touched by this instrument is declared to be larger and the other boy smaller. But such a procedure is cumbersome because there are many pairs of boys and we must scan through many records of individual boys before we can select the tallest. We could, of course, argue that a simpler solution would be to use an absolute measure of height, such as a ruler with feet and inches inscribed on it. But this procedure is not really simpler. Each boy must be compared against the ruler, and then the measurements themselves must be compared against each other in much the same way as the boys were to decide on the larger and smaller in each couple.

If we are simply interested in finding the tallest boy, then an alternative procedure may be used. Suppose we collect our group below our board which is horizontal and travels lightly up and down, and then ask all our group to stand up below it. Then the boy whose head touches the board when the whole group is standing up will be the tallest boy in the group. If then we call him out, the board will sink until it meets the head of the next tallest individual. If we introduce some other boys into the group, then if there is a taller boy in this group the board will be raised until it corresponds to his height. In such a system only the tallest individual will make contact with the board, and so he will himself have an immediate signal that he is the tallest boy.

Now suppose that instead of boys, we have signals, not varying in height, but in some other dimension (which we may continue to call "height") which corresponds to their importance to the organism. Suppose that each signal as it arrives is capable of pushing up some "level" to its own "height" (the height determined by its importance), then the most important signal arriving at any particular time will determine this level, analogous to the horizontal board in our example. It will then be the case that any signals which arrive then or after and are of lesser importance and so of smaller height will be below this level. However, if the signal of greater height ceases to be present, then the level will sink to the height reflecting the importance of one of the other signals which is arriving.

If we suppose that only signals whose height corresponds to the height of the level switch in further processes, such as motor output, memory storage, and whatever else it may be that leads to awareness, we have the outline of a system which will display the type of behavior we associate with attention. Only the most important signals coming in will be acted on or remembered. On the other hand, more important signals than those present at an immediately preceding time will be able to break in, for these will raise the height of the level and so displace the previously most important signals as the highest.

So far we have omitted any discussion of the role of general arousal in selective attention. Without such arousal, usually (but not invariably, Bradley and Elkes, 1953; Gastaut, 1954) indicated by characteristic patterns on the electroencephalogram, awareness of and behavioral responsiveness to peripheral stimulation are absent. Some degree of general arousal is thus necessary for attention to operate. Furthermore, individuals when aroused will attend to any incoming message, provided that it is not concomitant with a more important one, whereas when asleep they will only respond to very "important" messages, such as a person's own name (Oswald et al., 1960) or, in the case of a mother, the sound of her infant crying. And when drowsy, though responsive to a larger range of stimuli than when asleep, subjects will tend to "miss" signals which they would notice when fully awake.

The system which takes this into consideration is schematically represented in the diagram below (Fig. 1). Any given message will only be heeded

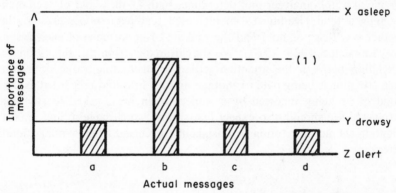

FIGURE 1. Diagram to illustrate operation of proposed system. (The interrupted horizontal line—1—represents the "level" of importance in the specific alerting system which is raised and lowered according to the incoming messages. The solid horizontal lines represent levels of general arousal. At X, the organism is asleep and none of the actual messages produce alerting. At Y, the organism is drowsy and only some incoming messages produce alerting. At Z, the organism is awake. All messages could be alerted to, but the specific alerting system allows only b to be heeded.)

if the horizontal line (Y) representing the degree of general arousal meets or crosses the vertical line, the height of which represents the "importance" of the message. Whether or not alerting will take place then depends both on the level of general arousal and on the importance of the message. Attention will not be paid to Message b though it is the most important of all incoming signals, when the level of general arousal is low (Position X). When the level of general arousal is at Z, which is very high, attention could be paid to all the signals a, b, c, d, and e. In fact, attention is paid only to b as a result of the operation of the specific alerting mechanism.

Further, it is supposed that a message will increase the level of general arousal in proportion to its importance and for various lengths of time in proportion to its importance, so that messages which would not have been heeded before will command attention if they follow in the wake of a more important message.

The mechanism whereby the weighting of importance of messages is carried out is given by Deutsch's (1953, 1956, 1960) theory of learning and motivation, and will be only briefly summarized here, since it is not the main point of the paper. It is assumed that on exposure to a succession of stimuli, link-analyzer units responsive to these stimuli will be connected together. Certain primary links, when stimulated by physiological factors, generate excitation, and this is passed on from link to link along the connections established by experience. Each link-analyzer unit will receive excitation depending first, on the state of the primary links to which it is connected, either directly or indirectly, and second, on the "resistance" of such a connection, which is determined by past learning. It is assumed that the amount of such excitation arriving at a link-analyzer unit determines both its threshold of excitability by incoming stimuli (leading to an increased readiness to perceive a stimulus whether it is there or not) and the ranking of importance of such a stimulus (e.g., Lawrence, 1949, 1950). We should predict from this theory an inverse correlation between the attention-getting or distracting value of a stimulus when attention is being paid to another, and its threshold (regarded as the likelihood of its being reported by a subject when he is asked to say what he perceives). We should also expect that stimuli which have a high importance weighting should more often be mistakenly perceived when similar stimuli are present.

Neurophysiological Correlates

We may ask how the suggested system would fit what is known of the physiological substrate of attentive behavior. One of the salient features of the system as proposed is that it assumes that all sensory messages which impinge upon the organism are perceptually analyzed at the highest level. It would therefore be of relevance to discuss the group of neurophysiological experiments the results of which have been claimed to demonstrate a neural blockage of "rejected" messages at the lower levels of the primary sensory pathways. Hernández-Peón, Scherrer, and Jouvet (1956) showed that the evoked response at the dorsal cochlear nucleus to clicks was reduced by the presentation of "distracting" olfactory and visual stimuli. A similar effect was found in the visual pathways (Hernández-Peón, Guzman-Flores, Alcarez, and Fernandez-Guardiola, 1957). Stimulation of the reticular formation could produce similar results, and it was supposed that such stimulation was treated as the presentation of a distracting stimulus. It has also been demonstrated by various workers (e.g. Galambos, Sheatz, and Vernier, 1956; Hernández-Peón and Scherrer, 1955) that responses to auditory clicks recorded from the dorsal cochlear nucleus (as well as other placements) diminish with repetition. Habituation to photic stimuli has been demonstrated for the retina (Palestini, Davidovich, and Hernández-Peón, 1959) and for the olfactory bulb (Hernández-Peón, Alcocer-Cuaron, Lavin, and Santibañez, 1957). It was therefore proposed that during inattention to a signal (either by distraction or habituation) information concerning this signal was blocked at the level of the first sensory synapse by means of "afferent neuronal inhibition." Recently, however, evidence has been produced indicating, at least for the visual and auditory pathways, that such changes in the evoked potential were due to peripheral factors, and represented simply a decrease in the effective intensity of the stimulus. Hugelin, Dumont, and Paillas (1960) report that when the middle ear muscles were cut stimulation of the reticular formation would not cause a diminution in the amplitude of the evoked responses. They report further that such contractions of the middle ear muscles which result from reticular stimulation produce a mean diminution of microphonic potentials of less than 5 decibels. The reduction in sensation brought about by these means therefore appears unimportant. Naquet, Regis, Fischer-Williams, and Ferrandez-Guardiola (1960) found that if the size of the pupil were fixed by local application of atropin the evoked potential recorded from placements below the cortex demonstrated a consistent amplitude.

The above findings do not, however, apply to changes in the cortical evoked response during distraction or habituation. Moushegian, Rupert, Marsh, and Galambos (1961) found that in animals in which the middle ear muscles had been cut, cortical evoked responses to clicks still demonstrated diminution during habituation and distraction, and amplification when the clicks were associated with puffs of air to the face. Naquet, in the experiment quoted above, reports that application of atropin to the pupil did not prevent a variation in cortical evoked responses, which diminished during desynchronization and were enhanced during synchronization of electrical rhythms, also changing in morphology.

Reports of changes in cortical evoked responses during habituation and distraction are many and varied, and it would be impossible in this space to describe the field in detail. Certainly disagreement exists over what occurs as well as over its interpretation. For instance, Horn (1960), recording flash evoked responses in the visual cortex of cats when resting, and when watching a mouse, found that the responses were reduced in amplitude when the cat was watching the mouse; when it ignored the mouse, responses remained of high amplitude. Further, after a series of tone-shock combinations, it was noted that the evoked response to flash was reduced after a series of tones only if there was "some visual searching component in the cat's response to the acoustic stimuli." Horn argues that attenuation of evoked responses in the cortex might be correlated with *greater* sensitivity in the appropriate region, rather than signifying a reduction in incoming information. However, other recent experimenters continue to maintain that evoked responses diminish in amplitude when attention is *not* being paid to the test stimulus. Garcia-Austt, Bogacz, and Vanzulli (1961) recorded scalp visual evoked responses in human subjects (who were able to give introspective reports) during presentation of flash stimuli. They report,

When the stimulus is significant and therefore attention is paid to it, the response is relatively simple and widespread. When, on the other hand, the stimulus is not significant and no great attention is paid to it, the response is reduced, complex, and localized.

It would seem that changes in the evoked potential at the cortex do indeed take place during habituation and attention shifts; but that what those changes exactly are, and what they represent, is not yet clear.

We should indeed expect, on the above theory of attention, changes in the cortical evoked potential when attention is being paid to a stimulus, reflecting the activation of various processes, such as motor output and memory storage. Pertinent to this assumption is the discovery by Hubel, Henson, Rupert, and Galambos (1959) of what they term "attention" units in the auditory cortex. By the use of microelectrodes implanted in unanesthetized and unrestrained cats, they obtained records from units which responded only when the animal was "paying attention" to the sound source. These attention units appeared to be both interspersed amongst the others and segregated from them. We may venture to interpret these results by supposing that the units in question formed part of the systems, discussed above, responsible for the appropriate motor response to stimulation or the committing of items to memory, and so forth, or that they lay on the pathway to these systems. Thus they would be inactive even if impulses evoked by auditory stimulation were reaching the cortex, provided that the animal was not also attending to the stimuli.

There is another theoretical assumption for which we might reasonably seek a neurophysiological counterpart. We suppose that a selection of inputs from a variety of sources takes place by comparison with a fluctuating standard. This implies the existence of an undifferentiated structure with widespread connections with the rest of the central nervous system. We are tempted, on account of the evidence for the diffuseness of its input, to identify the brain stem reticular formation as this particular structure. Potentials may be evoked throughout this structure by excitation of various sensory systems (French, Amerongen, and Magoun, 1952; Starzl, Taylor, and Magoun, 1951), and various cortical structures (Bremer and Terzuolo, 1954; French, Hernández-Peón, and Livingston, 1955). Occlusive and facilitatory interaction between responses evoked in the reticular formation from very different sources have further been observed (Bremer and Terzuolo, 1952, 1954; French et al., 1955). Single unit studies demonstrating a convergence of input from several sources have also been reported (Amassian, 1952; Amassian and DeVito, 1954; Hernández-Peón and Hagbarth, 1955; Scheibel, Scheibel, Mollica, and Moruzzi, 1955). A similar conclusion, that the reticular formation is capable of acting as a nonspecific system, can be based on neuroanatomical evidence.

Scheibel and Scheibel (1958) state on the basis of their extensive histological study:

The degree of overlap of the collateral afferent plexuses is so great that it is difficult to see how any specificity of input can be maintained, rather it seems to integrate and vector a number of inputs.

We have also postulated that the fluctuating level correlates with states of arousal. Again the brain stem reticular formation seems well suited to fulfill this function. Its importance in the regulation of states of arousal has been demonstrated both through work involving lesions (Bremer, 1935; French, 1952; French and Magoun, 1952; Lindsley, Schreiner, Knowles, and Magoun, 1949) and stimulation of this structure (Moruzzi and Magoun, 1949; Segundo, Arana, and French, 1955). Recently Moruzzi (1960) has shown that the lower brain stem may play an important role in the initiation of sleep. It also seems likely that the thalamic reticular system is involved in the regulation of states of arousal. Large bilateral lesions of the anterior portion of this system may produce coma analogous to that produced by lesions of the mid-brain (French et al., 1952) although the depth of coma so produced is less profound. Stimulation of portions of this system has also been shown to produce either sleep or arousal depending on the parameters of stimulation (Akimoto, Yama-guchi, Okabe, Nakagawa, Nakamura, Abe, Torii, and Masahashi, 1956; Hess, 1954).

The work of Adametz (1959), Chow and Randell (1960), and Doty, Beck, and Kooi (1959), who demonstrated that with different operational techniques and with assiduous nursing care massive lesions of the mid-brain-reticular formation need not produce coma, should, however, be considered. Chow, Dement, and Mitchell (1959) found also that massive lesions in the thalamic reticular system need not produce coma. Until reasons for these discrepant results are found we must regard our conclusions as to the role of the reticular system in attention as tentative.

Whatever the explanation of the findings on lesions in the reticular formation may turn out to be, it seems that, if we are right, some diffuse and nonspecific system is necessary as a part of the mechanism subserving selective attention. Such a system should be found to have afferent connections from all discriminatory and perceptual systems. Through these connections it should be influenced to take up a variety of levels; the level at any one time corresponding with the level of the "highest" afferent message from the discriminatory mechanisms. On its efferent side such a nonspecific system should again be connected with all discriminatory and perceptual mechanisms. Through such connections it would signal to them its own level. If this level of the nonspecific system was above that of a particular discriminatory mechanism, no registration in memory of motor adjustment would take place, if such a discriminatory mechanism was stimulated. Consequently, only that discriminatory mechanism being activated whose level was equal to that of the diffuse system would not be affected. In this way the most important message to the organism will have been selected.

References

Adametz, J. H. Rate of recovery of functioning in cats with rostral reticular lesions. *J. Neurosurg.*, 1959, **16**, 85–98.

Akimoto, H., Yamaguchi, M., Okabe, K., Nakagawa, T., Nakamura, I., Abe, K., Torii, H., and Masahashi, I. On the sleep induced through electrical stimulation of dog thalamus. *Folia psychiat. neurol. Jap.*, 1956, **10**, 117–146.

Amassian, V. E. Interaction in the somatovisceral projection system. *Proc. Ass. Res. Nerv. Ment. Dis.*, 1952, **30**, 371–402.

Amassian, V. E., and DeVito, R. V. Unit activity in reticular formation and nearby structures. *J. Neurophysiol.*, 1954, **17**, 575–603.

Bradley, P. B., and Elkes, J. The effect of atropine, hyoscyamine, physostigmine and neostigmine on the electrical activity of the brain of the conscious cat. *J. Physiol.*, 1953, **120**, 14–15.

Bremer, F. Cerveau isolé et physiologie du sommeil. *CR Soc. Biol., Paris,* 1935, **118**, 1235–1242.

Bremer, F., and Terzuolo, C. Rôle de l'écorce cérébrale dans le processus physiologique du réveil. *Arch. int. Physiol.* 1952, **60**, 228–231.

Bremer, F., and Terzuolo, C. Contribution à l'étude des mécanismes physiologiques du maintien de l'activité vigile du cerveau. Interaction de la formation réticulée et de l'écorce cérébrale dans le processus des réveil. *Arch. inter. Physiol.*, 1954, **62**, 157–178.

Broadbent, D. E. The role of auditory localization in attention and memory span. *J. exp. Psychol.*, 1954, **47**, 191–196.

Broadbent, D. E. *Perception and communication.* London: Pergamon, 1958.

Cherry, E. C. Some experiments on the recognition of speech with one and with two ears. *J. Acoust. Soc. Amer.*, 1953, **25**, 975–979.

Chow, K. L., Dement, W. C., and Mitchell, S. A., Jr. Effects of lesions of the rostral thalamus on brain waves and behavior in cats. *EEG clin. Neurophysiol.*, 1959, **11**, 107–120.

Chow, K. L., and Randell, W. Learning and EEG studies of cats with lesions in the reticular formation. Paper read at the first annual meeting of Psychonomics Society, Chicago, 1960.

Deutsch, J. A. A new type of behaviour theory. *Brit. J. Psychol.*, 1953, **44**, 305–317.

Deutsch, J. A. A theory of insight, reasoning and latent learning. *Brit. J. Psychol.*, 1956, **47**, 115–125.

Deutsch, J. A. *The structural basis of behavior.* Chicago: Univer. Chicago Press, 1960.

Doty, R. W., Beck, E. C., and Kooi, R. A. Effect of brain-stem lesions on conditioned responses in cats. *Exp. Neurol.*, 1959, **1**, 360–385.

Egan, J. P., Carterette, E. C., and Thwing, E. J. Some factors affecting multichannel listening. *J. Acoust. Soc. Amer.*, 1954, **26**, 774–782.

French, J. D. Brain lesions associated with prolonged unconsciousness. *AMA Arch. Neurol. Psychiat.*, 1952, **68**, 727–740.

French, J. D., Amerongen, F. K., and Magoun, H. W. An activating system in brain stem of monkey. *AMA Arch. Neurol. Psychiat.*, 1952, **68**, 577–590.

French, J. D., Hernández-Peón, R., and Livingston, R. B. Projections from cortex to cephalic brain stem (reticular formation) in monkey. *J. Neurophysiol.*, 1955, **18**, 74–95.

French, J. D., and Magoun, H. W. Effects of chronic lesions in central cephalic brain stem of monkeys. *AMA Arch. Neurol. Psychiat.*, 1952, **68**, 591–604.

Galambos, R., Sheatz, G., and Vernier, V. G. Electrophysiological correlates of a conditioned response in cats. *Science*, 1956, **123**, 376–377.

Garcia-Austt, E., Bogacz, J., and Vanzulli, A. Significance of the photic stimulus on the evoked responses in man. In Delafresnaye (Ed.), *Brain mechanisms and learning*. Oxford: Blackwell, 1961. Pp. 603–626.

Gastaut, H. The brain stem and cerebral electrogenesis in relation to consciousness. In Delafresnaye (Ed.), *Brain mechanisms and consciousness*. Springfield, Ill.: Charles C Thomas, 1954. Pp. 249–283.

Goldberg, J. M., Diamond, I. T., and Neff, W. D. Auditory discrimination after ablation of temporal and insular cortex in cat. *Federat. Proc.*, 1957, **16**, 47–48.

Goldberg, J. M., Diamond, I. T., and Neff, W. D. Frequency discrimination after ablation of cortical projection areas of the auditory system. *Federat. Proc.*, 1958, **17**, 216–255.

Gray, J. A., and Wedderburn, A. A. I. Grouping strategies with simultaneous stimuli. *Quart. J. exp. Psychol.*, 1960, **12**, 180–184.

Hernández-Peón, R., Alcocer-Cuaron, C., Lavin, A., and Santibañez, G. Regulación centrifuga de la actividad électrica del bulbo olfactorio. Punta del Este, Uruguay: Primera Reunión Cientifica de Ciencias Fisiólogicas, 1957. Pp. 192–193.

Hernández-Peón, R., Guzman-Flores, C., Alcarez, H., and Fernandez-Guardiola, A. Sensory transmission in visual pathway during "attention" in unanaesthetized cats. *Acta neurol. Lat.-Amer.*, 1957, **3**, 1–8.

Hernández-Peón, R., and Hagbarth, K. Interaction between afferent and cortically induced reticular responses. *J. Neurophysiol.*, 1955, **18**, 44–55.

Hernández-Peón, R., and Scherrer, H. Habituation to acoustic stimuli in cochlear nucleus, *Federat. Proc.*, 1955, **14**, 71.

Hernández-Peón, R., Scherrer, H., and Jouvet, M. Modification of electric activity in cochlear nucleus during "attention" in unanaesthetized cats. *Science*, 1956, **123**, 331–332.

Hess, W. R. The diencephalic sleep centre. In *J. F. Delafresnaye* (Ed.), *Brain mechanisms and consciousness*. Springfield, Ill., Charles C Thomas, 1954. Pp. 117–136.

Hirsh, I. J. The relation between localization and intelligibility. *J. Acoust. Soc. Amer.*, 1950, **22**, 196–200.

Horn, G. Electrical activity of the cerebral cortex of the unanesthetized cat during attentive behavior. *Brain*, 1960, **83**, 57–76.

Howarth, C. I., and Ellis, R. The relative intelligibility threshold for one's own name compared with other names. *Quart. J. exp. Psychol.*, 1961, **13**, 236–239.

Hubel, D. H., Henson, C. O., Rupert, A., and Galambos, R. Attention units in the auditory cortex. *Science*, 1959, **129**, 1279–1280.

Hugelin, A., Dumont, S., and Paillas, N. Tympanic muscles and control of auditory input during arousal. *Science*, 1960, **131**, 1371–1372.

Lawrence, D. H. Acquired distinctiveness of cues: I. Transfer between discriminations on the basis of familiarity with the stimulus. *J. exp. Psychol.*, 1949, **39**, 770–784.

Lawrence, D. H. Acquired distinctiveness of cues: II. Selective association in a constant stimulus situation. *J. exp. Psychol.*, 1950, **40**, 175–188.

Lindsley, D. B., Schreiner, L. H., Knowles, W. B., and Magoun, H. W. Behavioral and EEG changes following chronic brain stem lesions in the cat. *EEG clin. Neurophysiol.*, 1949, **1**, 455–473.

Moray, N. Attention in dichotic listening: Affective cues and the influence of instructions. *Quart. J. exp. Psychol.,* 1959, **11,** 56–60.

Moruzzi, G. Synchronizing influences of the brain stem and the inhibitory mechanisms underlying the production of sleep by sensory stimulation. *Int. J. EEG clin. Neurophysiol.,* 1960, Suppl. No. 13, 231–256.

Moruzzi, G., and Magoun, H. W. Brain stem reticular formation and activation of the EEG. *EEG clin. Neurophysiol.,* 1949, **1,** 455–473.

Moushegian, G., Rupert, A., Marsh, J. T., and Galambos, R. Evoked cortical potentials in absence of middle ear muscles. *Science,* 1961, **133,** 582–583.

Naquet, R., Regis, H., Fischer-Williams, M., and Fernandez-Guardiola, A. Variation in the responses evoked by light along the specific pathways. *Brain,* 1960, **83,** 52–56.

Oswald, I., Taylor, A., and Treisman, M. Discrimination responses to stimulation during human sleep. *Brain,* 1960, **83,** 440–453.

Palestini, M., Davidovich, A., and Hernández-Peón, R. Functional significance of centrifugal influences upon the retina. *Act. neurol. Lat.-Amer.,* 1959, **5,** 113–131.

Peters, R. W. Competing messages: The effect of interfering messages upon the reception of primary messages. *USN Sch. Aviat. Med. res. Rep.,* 1954, Project No. NM 001 064.01.27.

Poulton, E. C. Two-channel listening, *J. exp. Psychol.,* 1953, **46,** 91–96.

Scheibel, M. E., and Scheibel, A. Structural substrates for integrative patterns in the brain stem reticular core. In H. H. Jasper, L. D. Proctor, R. S. Knighton, S. Roberts, W. C. Noshay, C. William, and R. T. Costello (Eds.), *Reticular formation of the brain.* Boston: Little, Brown, 1958. Pp. 31–55.

Scheibel, M. E., Scheibel, A., Mollica, A., and Moruzzi, G. Convergence and interaction of afferent impulses on single units of reticular formation. *J. Neurophysiol.,* 1955, **18,** 309–331.

Segundo, J. P., Arana, R., and French, J. D. Behavioral arousal by stimulation of the brain in monkey. *J. Neurosurg.,* 1955, **12,** 601–613.

Sharpless, S., and Jasper, H. Habituation of the arousal reaction. *Brain,* 1956, **79,** 655–678.

Sokolov, E. N. Neuronal models and the orienting reflex. In Mary A. B. Brazier (Ed.), *The central nervous system and behavior: Transactions of the conference.* New York: Josiah Macy, Jr. Foundation, 1960. Pp. 187–276.

Spieth, W., Curtis, J. F., and Webster, J. C. Responding to one of two simultaneous messages. *J. Acoust. Soc. Amer.,* 1954, **26,** 391–396.

Starzl, T. E., Taylor, C. W., and Magoun, H. W. Collateral afferent excitation of reticular formation of brain stem. *J. Neurophysiol.,* 1951, **14,** 479–496.

Thompson, W. R., and Solomon, L. M. Spontaneous pattern discrimination in the rat. *J. comp. physiol. Psychol.,* 1954, **46,** 281–287.

Treisman, A. M. Contextual cues in selective listening. *Quart. J. exp. Psychol.,* 1960, **12,** 242–248.

Voronin, L. G., and Sokolov, E. N. Cortical mechanisms of the orienting reflex and its relation to the conditioned reflex. *Int. J. EEG clin. Neurophysiol.,* 1960, Suppl. No. 13, 335–346.

Webster, J. C., and Thomson, P. O. Responding to both of two overlapping messages. *J. Acoust. Soc. Amer.,* 1954, **26,** 396–402.

The Response of Reticular Units to Repetitive Stimuli

M. E. SCHEIBEL
AND A. B. SCHEIBEL

Reprinted from Arch. Ital. Biol, 1965, Vol. 103, pp. 279–299.

Introduction

In their study of habituation of the arousal reaction, Sharpless and Jasper (23) offered a significant physiological substrate for clinical observations that the individual, exposed to a non-conditioned, repetitive stimulus, shows progressive modification of its response. If the stimulus continues in unchanged form, the response becomes increasingly rudimentary and may disappear entirely. This process of habituation, adaptation, or attenuation of response has been sought and studied in a number of neural systems including the auditory (8), visual and proprioceptive (17), in the reticular formation (23), in individual units of somatosensory cortex (4), septal and hypothalamic nuclei (7), crustacean visual system (24) and frog tectum (12).

Responses of individual reticular units to repetitive stimulation seem to have been less adequately studied. With the exception of a passing reference by Huttenlocher to "attention units" (9), and some consideration of the attenuative properties of mesencephalic reticular elements by Bell and coworkers (2), we are unaware of any detailed studies besides our own (21).

It would therefore seem highly desirable to examine the properties of individual reticular units when exposed to iterative stimuli under a range of physiological conditions to determine whether behavior of the system complex (23) reflects the characteristics of its components.

The results of this investigation indicate that reticular units: a) show progressive decrement in response (habituation) to a stimulus repeated slowly over time; b) that underlying physiological processes such as sleep-wakefulness cycles may critically affect habituation of the unit; c) that an element habituated to one afferent stimulus remains accessible to other systems converging upon it and d) that pharmacological agents such as barbiturates and LSD 25 strongly affect unit patterns of response to the iterative stimulus.

Methods

The results to be discussed are drawn from analysis of approximately 90 bulbar and pontine units recorded in a series of 40 adult cats. Animals were anaesthetized with ether and tracheotomized, after which fine polyethylene catheters were inserted into at least one foreleg vein for subsequent drug injection. The system was kept patent by repeated small injections of warm Ringer or saline solution. After slipping a modified Sherringtonian electrode over one sciatic nerve, the dorsal surface of medulla and caudal pons was exposed. Varying amounts of posterior lobe of cerebellum were aspirated to facilitate exposure. Sigmoid (sensori-motor) cortex was then exposed over an area of 1 cm² and protected under warm paraffin oil. All potential pain and pressure points, and the cut skin edges were heavily infiltrated with procain after which the animal was maintained under repeated small doses of Flaxedil, artificially respired, and allowed to blow off ether over a period of 90 to 120 minutes. Body temperature, pulse rate, and pupil size were periodically monitored along with the EEG, led off bilaterally from stainless steel calvareal screws.

Single unit discharges were recorded with stainless steel needles insulated with Insulex except at the tip and electrolytically sharpened to tip diameters of 2 to 4 micra. In our experience, tips of this size are adequate for extracellular recording from elements of all cell populations likely to be found in the brain stem reticular formation. Potentials were led off in the usual manner through cathode followers to a. c. coupled preamplifiers (Grass), visualized on a double beam cathodo ray oscilloscope (Electron Tube Corp.), audio monitored when necessary, and recorded on 35 mm film with a Grass kymograph camera. The position of the recording tip was ultimately identified by depositing a trace of iron from the bare point and developing it with the Prussian blue method after which the blocks of tissue were fixed, sectioned, and stained by a rapid alcoholic silver method which allowed identification of our recording sites on the same day as the experiment (20).

During the course of the study we differentiated sleeping from waking states entirely on the basis of the EEG since the animal was immobilized with Flaxedil. By awake, we mean a preparation showing varying amounts of 8 to 11 per second alpha activity interspersed with periods of low voltage fast activity (presumably depending on the degree of vigilance at the moment), and moderately small pupils. Under the conditions of the experiment, we ran the risk of confusing a waking activated record with that of paradoxical (rhombencephalic) sleep (10). In our experience on the rare (two) occasions when we did recognize the latter, pupils appeared somewhat larger and the pulse was appreciably slower. Attempts to use the blood pressure as a further measure of rhombencephalic sleep gave erratic data but the absence of any significant fall, except when the preparation showed early deterioration, gave further credence to the almost complete absence of the paradoxical sleep stage during these experiments.

Accordingly, we use the term "sleeping stage" to refer to a preparation whose EEG showed the characteristic high voltage slow wave patterns frequently considered to represent the thalamic phase of sleep (10). All phenomena described as characteristic of the sleeping preparation will refer to this type of (slow wave) sleep.

Parameters of stimulation for sciatic nerve never exceeded 2 V in amplitude, 0.5 msec in pulse width and were limited to a maximal frequency of 1/sec. In 3 chronic freely moving preparations, these parameters were never found to cause obvious reactions of discomfort in the animal, nor did the monitored EEG reveal evidence of increasing synchronization or enhanced activation. Pompeiano and Swett (14) have reported EEG effects following cutaneous nerve stimulation of as little as 0.12 V. However, 6/sec frequencies were used and their records indicate a latency of 200 to 400 msec before development of EEG effects. At the voltage frequency parameters used in these studies, we have never noticed similar effects.

Results

During the course of these experiments we investigated the behavior of 133 units recorded at bulbar (51 units), pontine (39 units) and mesencephalic (19 units) levels, plus a smaller number located in pulvinar (11 units), lateral geniculate (7 units) and posterior ventral nuclear complex (6 units) to slow repetitive stimuli. The substance of this report concerns itself with the behavior of the 90 units led from bulbar and pontine reticular formation sites, in response to sciatic shocks repeated at 1 per second frequencies and to short bursts of cortical stimuli (100 per second, 12 to 20 shocks) administered at 5 to 20 second intervals.

The establishment of such units as reticular has been dealt with elsewhere (19) but depends, in part, on visual orientation of the electrode, demonstration of convergence of (bilateral) sensory modalities upon the unit isolated, clearcut inhibitory (occasionally facilitatory) response upon surface positive polarization of anterior lobe of cerebellum followed by marked rebound phenomena, and confirmation of position of the electrode tip by histological control.

The behavior of such reticular units when exposed to repetitive stimulation will be considered under the following categories: 1) response to sciatic stimulation in the waking state, 2) response to sciatic stimulation in the state of slow wave sleep, 3) response to cortical stimulation, 4) response to sciatic stimulation under barbiturate at varying dose levels, and 5) response to sciatic stimulation under the hallucinogen LSD 25.

1. Response to Sciatic Stimulation in the Waking State

Figure 1 illustrates the results of sciatic stimulation upon a typical "naive" unit of the medullary reticular formation, and upon the same unit subsequently habituated.* When the unit, firing "spontaneously" at a rate of 1 to 4 dis-

---

* A satisfactory descriptive term for that unit whose response pattern has been changed by previous exposure to the same stimulus is not easily selected. We will use the term "habituated" when referring to reticular units showing these changes, realizing that the word has somewhat different connotations when applied at the organismic level.

charges per second, is exposed to repetitive sciatic stimuli (2 V, 0.5 msec, 1/sec) there is marked enhancement of firing rate to values of 40 to 70 per second initially. Highest frequencies are achieved after the stimulus artefact with progressive decrement prior to the next stimulus as can be seen in *C* and *D* of Figure 1 and in *A* of Figure 8. Maximal firing frequencies are usually achieved within the first 3 or 4 responses to the iterative stimulus following which there is gradual decrease in the number of spike responses. In Figure 1 *D,* the driven response, although still visible, has almost reached background frequency levels. The main difference from the latter state rests in the residual tendency toward grouping of the few spike discharges in the early portion of each interstimulus period. Figure 2 shows graphically that the process of unit

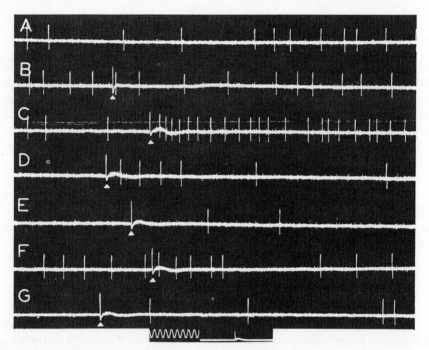

FIGURE 1. Habituation of a reticular unit to repetitive sciatic stimulation.

This figure summarizes the response of a typical bulbo-pontine reticular unit to repetitive sensory stimulation in the "naive" state and in the partly habituated state.

A. "Spontaneous" firing pattern. *B.* Unit is non-responsive to single cortical stimulus (2 V, 1 msec). *C.* First response of the "naive" unit to a series of sciatic stimuli (2 V, 1/sec, 0.5 msec) started at this point. *D.* Unit response pattern 2 minutes (120 shocks) after inception of stimulus. *E.* Unit response pattern 3 minutes (180 shocks) after inception of stimulus. *F.* After a 3-minute rest period, sciatic stimulus begins again (same parameters as before) and unit shows an abbreviated response. *G.* 0.5 minute later (30 shocks) unit is again virtually non-responsive to stimulus. The habituation effect appears to have been achieved approximately 6 times as fast on the second run as on the first.

In this and in all following spike figures, calibration is 60 cycles per second and 100 μV. Darts indicate stimulus artefacts and arrows, where present, indicate the same unit on two successive lines for orientation purposes where strips are continuous. The tips of some spike discharges have been retouched.

habituation appears to follow a cyclic pattern which is impressed on the overall descending curve. The cycles have an average period of about 4.5 seconds and the overall curve appears to approach asymptote between 1 and 2 minutes after inception of the stimulus. Figure 1 *E* shows that after 3 minutes of stimulation (180 shocks) the unit has apparently become unresponsive to the sciatic stimulus and may be considered habituated.

If stimulation is stopped at this point, the unit returns to its prestimulation "spontaneous" firing pattern over periods of from 10 to 60 seconds. If sciatic stimulation is started again after a resting period, driving effects of a more rudimentary nature are seen and the unit more rapidly traverses the habituation curve. In Figure 1 *F,* sciatic stimulation is reinstituted after a 3 minute rest and the unit is initially driven to frequencies of about 30 per second. This is about one half the frequency initially achieved by the "naive" unit. The total number of spikes per stimulus is now smaller and as seen in Figure 2 (dashed line), the habituation process appears essentially complete after 30 seconds.

As long as the animal continues electroencephalographically awake and in good physiological condition, this procedure can be repeated at intervals.

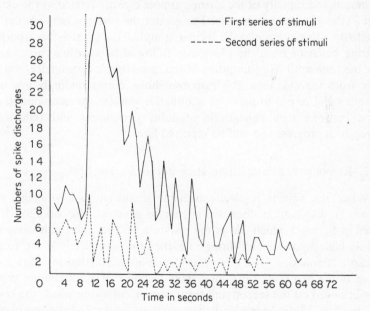

FIGURE 2. Contrast in habituation patterns of a bulbar reticular unit exposed to repetitive sciatic stimuli for the first time, and after previous exposure.

In both curves, the first nine seconds represent "spontaneous" firing. Sciatic stimulation starts at the tenth second indicated by the vertical dotted line. The continuous line graphs the response of the reticular unit exposed for the first time to repetitive sciatic stimulation (2 V, 1/sec, 0.5 msec). The dashed line follows the course of the same unit, exposed to a second series of repetitive sciatic stimuli (same parameters) following a 3-minute rest period. The oscillation-like variations in the number of spike discharges per stimulus during the period of habituation seem characteristic for this process.

In each block of reticular unit responses there is a smaller initial driving response, and a more rapid return toward asymptote, assuming that stimulus parameters remain the same and the interval between blocks of stimuli is not appreciably lengthened. In some well-habituated units, the ultimate response pattern resembles strip *B* in Figure 8 where there is no discernible response even to the first of a series of sciatic stimuli.

As increasing time is allowed to elapse between blocks of sciatic stimuli, the unit becomes progressively less habituated, and upon resumption of sciatic stimulation after 10 to 30 minutes, unit response is initially more active. Although there is wide variation in reticular unit recovery periods, and the number of units that can be followed over sufficiently long periods is limited, our experience indicates that intervals of from 30 to 150 minutes appear adequate for return of full responsiveness to most reticular units. About 75% of reticular elements recorded with the technique described above show some variation of the kind of habituation phenomena just described.

If the parameters of stimulation are charged during the course of the habituation process, unit firing behavior changes in the direction of the prestimulus period, as habituation appears to be partially or completely lost. The amount and rapidity of the change appear directly related to the extent of change in the stimulus parameters. The greater the variance between the newly selected stimulus pattern and the former stimulus, the greater the departure in unit firing behavior from the previously followed habituation curve, and the longer the time until its resumption. If the new stimulus parameters vary only slightly from the old, then unit response shows correspondingly less change and more rapid return to previous habituation curves. An examination of the relation between such changes in stimulus parameters and reticular unit response is in progress and will be reported later.

2. Response to Sciatic Stimulation in the Sleeping State

When the animal is electroencephalographically asleep (high voltage slow wave), habituation does not appear to develop. The situation is summarized in Figure 3 which shows the response of 2 reticular units, one with a relatively high "spontaneous" firing rate, the other completely silent, to repetitive sciatic stimulation. There is no evidence of habituation in either case. In the case of the first unit, a maximal spike response of 50 discharges per stimulus is achieved on the second and third stimuli, following which the response curve drops to 35 discharges and then oscillates unevenly between 36 and 54 discharges per sciatic stimulus. Variation in the response sequence is greater than in the wakeful state and a cyclic organization of successive responses is less obvious. In the case of the unit initially silent in the unstimulated state, it can be seen that maximal unit response of 20 discharges per stimulus is achieved during the third and fourth stimuli following which the discharge pattern oscillates between 10 and 20 spikes per stimulus in a pattern but little more regular than the one above.

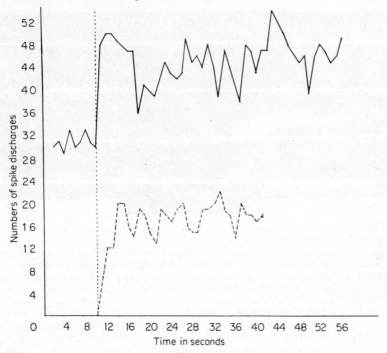

FIGURE 3. Lack of habituation in 2 bulbar reticular units during slow wave sleep.

The first 9 seconds trace the unit during the unstimulated condition. Sciatic stimulation (2 V, 1/sec, 0.5 msec) begins at the tenth second (dotted vertical line). The solid line traces the course of a unit whose "spontaneous" firing rate is rather high, averaging 30 discharges per second. The dashed line graphs the pattern of a unit which shows no firing activity during the unstimulated state.

3. Response to Cortical Stimulation

In almost all cases we have found that cortical modulation of reticular units can only be demonstrated with rapid bursts of cortical stimuli (18). Strip *B* of Figure 1 indicates that individual cortical stimuli (2 V, 1 msec), unlike sciatic shocks, are totally without effect on reticular units. Groups of 10 or more stimuli at frequencies of about 100 per second are very much more effective in initiating massive driving responses of many reticular units (Fig. 4) although about 20% of reticular units seem completely inaccessible at all times to cortical driving. In Figure 4, an almost total lack of response of the unit to sciatic stimulation indicates an advanced degree of habituation to this input. A group of 17 stimuli (1 V, 100/sec, 1 msec) applied to anterior sigmoid gyrus initiates an active reticular response. The unit is driven to a frequency of about 60/sec following a latent period of approximately 50 msec. During the period of cortical stimulation (170 msec) there is little or no change in unit behavior as it can be followed through the stimulus artefact. In strip *D,* cortex is again stimulated with 24 shocks delivered with the same parameters. The reticular unit is actively inhibited during this period. After a

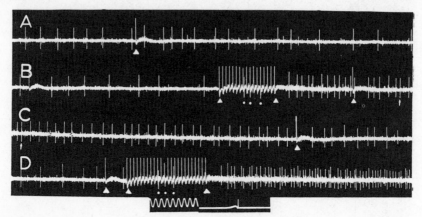

FIGURE 4. Responsiveness of a bulbar reticular unit, habituated to repetitive sciatic stimuli, to short bursts of cortical stimuli.

Strip A and the first half of strip B demonstrate the non-responsiveness of the unit to repetitive sciatic stimulation (2 V, 1/sec, 0.5 msec) following habituation to this stimulus modality. In strip B, the unit is exposed to a short burst of cortical stimulation (anterior sigmoid, 17 shocks, 1 V, 100/sec, 1 msec) which exerts a marked driving effect upon the unit. A similar, although somewhat longer duration stimulation (24 shocks) has an even more intense driving effect on the unit which reaches firing frequencies of over 100/sec. The sciatic stimulus which continues during this period remains without effect except for a brief period of inhibition immediately following the shock artefact. Dots indicate the reticular spike discharges occurring during the period of cortical stimulation. In the case of this unit, as with most reticular units studied, cortical stimulation produced a temporary inhibitory effect on the unit discharge pattern during the actual period of stimulation.

quiet period of about 50 msec following the last cortical shock, the driving response is seen once more during which firing frequencies as high as 120 to 140 per second are achieved.

Although the cortical stimulation burst is a technically unwieldy stimulus to handle in the repetitive mode, a number of runs have been made during which groups of 10 to 20 stimuli (100/sec, 1 V, 1 msec) were applied to sigmoid cortex every 2 seconds. Under these conditions, habituation of the reticular unit to this stimulus was also achieved though after longer periods averaging about 10 minutes to asymptote.

Brief periods (1/4 to 1 second) of surface positive polarization when applied to sensorimotor cortex regularly, every 5 to 20 seconds, also drove about 60% of bulbar reticular units and resulted in eventual habituation after periods of from 5 to 20 minutes. Because of several interesting collateral features of this type of stimulation, this part of the program remains under investigation and will be reported later.

4. Response to Repetitive Sciatic Stimuli Under Barbiturate

The nature of reticular unit response to repetitive stimulation under barbiturate depends significantly on the dosage used. With anaesthetizing doses of 30 mg per kg or more, there is partial or complete cessation of "spontaneous" reticular firing. Complete unit silence usually reflects higher dosage levels or greater individual sensitivity on the part of the animal. In this condition it may be impossible to drive the unit with any mode or intensity of stimulus for periods of from 30 to 60 minutes. The first signs of lightening of the anaesthetic level usually consist in the appearance of occasional "spontaneous" discharges and sporadic response to repeated sciatic stimuli.

The response to small and intermediate dose levels of Nembutal (up to 10 mg per kg) is characteristic and often quite dramatic. Figure 5 shows a typical group of reticular responses to sciatic stimulation (2 V, 1/sec, 0.5

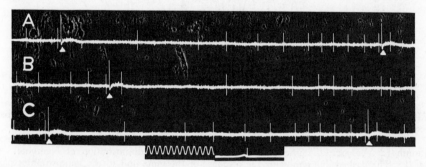

FIGURE 5. Paradoxical driving effect of repetitive sciatic stimuli on reticular unit after administration of barbiturate.

Following administration of Nembutal (10 mg/kg) the usual firing pattern of the unit is significantly changed in that slowest firing frequencies occur in the first few hundred milliseconds following each sciatic stimulus. Frequencies then increase and achieve their maximal rate just before the next sciatic shock.

msec). Following each stimulus there is a silent period of from 200 to 500 milliseconds. Unit firing begins thereafter and may achieve levels of 30 or more per second in the last 100 or 200 msec period before the next sciatic shock. In effect, the arrangement of the spike firing sequence is the reverse of that in the non-nembutalized preparation (compare strips A and C of Fig. 8) and is therefore called a paradoxical response. The possible significance of this pattern will be discussed below.

Figure 6 epitomizes unit response to sciatic stimulation at 2 epochs following administration of a 10 mg per kilo dose of Nembutal. Sciatic stimulation (2 V, 1/sec, 0.5 msec) is started 10 minutes after intravenous drug administration and the ensuing record is similar to that of the sleeping animal in that no habituation occurs. However, there is relatively less initial increment in spike discharge rate, and the fluctuations of unit response appear wider, approaching 15 to 20 discharges per cycle. This response fluctuation or Nembutal "rolling" effect is also observed in the spontaneously active unit under light Nembutal and clearly relates to some action of the barbiturate on unit firing control mechanisms, whether intraneural or extraneural (see discussion).

As barbiturate dose levels are fractionally increased, the number of spontaneous or driven unit responses progressively decreases, culminating in complete silence as described above for doses above 10 mg per kilo.

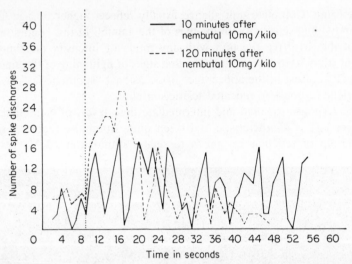

FIGURE 6. Effect of small doses of barbiturate on the habituation response of a bulbar reticular unit.

The solid line represents the response of a bulbar reticular unit to repetitive sciatic stimuli (2 V, 1/sec, 0.5 msec) 10 minutes after I. V. administration of Nembutal 10 mg/kg. The dashed line represents the response of the same unit to the same stimulus pattern 120 minutes after administration of the drug. The dotted vertical line indicates onset of the repetitive stimulus. In the first instance, habituation of the unit response does not develop. In the second instance, it does. The solid line graph also illustrates how small amounts of barbiturate enhance the cyclic variation in unit response to a repetitive stimulus. In this case, the variation in number of spike discharges between pairs of stimulus-response sequences averaged 12 discharges. This is more than twice the response variation in the non-barbiturized preparation.

5. Response to Sciatic Stimulation Under LSD 25

Small amounts of LSD 25 (0.05 mg) injected intravenously produce an interesting change in the character of the majority of reticular unit discharge patterns (14 out of 20 units) within 7 to 10 minutes of the injection. In the case of the spontaneously firing unit, the responses become increasingly irregular in time and begin to appear in bursts or clusters of 3 to 6 spikes presented at frequencies of 30 to 60 per second. When sciatic stimulation (2 V, 1/sec, 0.5 msec) is begun, the response pattern continues but the bursts of spike discharges are somewhat longer in duration, containing 4 to 10 spikes per stimulus. These bursts may follow closely upon the stimulus (Fig. 7) or may appear during the interstimulus intervals. Additionally, between 30 and 40% of sciatic shocks are without apparent effect upon the unit. No habituation occurs during the LSD effects which may last for 1 to 4 hours. As the drug effect wanes, the number of "spontaneous" burst-like responses per unit time decreases while the number of individual spike responses increases until the original "spontaneous" firing pattern is again resumed.

Upon occasion we have noticed a similar tendency of bulbo-pontine re-

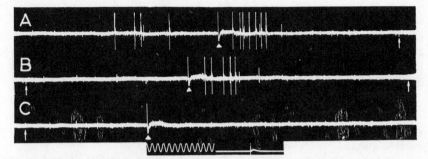

FIGURE 7. Effect of LSD 25 on reticular unit response to sciatic stimulation.

Following I. V. administration of 0.05 mg of LSD 25, the behavior of the majority of bulbo-pontine reticular units is markedly altered. Strip A shows that the responses of such units are quite characteristically grouped into short bursts, whether "spontaneous" or evoked. The first 4 responses are grouped somewhat loosely into a "spontaneously derived" burst while the group of 7 discharges that follow apparently represent a response to the sciatic stimulus (dart) which is repeated once per second (2 V, 0.5 msec). The next sciatic stimulus provokes a similar response while the stimulus following that produces no response by the unit. This highly erratic burst-type discharge pattern under LSD 25 is typical for the majority of bulbar reticular units.

ticular unit firing to be characterized by brief discrete bursts rather than by the more usual continuous trains of discharges, upon administration of small amounts of chloralose. However, under these conditions, the unit was invariably responsive to stimuli such as sciatic shocks rather than unpredictably so as with LSD 25.

Of the 6 remaining units out of our experience with 20, which did not respond with erratic burst type discharges to LSD 25 in the presence or absence of sciatic stimulation, 4 became completely nonresponsive after administration of the drug, and 2 showed no obvious changes in their firing pattern, both in the unstimulated and the stimulated state.

6. Cessation of Stimulation in the Partly Habituated Unit

When the iterative stimulus is abruptly stopped before habituation of unit response is complete, 80% of units (12 out of 15) show an interesting phenomenon suggesting that some degree of time-locked patterning develops in unit firing, even after as few as 30 to 40 stimulus shocks (sciatic stimuli, 2 V, 1/sec, 0.5 msec). An example of this phenomenon is shown in Figure 9. Following cessation of the sciatic stimulus to which the unit was still somewhat responsive, a definite bunching of spike discharges continued to be evident approximately once each second for from 3 to 6 seconds. However, the spike "response" to the first missed stimulus reached maximal firing frequency 300 msec later, rather than in the first or second 100 millisecond period as is usual for the reticular unit response to sciatic stimuli. Maximal "response" to the second missed stimulus showed further shift, occurring in the fourth 100 msec period, while the third "response" was maximal 500 msec after the missed

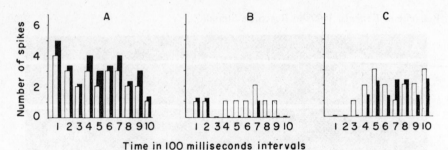

Time in 100 milliseconds intervals

FIGURE 8. Histogram comparing firing activity of a bulbar reticular neuron during 2 consecutive 1-second periods under varying conditions.

The same stimulus (sciatic nerve, 2 V, 1/sec, 0.5 msec) is used in all three. In each case, the white bars represent the first of the two consecutive runs; the black bars, the second.

A. Represents the number of spike responses in the 10 consecutive 100-msec periods following the sciatic stimulus in the unhabituated reticular unit. B. Illustrates the same sequence for 2 consecutive 1-second periods in the habituated unit. In C, Nembutal, 10 mg/kg had been administered I. V. 15 minutes earlier. This pair of 1-second spike sequences illustrates the "paradoxical" response with the spike firing at its lowest ebb (smallest number per 100-msec period) just after the stimulus and achieving maximal response much later in the interstimulus period.

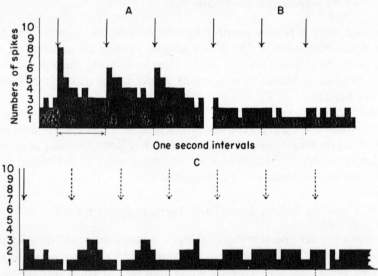

One second intervals

FIGURE 9. Histogram illustrating 3 epochs in the process of habituation and dishabituation.

A. Illustrates the first three exposures of a bulbar reticular unit to repetitive sciatic stimulation (2 V, 1/sec, 0.5 msec) marked by the solid vertical arrows above. B. Illustrates the apparent non-responsiveness of the unit habituated to the stimulus over a period of 60 shocks. C. Illustrates a frequently noted phenomenon in the partly habituated reticular unit immediately after the repetitive stimulus is stopped. The last sciatic shock, marked by the solid vertical arrow, is accompanied by a moderate increase in spike discharges. At the times of the first three missed sciatic shocks (dashed vertical arrows) there is enhancement of unit discharge as if the shock had actually been administered, though with increasing latency. Thus the response to the first missed shock is maximal after 300 msec, that to the second, after 400 msec, and that to the third, after 500 msec. There is no further evidence of time-locked firing sequences after this.

stimulus. In one case, following 75 sciatic stimuli, a pontine unit showed 6 consecutive "responses," the "responsive burst" occurring almost 750 msec after the sixth missed stimulus. The effects of the sleep-wakefulness cycle on this phenomenon are under investigation.

Discussion

The conditions in this initial group of experiments were rigorously limited to allow us to determine, in as simple a context as possible, whether habituation of bulbo-pontine reticular units could be demonstrated, and if so, what the general features of the response might be.

Two stimulation sites were selected since earlier work (19) had shown these to be among the most effective for influencing the behavior of maximal numbers of reticular elements. The sciatic nerve represented a broadly effective, if shot gun method for stimulating a majority of reticular units from a peripheral site. No differentiation among fiber populations in this mixed nerve was made and it is likely that a combination of types I, II, and III fibers were stimulated. However, the relatively low stimulating voltages (1–2 V) and fairly brief pulse durations (0.5 msec) employed together with the rapid rise times of our essentially square wave stimulus pulses suggest that the smaller, poorly myelinated or unmyelinated components of the type III population were less fully represented than the larger fibers. The communications by Pompeiano and Swett (15, 16) should be consulted for a discussion of some of these problems. Since the small fiber group is largely limited to the lateral division of the dorsal root and to the spino-thalamic projection, it seems likely that most of our reticular unit driving effects came from collaterals and/or terminals of spino-cervico-thalamic (5) and spino-reticular (3, 13, 19) systems since there is no evidence of reticulo-petal collaterals from the medial lemniscal system (3, 19, 22, etc.). Analysis of the effects of repetitive stimulation of individual muscle and cutaneous nerves upon the same reticular units is clearly indicated.

Our mode of cortical stimulation (100/sec, 1 V, 0.5 to 1 msec, 10 to 20 shock trains) was also grossly unphysiological. However, it served a purpose by providing a readily measured and monitored technique for activating a maximal number of units beneath the stimulating electrodes. Utilization of the less-artefact-laden technique of cortical polarization seems indicated for more extensive analyses of this sort and is being used in ongoing investigations.

The demonstration of habituation to repetitive sensory stimulation in a significant number of bulbar and pontine reticular units raises questions as to the mechanisms involved. Habituation has been described in a number of brain stem, subcortical, and cortical centers, but seldom in the units of primary sensory systems. Where the gracile-cuneate recordings of Perl, Whitlock, and Gentry (13) indicate habituation, their points of stimulation were found largely limited to the periphery of receptive fields, suggesting possibilities for convergent circuitry in sensory nuclei.

As a working hypothesis, we suggest, with Bell and coworkers (2) that habituation arises outside of primary afferent systems and is in fact related to multisynaptic linkages characterized by significant degrees of convergence and integration. Several factors seem to point to its genesis in a dynamic interplay between facilitatory and inhibitory components which apparently are differentially affected by physiological and pharmacological states.

Although there is some variation in the number of spikes discharged per unit time by any "spontaneously" firing reticular unit, the habituation curve seems characterized (Fig. 2) by oscillatory variations of at least 10 discharges per second in amplitude and 4.5 seconds in period. As the curve approaches asymptote, the rhythmic fluctuations in spike frequency decrease, perhaps as inhibitory damping becomes more active.

Short bursts of cortical stimulation are interesting in that unit firing activity, depending on ongoing firing rates, is moderately to profoundly inhibited during the actual period of stimulation (Fig. 4). There is an additional quiet period of at least 50 msec before the massive facilitation of unit firing becomes apparent, resembling in many respects the intense rebound phenomena that follow cerebellar inhibition of reticular unit activity (19).

There is noticeable similarity in reticular unit response to repetitive sensory stimuli under conditions of slow wave sleep and light barbiturate anaesthesia. In both cases, habituation to the stimulus does not occur and there is continuous, often enhanced firing variability from stimulus to stimulus. Absence of habituation and increase in the cyclic swing of unit responsiveness both seem to imply change in the balance of factors controlling cell responsiveness, possibly a decrease in the level of inhibitory tone. Huttenlocher (9) has suggested an increase in excitability of many brain stem units during slow wave sleep while Evarts (6) points to the increased range of reticular unit responsiveness during wakefulness as evidence for enhanced activity of inhibitory mechanisms.

In the case of light doses of barbiturate, it would appear that certain inhibitory systems are selectively inactivated, initially, as evidenced by loss of habituation phenomena. Indeed both animals and man may go through a transient phase of excitement during early stages of barbiturate anaesthesia. On the other hand, it appears that certain types of inhibitory activity may be enhanced by barbiturate as evidenced by the high degree of spike firing suppression in the period immediately after each stimulus (Fig. 5 and strip C of Fig. 8). With increasing amounts of the drug, spike firing becomes more erratic, decreases in total amount, and finally ceases altogether. At this point we must assume that facilitatory (driving) mechanisms have also failed. The structural locus for these developments remains unknown. Recent investigations of Løyning, Oshima and Yokota (11) on monosynaptic spinal reflex pathways suggest that "barbiturates act mainly on the afferent nerve terminals by reducing their spike amplitude resulting in less transmitter release and a reduced synaptic potential" (p. 425). Although there is, as yet, no similar evidence in the reticular formation, the Golgi method reveals great structural similarity between terminations of the large (primary afferent) monosynaptic fibers in the cord, and many of the terminals reaching bulbo-pontine reticular cells (22). On this basis, we might hypothesize that the progressive failure of the subsumed inhibitory and facilitatory systems projecting upon the reticular cell was due in large measure to decreasing availability of synaptic transmitter substances. Following this reasoning, if we then assume that the paradoxical driving effect discussed above is due to delayed resynthesis of the facilitatory transmitter, it should be possible to remove all unit response either by fractional increase in barbiturate dosage (which has been done) or by small progressive increments in the frequency of the stimulus which the reticular unit is asked to follow.

Unit response to LSD 25 is characterized by burst type discharges which may or may not follow the sensory (sciatic) stimulus. The fact that this paroxysm-like activity of the reticular element may be seen without sensory driving recalls recent data of Adey (1) suggesting that LSD 25 may trigger EEG seizure activity in hippocampus. The addition of repetitive sensory stimulation increases the total number of such unit bursts. Those that clearly follow the stimulus seem somewhat longer in duration and contain larger numbers of spikes (Fig. 7), yet only 60% of sciatic stimuli produce an answering reticular

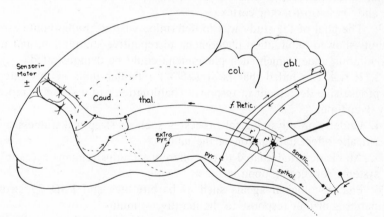

FIGURE 10. Schematic diagram showing a few of the axon circuit systems possibly involved in the interacting facilitatory-inhibitory mechanisms underlying processes of habituation.

Bulbo-pontine reticular cells, r^1 and r^2, of the sort from which the above recordings were probably derived, receive sensory information from the periphery via collaterals and/or terminals from spinoreticular (spretic.) and spinothalamic (spthal.) fibers. Descending impulses from higher centers reach the cells over components of the pyramidal (pyr.) tract, through multisynaptic cortico-caudate (caud.) and extra-pyramidal (extra pyr.) loops and via cerebellofugal systems driven by cortical, extra-pyramidal, reticular, vestibular, etc., mechanisms. In addition, the individual components of the reticular formation play upon each other, adding to the complexity of the polysynaptic mechanisms involved.

burst. It would seem as if LSD 25 partially decouples the reticular response from the sensory input. The known clinical effects of this drug include distortions and misinterpretations of perceptions, disturbances which might be expected if the usual neural equivalents of known sensory inputs had become erratic and unpredictable.

Insufficiency of data limits us to a phenomenological analysis of reticular unit function, nor is it even possible to state whether the interplay of inhibitory and facilitatory effects discussed above rely mainly on metabolic processes within the individual neuron, or relate significantly to the circuit arrangements within which the cell finds itself. The latter possibility motivates inclusion of Figure 10 which shows a grossly oversimplified scheme of some connections relating to 2 reticular cells of the type from which we may have been recording. The multiplicity and heterogenous nature of the contributing systems offer a significant substrate of possibilities within which the effects described above might eventually be understood.

Summary

1. The behavior of 90 bulbar and pontine units have been studied in the reticular formation of 40 cats subjected to repetitive stimulation of sciatic nerve and/or sensori-motor cortex.

2. The goal of the study was to determine whether bulbo-pontine reticular units showed habituation phenomena to repetitive stimulation, and if so, the conditions under which such phenomena could be demonstrated.

3. It was concluded that most (75%) reticular units in this category show progressive decrement in response (habituation) to a stimulus repeated slowly over time.

4. Underlying physiological processes such as sleep-wakefulness cycles may critically affect habituation of the unit.

5. An element habituated to one afferent stimulus remains accessible to other systems converging upon it.

6. Pharmacological agents such as barbiturates and LSD 25 strongly affect patterns of unit response to the iterative stimulus.

7. Variations in unit responsiveness under these conditions are discussed in the context of changes in the balance of facilitatory and inhibitory forces playing upon the unit which normally maintain it at some level of dynamic equilibrium.

Acknowledgements

We wish to thank Dr. K. Tasaki, Dept. of Physiology, Sendai University Medical School, Japan, for help with some of the early experiments.

Bibliography

1. Adey, W. R. Unpublished work.
2. Bell, C., Sierra, G., Buendia, N. and Segundo, J. P. Sensory properties of units in mesencephalic reticular formation. *J. Neurophysiol.,* **27:** 961–987, 1964.
3. Bowsher, D. Projection of the gracile and cuneate nuclei in Macaca mulata: and experimental degeneration study. *J. comp. Neurol.,* **110:** 135–156, 1958.
4. Brooks, V. B., Rudomin, P. and Slayman, C. L. Sensory activation of neurons in the cats' cerebral cortex. *J. Neurophysiol.,* **24:** 286–301, 1961.
5. Demirjian, C. and Morin, F. Microelectrode analysis of the thalamic projections of the lateral cervical nucleus. *Anat. Rec.,* **148:** 275, 1964.
6. Evarts, E. V. Effects of sleeping and waking on activity of single units in the unrestrained cat. Pp. 171–182. In: C. Wohlstenholme and M. O'Connor (Eds.), *The nature of sleep,* Boston, Little, Brown and Co., 1961.
7. Gross, B. A. and Green, J. D. Activity of single neurons in the hypothalamus, effect of somatic and other stimuli. *J. Physiol.,* **148:** 554–569, 1959.
8. Hernández-Peón, R., Scherrer, H. and Jouvet, M. Auditory potentials at cochlear nucleus during acoustic habituation. *Acta neurol. latinoamer.,* **3:** 144–156, 1957.
9. Huttenlocher, P. R. Evoked and spontaneous activity in single units of medial brain stem during natural sleep and waking. *J. Neurophysiol.,* **24:** 451–468, 1961.
10. Jouvet, M. Recherches sur les structures nerveuses et les mecanismes responsables des defferentes phases du sommeil physiologique. *Arch. ital. Biol.,* **100:** 125–206, 1962.
11. Løyning, Y., Oshima, T. and Yolota, T. Site of action of thiamylal sodium on the monosynaptic spinal reflex pathway in cats. *J. Neurophysiol.,* **27:** 408–428, 1964.
12. Lettvin, J. Y., Maturana, H. R., Pitts, W. H. and McCulloch, W. S. Two remarks on the visual system of the frog. Pp. 757–776. In W. Rosenblith (Ed.), Cambridge, Mass. and New York, M.I.T. Press and John Wiley, 1961.
13. Mehler, W. R., Feferman, M. E. and Nauta, W. H. Ascending axon degeneration following antero-lateral cordotomy. An experimental study in the monkey. *Brain,* **83:** 718–750, 1960.
14. Perl, E. R., Whitlock, D. C. and Gentry, J. R. Cutaneous projection to second order neurons of the dorsal column system. *J. Neurophysiol.,* **25:** 337–359, 1962.
15. Pompeiano, O. and Swett, J. E. EEG and behavioral manifestations of sleep induced by cutaneous nerve stimulation in normal cats. *Arch. ital. Biol.,* **100:** 311–342, 1962.
16. Pompeiano, O. and Swett, J. E. Identification of cutaneous and muscular afferent fibers producing EEG synchronization or arousal in normal cats. *Arch. ital. Biol.,* **100:** 343–380, 1962.
17. Roger, A., Woronin, L. G. and Sokolov, J. N. Elektroenzephalographische Untersuchung der zeitweiligen Vorbindung beim Erlöschen des Orientierungsreflexes beim Menschen. *Pawlow-Zeitschrift für höhere Nerventätigkeit,* **8:** 1–15, 1958.
18. Rossi, G. F. and Brodal, A. Terminal distribution of spinoreticular fibers in the cat. *Arch. Neurol. Psychiat., Chicago,* **78:** 439–453, 1957.
19. Scheibel, M., Scheibel, A., Mollica, A. and Moruzzi, G. Convergence and in-

      teraction of afferent impulses on single units of reticular formation. *J. Neurophysiol.*, **18:** 309–331, 1955.
20. Scheibel, M. and Scheibel, A. Histological localization of microelectrode placement in brain by ferrocyanide and silver staining. *Stain Technol.*, **31:** 1–5, 1955.
21. Scheibel, M. and Scheibel, A. Adaptation of reticular units to repetitive stimulation. *Anat. Rec.*, **145:** 348, 1963.
22. Scheibel, M. and Scheibel, A. Unpublished data.
23. Sharpless, S. K. and Jasper, H. H. Habituation of the arousal reaction. *Brain*, **79:** 655–680, 1956.
24. Waterman, T. H. and Wiersma, C. A. G. Electrical responses in crustacean visual system. *J. cell. comp. Physiol.*, **61:** 1–16, 1963.

Neurophysiological Correlates of Habituation and Other Manifestations of Plastic Inhibition (Internal Inhibition)

RAÚL HERNÁNDEZ-PEÓN

Reprinted from *Electroencephalography and Clinical Neurophysiology*, 1960, Vol. 13 (Supplement), pp. 101–114.

Learning not to respond to a stimulus which previously evoked a behavioural response is defined as negative learning. It must be distinguished from positive learning which involves the acquisition of a response to a stimulus which did not elicit it before. The elimination of irrelevant responses depends upon central processes actually preventing their appearance which otherwise would occur. This enduring active process, which I will attempt to discuss today, will be referred to as *"plastic inhibition."*

Plastic inhibition is probably the primary and most important manifestation of learning without which animal behaviour would be disorganized, and adaptation of the organism to the external environment would be impossible. Even the acquisition of new responses by *plastic association* (Hernández-Peón, 1957) is accompanied by elimination of a great number of irrelevant responses. Selectivity of Pavlov's conditioned reflexes during late stages of conditioning probably involves a great deal of plastic inhibition.

Although plastic inhibition is probably a single process operating in the same way both for inborn and for acquired responses, for semantic purposes it may be convenient to conserve the terms *habituation* and *extinction* (as originally proposed by Dodge and by Pavlov) in order to differentiate the disappearance of inborn and of acquired or conditioned responses, respectively. In making such a distinction I am aware of the difficulties in deciding whether certain responses are the result of learning, or of maturation of the central nervous system.

Habituation

Thorpe (1950) has defined habituation as "a simple learning not to respond to stimuli which tend to be without significance in the life of the animal; a tendency merely to drop out responses." Since waning of a response may be the result of sensory adaptation at the receptor organ, or fatigue at any level of neural circuits including the effector organs, it is convenient to emphasize the enduring effects of habituation produced by intermittent stimulation even though it is repeated at intervals of minutes, hours or days. Such a long maintained waning of response clearly distinguishes habituation from adaptation and fatigue. Moreover, as it will be shown later, the fact that the enduring waning does not occur in functionally isolated neural circuits implies that habituation requires elements other than the conducting system involved. Therefore, the assumption made by Thorpe that habituation is correlated with a change in the central nervous system is supported by experimental observations.

Common experience proves the effects of habituation both in effector responses, as well as on the sphere of sensory perception. However, until electrophysiological methods were used for the investigation of plastic phenomena, habituation had been studied only through its manifestations on the motor outflow. More recently, by recording the electrical activity of the brain, habituatory changes have been detected at practically all the levels of the central nervous system including the lowest levels of sensory pathways. These changes may be grouped as follows: 1) habituation at specific sensory systems, and 2) habituation at polysensory or non-specific sensory systems.

The personal observations to be described and discussed in this communication were obtained in collaboration with Drs. Alcaraz, Alcocer-Cuarón, Brust-Carmona, Buser, Davidovich, Fernández-Guardiola, Jouvet, Guzmán-Flores, Lavín, Marcelin, Miranda, Palestini, Santibañez, and Scherrer, to whom I wish to express my acknowledgment. Only a small part has already been reported, and the details of most of the experimental material will be published elsewhere.

Habituation at Specific Sensory Systems
(Afferent Neuronal Habituation)

The term specific sensory systems refers to the classical paucisynaptic afferent pathways (Pavlov's analyzers) which carry sensory impulses of a single modality from the receptors up to the corresponding cortical receiving area.

Material and Method

Electrical recordings were made in awake freely moving cats with electrodes permanently implanted in various brain structures. Bipolar electrodes 0.6 mm. in diameter were introduced with the aid of a stereotaxic instrument in the dorsal cochlear nucleus, in the optic tract, in the olfactory bulb, in the spinal fifth sensory nucleus, in the lateral geniculate body, and in the visual, auditory and somatic sensory cortical areas. Only one sensory pathway was explored in each cat. Evoked potentials were recorded in the sensory pathways by means of a cathode-ray oscilloscope or of an ink-writing electroencephalograph. The sensory stimuli used for evoking those potentials were always brief in duration: clicks, flashes of light, puffs of air with different odours, and single square weak electrical pulses applied to the skin.

Results

Acoustic Habituation

In 1951 Artemiev observed in awake cats that auditory evoked potentials recorded from the auditory cortex vanished rapidly as the acoustic stimulus was successively repeated. In contrast, in the anesthetized animal the amplitude of the cortical auditory potentials remained remarkably stable. Undoubtedly, the phenomenon observed by Artemiev was the cortical manifestation of habituation in the auditory pathway.

These observations seemed to support Pavlov's interpretation that "extinction" is the result of cortical inhibition. But although cortical recordings alone usually satisfy interpretations ascribing federal privileges to the cortex, they do not permit any conclusion as to the original site of the observed phenomenon. In fact, all subcortical changes of electrical activity have their cortical counterpart which, therefore, are only manifestations of the corresponding subcortical phenomena.

The finding that sensory transmission at the spinal cord (Hagbarth and Kerr, 1954), at the gracilis nucleus (Hernández-Peón, Scherrer and Velasco, 1956), at the spinal fifth sensory nucleus (Hernández-Peón and Hagbarth, 1955), at the retina (Granit, 1955; Hernández-Peón, Scherrer and Velasco, 1956), and at the lateral geniculate body (Hernández-Peón, Scherrer and Velasco, 1956) is greatly modified by electrical stimulation of central structures including the reticular system of the brain stem led us to test whether those centrifugal mechanisms, acting at low levels of sensory pathways, would be involved in sensory habituation. Indeed, in 1955 Hernández-Peón and Scherrer observed that monotonous repetition of an acoustic stimulus resulted in persistent diminution and eventual disappearance of the evoked potentials recorded from the dorsal cochlear nucleus. The pioneer work of these authors has been confirmed by Galambos *et al.* (1956) and extended by Hernández-Peón, Jouvet and Scherrer (1957). The decrement of the evoked potentials was progressive but followed a waxing and waning course.

Recovery of the diminished auditory potentials (*dishabituation*) was obtained a) after a more or less prolonged period of rest; b) by application of an extraneous acoustic stimulus; c) by repeated association of the habituatory clicks with a nociceptive stimulus (electric shock to a leg of the animal) according to the classical Pavlovian conditioning technique; d) under barbiturate anesthesia; and e) by an extensive lesion of the mesencephalic tegmentum which rendered the cat unconscious. Although afferent neuronal habituation at the cochlear nucleus disappeared during unconsciousness elicited by anesthetics or by brain stem lesions, it must be pointed out that the auditory electrical responses which waned by habituation, remained absent during light physiological sleep.

It is evident, therefore, that during acoustic habituation in the awake animal, sensory blockade takes place as far down as the first synapse of the auditory pathway. It is logical that the auditory signals will be reduced or suppressed in the cortex when their entrance to the brain is blocked. But the above mentioned finding does not preclude that sensory inhibition might also take place at higher levels of the auditory pathway. By recording simultaneously from the auditory cortex and from the cochlear nucleus, Lifschitz (1958) has recently observed that habituation, as judged by the decline of the evoked potentials, occurs faster at the auditory cortex than at the cochlear nucleus. This observation indicates that during habituation, sensory inhibition takes place at different levels of the specific afferent pathways, and that higher stations (cortex) are more susceptible than the lower synapses. As it will be seen below, similar observations have been made in other sensory paths.

Photic Habituation

In order to explore the effects of habituation in the visual pathway, Hernández-Peón *et al.* (1956, 1958) recorded from the optic tract, from the lateral geniculate body and from the visual cortex, the potentials evoked by flashes of light repeated at irregular intervals of 8 to 10 seconds. Repetition of the photic stimuli led to an oscillating but progressive diminution of the cortical and thalamic potentials without apparent modification of the retinal evoked discharges. The effects of habituation appeared first in the late evoked waves, and like those in the cochlear nucleus, they persisted long after several thousands of stimuli. Dishabituation was obtained 1) after an adequate period of rest; 2) by presentation of extraneous acoustic or visual stimuli; and 3) under barbiturate anesthesia. In the monkey, Ricci, Doane and Jasper (1957) have observed habituation in the visual cortex at the unitary level with micro-electrode recordings. But the effects of habituation are not only restricted to the cortical and thalamic stations of the visual pathway. Palestini, Davidovich and Hernández-Peón (1958) have recently obtained evidence of retinal habituation. The late evoked activity of optic tract potentials was reduced by regular monotonous repetition of flashes of light. The decrease of retinal discharges cannot be ascribed to retinal chemical changes involved in adaptation to light since they reappeared ((dishabituation) by introducing extra photic stimuli, thus changing the rhythm of stimulation.

Olfactory Habituation

Fading of the sensation of smell by continuous or repeated presentation of the same odour is a commonly experienced phenomenon which is usually referred to as olfactory adaptation. However, this phenomenon cannot be accounted for by failure of the olfactory receptors. Not only olfactory receptors are very resistant to adaptation (Ottosson, 1956), but the transient effects of receptor adaptation do not explain the persistent failure of olfactory sensation. Since central factors must be involved, this phenomenon is better identified with habituation. In order to test whether habituation occurs in the olfactory pathway, Hernández-Peón, Alcocer-Cuarón, Lavín and Santibañez (1957, 1958) recorded from the olfactory bulb the electrical activity evoked by olfactory stimuli (puffs of air with different odours) delivered through a nasal catheter chronically implanted. Indeed, these authors found that the induced activity in the olfactory bulb of awake cats diminished with repetition of the same olfactory stimulus. That waning of the evoked responses was centrally determined has been shown by their recovery (dishabituation) in the following circumstances: a) after a variable period of rest; b) by presentation of extraneous alerting stimuli (acoustic or nociceptive); c) by brief electrical stimulation of the mesencephalic reticular formation; d) by restoring meaning to the odour to which the cat had become habituated; e) under barbiturate anesthesia; and f) after lesions involving the mesencephalic tegmentum. In the two latter conditions, the olfactory evoked potentials in the olfactory bulb were remarkably stable. It must be pointed out that lesions involving the pontine tegmentum did not prevent habituation of induced activity in the olfactory bulb.

Tactile Habituation

By electrophysiological recordings, Hagbarth and Kugelberg (1958) have shown that abdominal skin reflexes in man diminished with repetition of the same tactile stimulus. Since habituation of this spinal reflex was specific for the stimulated skin area, and the motoneurons of the habituated reflex were still discharged by neighbouring skin afferents, the Swedish authors have rightly concluded that the plastic changes took place in the spinal internuncial system. The effects of habituation to tactile stimuli have been recently explored in the trigeminal pathway of cats by Hernández-Peón, Davidovich and Miranda (1958). The potentials evoked by weak electrical stimuli, or by puffs of air delivered to the skin of the face were recorded both at the spinal fifth sensory nucleus, and at the face area of the primary somatic sensory cortex (Fig. 1). In both places, the evoked potentials diminished in amplitude with regular repetition of the tactile stimulus at intervals of 1 to 3 seconds. But the cortical potentials disappeared faster than those from the medulla. Habituation at the medullary trigeminal synapse presented similar characteristics to those observed in other sensory pathways. Dishabituation was produced a) after a period of rest; b) by presentation of an extraneous acoustic stimulus; c) by changing briefly the rhythm or the intensity of the habituatory tactile stimulus; d) by brief electrical stimulation of the mesencephalic reticular formation; and e) under barbiturate anesthesia. In contrast to the recovery and remarkable constancy of the tactile medullary potentials under anesthesia (Fig. 2), the potentials extinguished by habituation remained absent during physiological sleep (as judged by the behavioural attitude of the cat, and by the electrocorticographic pattern of sleep), as illustrated in Figure 1.*

Comments

From the presented evidence, it is obvious that the amplitude of afferent signals along specific sensory pathways is reduced by previous exposure of the animal to repetition of the same indifferent stimulus. By indifferent is meant a stimulus which the animal faces with impassibility. It is also clear that sensory signals diminish at all the levels of the central nervous system, from the first sensory synapse up to the cortex. However, there are differences between the rate of establishment of habituation at different levels, being faster at the cortex, and slower at the first sensory synapse.

Afferent neuronal habituation at the cochlear nucleus, at the retina, at the olfactory bulb, and at the spinal fifth sensory nucleus can be accounted for by centrifugal plastic inhibition acting at those peripheral sensory synapses (Hernández-Peón, 1955, 1957). There is anatomical evidence of centrifugal fibres terminating in all those lower sensory centers (Cajal, 1904; Lorente de Nó, 1933; Brodal, 1957), but their origin remains unsettled. Physiological experiments have shown that electrical stimulation of the brain stem reticular system blocks afferent volleys at these second order sensory neurons. These findings, together with the observations that functional integrity of the same central region of the brain stem is required for the establishment of afferent neuronal habituation at that level, strongly suggest an important role of the

* Editor's note: Figures 1–7 have been deleted from the text of this article. The reader is referred to the original source for these illustrations.

reticular system in this phenomenon; but, they leave undecided the role which higher structures might have on the postulated plastic sensory inhibition. Experiments on decorticated animals are needed in order to elucidate this question.

Although it has been generally assumed that habituation requires cortical participation, it seems likely to me that the cortex will be found to be unnecessary for afferent neuronal habituation to simple stimuli, as it has been found in other manifestations of habituation. Brust-Carmona (1958) and Brust-Carmona and Hernández-Peón (1956) have observed habituation of post-rotatory nystagmus in decorticated cats, and in cats with complete transection of the brain stem at the mesencephalon. King (1926) has also observed habituation of post-rotatory nystagmus in decerebrate squabs. As it will be mentioned later, Sharpless and Jasper (1956) found habituation of arousal to simple tones after bilateral removal of the auditory cortex. Therefore, the conclusion seems warranted that at least certain types of habituation do not require diencephalic and telencephalic structures.

The hypothesis that the plastic sensory inhibition responsible for afferent neuronal habituation probably originates in the central core of the brain stem does not imply equipotentiality of all the regions of the reticular system for all the sensory paths. It seems likely that different levels of the brain stem are more related to some and not to other afferent pathways. For instance, as it has been mentioned, pontine lesions did not affect olfactory habituation (Hernández-Peón, Alcocer-Cuarón, Lavín and Santibañez, 1958), but eliminated and prevented habituation of post-rotatory nystagmus (Brust-Carmona, 1958). On the other hand, mesencephalic lesions which eliminated acoustic and olfactory habituation did not prevent habituation to vestibular stimulation.

The finding that afferent neuronal habituation persists during physiological sleep is not in contradiction with the view which postulates the reticular system as a source of centrifugal sensory inhibition. Many reticular neurons which are depressed by anesthetics must remain active during physiological sleep.

Monotonous repetition of the testing stimulus on a uniform external environment seemed to be necessary for the establishment and maintenance of habituation. Any variation in the intensity or rhythm of the habituatory stimulus, or the presentation of other stimuli either of the same or different modalities disrupts the accumulation of the habituatory plastic sensory inhibition. This kind of dishabituation will be referred to as "dishabituation by diaphoro-stimulation" ($\varsigma\delta\mu\iota\phi\rho\rho\sigma$ = different) of homosensory or heterosensory nature. The similarity between dishabituation by diaphoro-stimulation with "disinhibition" of conditioned responses observed by Pavlov in the same circumstances must be emphasized. In this case, the paradoxical effect of the "activating" stimuli (which are known to produce "external inhibition" and suppression of afferent signals at the first sensory synapse) is to release the postulated plastic inhibitory influence. Dishabituation by heterosensory diaphoro-stimulation can only be produced by means of central processes through synaptic pathways. This observation not only substantiates the central nature of habituation, but it rules out the possibility of presynaptic post-stimulatory phenomena of the type of post-tetanic potentiation for explaining dishabituation. Furthermore, as the term describes, post-tetanic potentiation follows repetitive stimulation, and the degree and duration of enhancement are proportional to the number of stimuli. Contrariwise, in our experiments, repetition of the dishabituating stimulus produced loss of its efficacy. A plausible explanation for this kind of dishabituation is that sudden and intense excitation of the reticular system would derange some dynamic and delicate equilibrium of inhibitory neurons which would be necessary for maintenance of plastic inhibition. In favor of this hypothesis we have made the observation that brief, intense electrical stimulation of the mesencephalic reticular formation, producing alertness, brought about dishabituation of sensory neurons.

Since intermittent sensory stimulation elicits persistent inhibition of specific sensory neurons, it should be expected that maintained stimulation will produce similar effects. If this inference proves to be true, recurrent inhibition of sensory neurons must be taken into consideration for explaining post-excitatory fading of sensation ("auditory fatigue," "adaptation to light," "olfactory and tactile adaptation") which is usually assumed to result exclusively from fatigue or adaptation at the receptor level.

From teleological reasoning, centrifugal inhibition of non-significant sensory signals at their entrance to the central nervous system is a useful mechanism for the individual. It is likely that the regulation of that mechanism is altered in some pathological states. For instance, failure of afferent neuronal habituation, resulting in excessive entrance of sensory signals to the brain, would explain the unusual responsiveness of neurotic patients, and their heightened perception of non-significant stimuli.

Habituation at Polysensory or Non-Specific Sensory Systems (Neuropil Habituation)

Under the term "polysensory system" I include all central structures outside the specific sensory pathways receiving afferent signals of more than one sense modality. Extending from the spinal cord up to the cortex, this system of sensory convergence includes spinal internuncial neurons, the reticular system of the brain stem, as well as subthalamic, septal, caudate, hippocampal, amygdaloid, etc. afferent neurons.

Material and Method

The background and evoked electrical activity to be described was recorded with the same technique previously stated, and the results were obtained in cats with electrodes permanently implanted in the mesencephalic reticular formation, in the olfactory bulb, in the septal region, in the sensorimotor cortex, and in the visual cortex.

Results

Habituation at non-specific sensory systems ("neuropil habituation") has common characteristics with afferent neuronal habituation. Both are developed following a waxing and waning course; both are long persisting and cumulative; both have certain specificity for the habituatory stimulus; both are observed at cortical and subcortical levels of the central nervous system; both are best seen with low intensities of stimulation; and both are eliminated and prevented by pharmacological actions. The main difference between habituation at specific and non-specific sensory systems lies in the greater susceptibility of the latter structures.

Habituation at the brain stem will be manifested in such functions as arousal, ascending diffuse sensory conduction, and in some autonomic and somatic activities. Perhaps, the well known effects of habituation to alerting stimuli on muscular, cardiac and sudomotor activities are the translation of plastic inhibition of polysensory structures at the brain stem level.

Habituation of Non-specific Evoked Potentials

As it is well known, long latency responses to various sense modalities are obtained from the polysensory system. During simultaneous recordings of evoked potentials from the mesencephalic reticular formation and from first sensory relays, it can often be seen that the reticular potentials decline faster than the specific sensory signals. In their experiments on facial tactile habituation, Hernández-Peón, Davidovich and Miranda (1958) observed that the reticular potentials evoked by tactile stimuli disappeared faster than those from the spinal fifth sensory nucleus. Cortical evoked responses recorded in regions other than the corresponding specific projection area also disappear at a faster rate than the primary cortical potentials. For instance, auditory evoked potentials recorded from the sensorimotor cortex disappear with few repetitions of the acoustic stimulus. Very often, after two or three presentations of the stimulus, the cortical evoked responses disappear completely. This is one of the fastest examples of habituation.

As in the specific sensory systems, non-specific evoked potentials extinguished by habituation recover their original amplitude (dishabituation) a) after a prolonged period of rest; b) by introducing an extraneous alerting stimulus; c) by briefly raising the intensity of the habituatory stimulus; d) following several associations of the habituatory stimulus with a nociceptive stimulus (electric shock to a leg of the animal) according to the classical Pavlovian conditioning technique; and e) under chloralose anesthesia.

Barbiturates eliminate afferent neuronal habituation, but they also eliminate non-specific reticular and cortical sensory responses. Chloralose has different central effects. Lifschitz (1958) has shown that chloralose enhances not only the auditory potentials from the cochlear nucleus, but also those recorded from the mesencephalic reticular formation and from the sensorimotor cortex. Furthermore, during chloralose anesthesia the amplitude of all those evoked responses remain remarkably constant.

The excitability of polysensory structures varies according to the significance of the stimulus. It decreases during habituation, and it is greatly enhanced during the early stages of Pavlovian conditioning. This is clearly shown in the following experiments made by Buser, Jouvet and Hernández-Peón (1958). These authors recorded auditory potentials evoked by clicks in the mesencephalic reticular formation. At the beginning, when giving a pair of clicks at an interval of 300–600 msec. the potentials evoked by the second click were always smaller than the potentials evoked by the first click. After obtaining a good number of control records, the cat was conditioned to an unavoidable electric shock delivered to a leg, using the pair of clicks as conditional stimulus. After several click-shock associations, the amplitude of the paired auditory evoked potentials increased; but it was noted that the second potential in each pair very often equaled the size of the preceding potential. This, indeed, was an extraordinary finding. Furthermore, the early reticular hyperexcitability produced by conditioning, sometimes proved to be very resistant to extinction (Fig. 3). These experiments provide evidence of plastic modification of the recovery cycle of reticular neurons during the early stages of conditioning.

Habituation of the Arousal Reaction

Habituation of the electrocorticographic arousal reaction, which has been excellently studied by Sharpless and Jasper (1956), can be recorded not only at the cortex, but practically at all the levels of the central nervous system. The recent disclosure of centrifugal activation of the olfactory bulb during arousal, produced by all kinds of sensory stimuli (Lavín, Alcocer-Cuarón and Hernández-Peón, 1959), enabled us to demonstrate the effects of habituation in this peripheral sensory structure (Hernández-Peón, Lavín, Alcocer-Cuarón and Marcelin, 1960). The first presentation of an alerting stimulus to the cat elicits in the olfactory bulb intermittent bursts of fast rhythmic activity (34–48/sec.) (Fig. 4). The amplitude and persistence of these "arousal discharges" are related to the degree of alertness of the animal, and they rapidly diminish with few repetitions of the stimulus. There is little doubt that the mesencephalic reticular formation plays an important role in the generation of the arousal discharges of the olfactory bulb, since they are reproduced by electrical stimulation of this region, and they disappear after making a lesion in the mesencephalic tegmentum.

But with monotonous repetition, an indifferent stimulus not only fails to elicit the electrographic manifestations of arousal, but later on, it induces cortical slow waves (Fig. 5). Palestini, Davidovich, Alcocer-Cuarón and Hernández-Peón (1958) have observed in the visual cortex that long continued repetition of flashes of light, every 2 seconds, resulted in the appearance of spindle bursts following the evoked potentials (Fig. 6). And, if after a long regular intermittent stimulation, the photic stimuli were interrupted, those spindle bursts continued for a few seconds at approximately the same intervals of the previous stimulation. It seems as though some triggering system would continue to discharge at the imposed rhythm.

Comments

All the above mentioned electrical manifestations of habituation might well be the expression of inhibition affecting some elements of the reticular system of the brain stem, which at the same time forms part of the polysensory system, conducting all kinds of sensory signals throughout the brain. Inhibition of the rostral portion of the arousal system at the mesencephalon would explain both the failure of arousal and the triggering of spindle bursts by the habituatory stimulus. Similar spindle bursts are triggered by single shocks applied to the nucleus ventralis anterior of the thalamus, the excitability of which is greatly enhanced by barbiturate anesthesia and by a midbrain transection (Scherrer and Hernández-Peón, 1955). If the mesencephalic portion of the reticular system exerts a tonic ascending inhibitory influence upon the diffuse thalamic system, it can be understood that functional depression of the mesencephalic structures produced either by anesthetics, by lesions, or by an active inhibitory process will result in hyperexcitability of the thalamic spindle-triggering system.

We can only speculate at the present moment as to the origin of the possible inhibitory influence affecting elements of the rostral portion of the reticular system. A number of experimental data in the literature favors the hypothesis that some supramesencephalic structures, including the limbic system, may exert inhibitory effects upon the arousal system. On the other hand, the recent and important observations of Batini, Moruzzi, Palestini, Rossi and Zanchetti (1958) have shown that a midpontine transection of the brain stem gives rise to a state of hypervigilance. This finding suggests that ascending influences arising at lower (pontine and bulbar) levels of the reticular formation would inhibit the rostral portion at the mesencephalon. A third possibility is that habituatory inhibition would proceed from neighbouring neurons reciprocally connected. The plastic changes in the recovery cycle of reticular potentials demonstrated by Buser, Jouvet and Hernández-Peón (1958) during conditioning, indicates that a great deal of central post-excitatory depression which is usually ascribed to occlusion and refractoriness, can be better accounted for by active inhibition. According to this new concept, and extending it to all the central nervous system, the discharge of central neurons brings about a decreased excitability of the same neurons by a feedback inhibitory mechanism. Habituation would result from the accumulation of self-inhibition.

It is logical that removal or loss of plastic inhibition in the polysensory system will bring about a state of diffuse central hyperexcitability in which a single afferent volley will discharge a great number of neurons throughout the brain. Such seems to be the central action of chloralose, and perhaps some convulsant drugs (Metrazol, for instance) may act in the same way. It can also be conjectured that massive activation of internuncial systems consecutive to lack of their tonic inhibition, would explain generalized discharges of moto-neurons, as those observed in myoclonic jerks produced by all varieties of sensory stimuli.

Extinction

Similar effects to those produced by habituation have been observed in specific and non-specific sensory systems, during extinction of electrical responses obtained as a result of Pavlovian conditioning.

Material and Method

Cats with electrodes permanently implanted in the optic tract, in the visual cortex, and in the mesencephalic reticular formation were conditioned according to the following technique: series of 4 flashes of light at a rate of 1/sec. were used as conditional stimuli. The unconditional stimulus was an unavoidable electric shock applied to a leg of the cat during the 4th flash. The flashes-shock associations were repeated at irregular intervals of one to two minutes.

Results

After a variable number of flashes-shock associations, some changes appeared in the photic potentials from the optic tract, from the visual cortex and from the mesencephalic reticular formation. These changes were more evident in the late evoked activity. The amplitude increased, particularly in the responses to the third and fourth flashes. It should be noted that the effect of conditioning in the sensory pathway activated by the conditional stimulus appeared much earlier than the flexor motor conditioned response.

By cessation of reinforcement, the plastically facilitated photic responses diminished in amplitude even beyond the size of the first non-conditioned responses. Moreover, in this state, a single electric shock to the leg was capable of restoring firmly the enhanced conditioned potentials.

It is evident that the above mentioned effects observed at the retina, at the visual cortex, and at the mesencephalic reticular formation are entirely comparable to those described by Pavlov as "extinction" and "disinhibition" of salivary and flexor conditioned responses.

In the visual cortex, in addition to the changes of evoked potentials, bursts of slow waves were triggered by the non-reinforced photic stimuli (Fig. 7). These bursts started with the 4th flash, and later on they were triggered by the third, the second, and the first flashes. Similar bursts developed during internal inhibition produced by delayed association, i.e., by delivering the electric shock some seconds after the 4th flash.

Comments

Pavlov reached the conclusion that extinction results from an active inhibitory process (internal inhibition) taking place at the cortex, and that the non-reinforced conditional stimulus acquires inhibitory properties. The modifications produced in the optic tract and cortical potentials by cessation of reinforcement are in line with the general properties of internal inhibition described by Pavlov. But at the same time, such results demonstrate that internal inhibition may affect subcortical levels of afferent pathways as far down as second order sensory neurons. It is evident that extinction of conditioned optic tract potentials does not result from simple vanishing of centrifugal retinal facilitation. The rapid and persistent recovery of enhanced retinal discharges after a single unconditional nociceptive stimulus (disinhibition) strongly indicates how firmly plastic association had been established by conditioning. Therefore, the conclusion seems warranted that application of non-reinforced conditional photic stimuli leads to the development of centrifugal inhibition upon the retina itself. According to this view, the non-reinforced stimulus acquires inhibitory properties on its own signals at second order sensory neurons, thus reducing their entrance to the brain. But the inhibition elicited by the non-reinforced stimulus probably involves many other parts of the central nervous system. The cortical slow waves observed during extinction might be a sign of inhibition of some elements of the brain stem arousal system.

The following diagram (Fig. 1) summarizes my present working hypothesis concerning some demonstrated sites of action and some hypothetical sites of origin of plastic inhibition, responsible for habituation and extinction, occurring both at specific and non-specific sensory systems. Whereas the mesencephalic portion of the reticular system seems to be a probable source for centrifugal inhibition acting at the first sensory synapse of specific afferent pathways, some experimental data suggest that inhibition acting upon rostral portions of the arousal system may arise at lower levels (pontine and bulbar) of the reticular system itself, and at some higher regions of the brain.

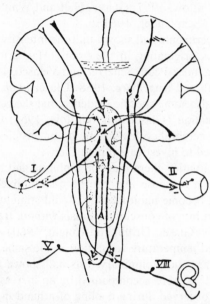

FIGURE 1. Diagram showing the plastic inhibitory influences involved in habituation and extinction. Centrifugal inhibition from the upper part of the brain stem reticular system blocks afferent transmission at the olfactory bulb (I), at the retina (II), at the spinal trigeminal sensory nucleus (V), and at the cochlear nucleus (VIII). The arrows terminating in the rostral portion of the arousal system represent possible inhibitory influences coming from the limbic system and from lower levels of the reticular system itself.

Influence of the Cerebral Cortex on Habituation

E. M. GLASER AND J. P. GRIFFIN

Reprinted from *Journal of Physiology*, 1968, Vol. 160, pp. 429–445.

If sensory stimuli are repeatedly applied to intact animals or to people at intervals of minutes, hours, or days, then the responses to those stimuli gradually diminish or disappear. This is a result of habituation, and there is reason to believe that it is a fundamental physiological mechanism of adaptation (Glaser and Whittow, 1953) but it has been known to psychologists for a long time (see Humphrey, 1933; Davis, 1934). The problem has been previously discussed (Glaser and Whittow, 1957; Glaser, Hall and Whittow, 1959) and reviewed (Glaser, 1958; Scholander, 1961).

A number of experiments had shown that the intensity of responses could be altered by impulses originating in the brain (Hagbarth and Kerr, 1954; Galambos, 1956; Hernández-Peón, Scherrer and Velasco, 1956; Sharpless and Jasper, 1956, Hagbarth and Kugelberg, 1958; Glaser *et al.* 1959; Scholander, 1960) and there was also some specific evidence that the cerebral hemispheres might influence habituation (Glaser and Whittow, 1957; Glaser, 1958), but the part played by the cerebral cortex was by no means clear. The present experiments were designed to investigate this further.

In studies of habituation there must be a precise and reproducible stimulus which gives rise to a response that can be quantitatively assessed. It was known that rats could become habituated to a cold stimulus, and a technique for measuring the heart rate of conscious animals without trauma was available (Glaser and Yap, 1959; Glaser, Griffin and Knight, 1960). It was known also that the rat's tail served temperature regulation in the same way as the human hand (Knoppers, 1942), and preliminary tests had shown that immersions of rats' tails in water at 4° C were accompanied by an increase of the heart rate which resembled that observed during cooling of a hand in a previous experiment on habituation (Glaser and Whittow, 1957). This meant that the cooling of rats' tails could provide a suitable stimulus, while measurements of the heart rate would provide a suitable response. Some of the results have already been briefly reported (Glaser and Griffin, 1961).

Methods

Procedure

Female Wistar rats with initial weights of 120–130 g were used. Throughout the experiment the rats lived in the room in which the tests were carried out and which was kept at a temperature of 20–22·5° C (dry bulb) and 16·5–18·5° C (wet bulb). In all experiments each rat was held vertically without much restraint in a copper-wire tube from which its tail protruded through a rubber stopper to a constant level; the top of the tube was open and lined with rubber, comfortably supporting the animal's head and neck, so that its eyes and nose were outside the tube. Platinum-wire electrodes of 26 s.w.g. were inserted into the skin of the animals' backs under light ether anaesthesia, or while the animals were under pentobarbitone anaesthesia for operations on the brain, and screened electrocardiogram (e.c.g.) leads were clipped to these electrodes before each test. The electrodes remained there throughout the experiment, and they rarely needed replacing, as the animals took no notice of them.

Previous experiments had shown that placing rats in the vertical position caused a rise of their heart rates even after 30 min were allowed for immediate postural adjustments, but when the rats were put into that position every day for several days the rise of their heart rate became gradually less, which suggested that habituation to the vertical position had taken place (Glaser and Yap, 1959). It has also been observed in man that experimental procedures produced responses which diminished with habituation (Glaser, 1953; Glaser and Whittow, 1954). The rats were therefore placed vertically in the copper wire tubes for 2½ hr daily on 14 consecutive days while their tails were immersed to a constant level in water at 31° C, and every rat was trained to the basic experimental conditions in this way. Operations on the brain were done 7 days before this habituation to the experimental conditions was begun.

Immersions of the tails at 4° C were only carried out after training the rats to the experiment over 14 days. Base-line readings of the heart rate were taken each day before the tail was cooled and after the rats had been under the basic experimental conditions for 45 min with the tails at 31° C. All immersions of the tail at 4° C lasted for 10 min and they were always repeated six times daily with intervals of 10 min during which the tails were at 31° C.

Measurements

The heart rate was counted by decade scalers into which the amplified and discriminated R spike of the e.c.g. signal was fed. An automatic time switch gave readings over 15 sec, which meant that there was no subjective elements in these counts. Signals were monitored on cathode-ray tubes and on the scalers (Glaser *et al.* 1960).

The oxygen consumption of conscious rats was measured in a respirometer, as described by Davis and Van Dyke (1932), and the readings were taken by someone otherwise unconnected with the experiment who did not know what operations had been carried out on any particular animal.

The skin temperature was measured by copper-constantan thermocouples looped around the tail at a constant distance from its tip and closely adhering to the skin. The temperature was read on a calibrated potentiometer to $0 \cdot 1°C$ and the reference junction was in melting ice.

Operations

Pentobarbitone anaesthesia was used. The fronto-parietal suture was located on the skull, and the site of operations was related to this. Lesions were produced by undercutting the cerebral cortex with a mounted sharpened needle inserted through burr holes, after which the separated brain tissue was removed by gentle suction. Stimulation of the brain surface was done by concentric stainless-steel electrodes, as described by Galambos (1956). Burr holes were made 7 days in advance under general anaesthesia and the electrodes inserted on the day of the experiment with local anaesthesia of the skin. The resistance of the electrodes in open circuit was 20–50 MΩ. After recovery from the immediate effects of operation, the operated rats ate, drank, gained weight, and cleaned themselves in the same way as the unoperated controls.

Histological Studies

All operated brains were removed, fixed in formol-saline, and mounted in paraffin; serial sections were stained either by haematoxylin and orange C or by luxol fast blue and cresyl violet (Klüver and Barrera, 1953). Every section was independently checked by a neuropathologist who was specially interested in the rat's brain but otherwise unconnected with the experiment, and rats were allocated to different groups according to his assessment based on the presence of changes during the animal's lifetime, such as pigment phagocytosis, gliosis, and demyelination.

Results

Habituation to the Experimental Conditions

When the rats were first placed vertically in the copper-wire tubes with their tails at 31° C, a steady state of the heart rate was achieved after 45 min in the tubes. On successive days the heart rate became gradually lower. This is shown in Figure 1, which gives the results from a batch of eight normal rats placed in the vertical position for 2½ hr daily over 14 consecutive days while their tails were at 31° C. On the 1st day the mean heart rate was 437 beats/min after 45 min and 429 beats/min after 2½ hr; on the 14th day it was 398 beats/min after 45 min and 396 beats/min after 2½ hr. The gradual fall of the heart rate over 14 days followed the same pattern as habituations previously observed (Glaser and Whittow, 1957; Glaser *et al.* 1959; Glaser and Lee, 1959). The finding that the heart rates were similar at 45 min and at 2½ hr also meant that base-line readings obtained at 45 min were relevant to experiments lasting for another 1½ hr.

Figure 2 shows the basic heart rates of rats with and without different lesions of the brain surface after 14 days' training to the experimental conditions, and it also shows that once habituation had taken place to the experimental conditions the basic heart rate was not affected to any relevant extent by immersions of the tails at 4° C on preceding days. Before the first immersion of the tails at 4° C (after 14 days' habituation to the experimental conditions), the mean basic heart rates of normal control rats, of animals with unilateral lesions of the frontal area, and of animals with lesions of the occipito-parietal region were within the mean range of 380–410 beats/min, and there was no further fall during the next 10 days, though there were some day-to-day fluctuations. In nine rats with superficial bilateral lesions of the frontal areas the mean basic heart rate was 461 beats/min after 14 days' training to the experimental conditions and 458 beats/min 10 days later.

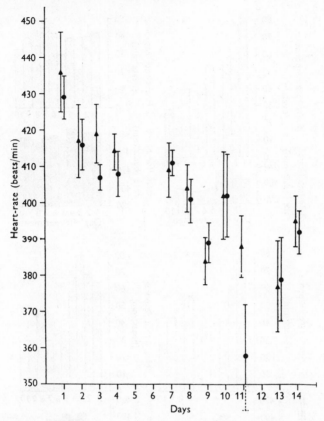

FIGURE 1. Habituation to the basic experimental conditions. Mean heart rates, with standard deviations, of eight rats on 14 successive days, after 45 min and 2½ hr in vertical, rubber-lined tubes, with the tails at 31°C. ▲ 45 min, ● 2½ hr.

OXYGEN CONSUMPTIONS OF NORMAL RATS AND OF RATS WITH BILATERAL FRONTAL CORTICAL LESIONS.   In order to find out whether the higher heart rates of rats with bilateral frontal cortical lesions were caused by some metabolic change or by an inability to adjust to the basic experimental conditions, the oxygen consumptions were measured in a respirometer, with the rats either unrestrained or held vertically in the tubes. Errors from habituation to the respirometer were avoided by comparing operated and unoperated rats of the same weight which had and which had not been trained to the experimental conditions.

When unoperated rats and rats with bilateral frontal cortical lesions were not under the basic experimental conditions their mean oxygen consumption was 2–2·16 l./kg/hr both before and after training to the experiment. Under the experimental conditions the mean oxygen consumption of all untrained rats increased by 40–44%, but after 14 days' training this increase was only 11% in control rats, whereas in rats with bilateral frontal lesions it remained at 45% (Table 1).

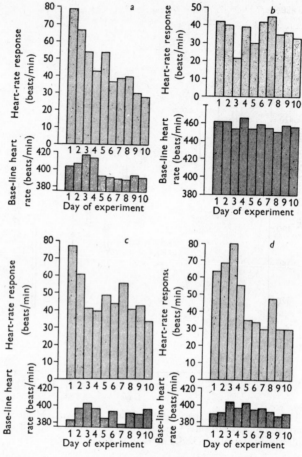

FIGURE 2. Responses of the heart rate to immersions of the tails at 4°C. *a*, Mean of ten normal control rats; *b*, mean of nine rats with bilateral frontal cortical lesions; *c*, mean of six rats with occipito-parietal lesions; *d*, mean of five rats with unilateral frontal lesions.

Habituation to Repeated Immersions of the Tail at 4° C

Figure 2 shows the mean increases of the heart rate observed in rats with and without lesions of the cerebral cortex while their tails were being immersed at 4° C six times daily for 10 min at a time on 10 consecutive days, and it shows that the heart rate of all operated and unoperated animals increased when their tails were being cooled; this increase became gradually less if the frontal cortex was intact at least on one side of the brain, but it remained about the same during 10 days if the frontal cortex was bilaterally damaged.

The animals were tested in ten batches, each of which contained two operated rats and one normal control. The mean heart rate of ten normal

Table 1.

Oxygen consumption of rats with bilateral frontal cortical lesions and of normal controls (standard errors of means are given in brackets).

	No.	Mean weight (g.)	Mean O_2 consumption (l./kg/hr)		
			Outside tubes	Inside tubes	Difference (%)
Without training to experiment					
Operated rats	6	134 (± 3·5)	2·16	3·09	44 (± 5·1)
Controls	6	136 (± 2·0)	2·12	2·93	40 (± 5·3)
After 14 days' training to experiment					
Operated rats	5	142	2·13	3·13	45
Controls	6	137 (± 4·4)	2·00	2·13	11 (± 8·7)

control rats rose by 79 beats/min over its basic level on the 1st day of cooling at 4° C, and this increase became gradually less, until it was only 28 beats/min on the 10th day, the difference between the means on the 1st and 10th day being significant ($t = 9·888$; $P < 0·001$). Rats with lesions of the occipito-parietal cortex gave results which were indistinguishable from the normal controls, the mean increase of the heart rate being 77 beats/min on the 1st day and 34 beats/min on the 10th day of immersion of the tail at 4° C ($t = 9·225$; $P < 0·001$). Rats with one-sided lesions of the frontal area gave results which resembled those obtained in normal controls, showing a mean increase of 64 beats/min on the 1st day and 30 beats/min on the 10th ($t = 5·605$; $P < 0·001$). In all these three groups of rats the actual heart rates while the tail was being cooled were 455–480 beats/min on the 1st day and 410–430 beats/min on the 10th day.

Rats with bilateral lesions of the frontal areas had higher initial heart rates under the basic experimental conditions (see above) and they showed a smaller relative response to cooling of their tails than other rats, the mean increase of the heart rate being 42 beats/min on the 1st day, but the actual heart rate was 20–30 beats/min higher in these than in other rats. Subsequently neither the absolute heart rate nor the relative increase above the base level showed any tendency to diminish while the tail was being cooled, and the absolute heart rate remained in the vicinity of 500 beats/min.

There were some superimposed irregular variations of the responses, which resembled daily variations of the heart rate under the basic experimental conditions, but analysis of variance showed that the results were not influenced by any variations of technique or of environment. Analysis of variance showed also that there were no significant interactions of any variables with different immersions of the tail at 4° C on the same day.

Measurements of the skin temperature of the tail showed that equilibrium was always reached after 5 min at 4° C and that the tail temperature during and before immersions at 4° C did not change over 10 days, which conforms with similar observations made on the human hand (Glaser and Whittow, 1957). Histological examination of the tails at the end of the experiment showed no evidence of tissue damage through cold injury.

SITES OF LESIONS.   Figures 3–5 show the extent of lesions in the twenty operated rats. The amount of brain tissue removed from the occipito-parietal area in some of the rats which did habituate to cooling of their tails was greater than the amount removed from both sides of the frontal area in

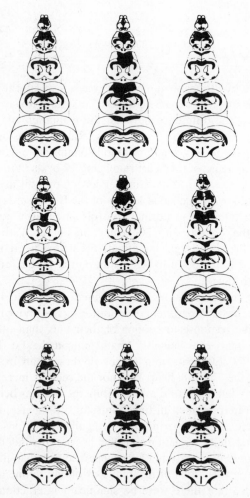

FIGURE 3. Sites of bilateral frontal lesions drawn from serial sections of the brain.

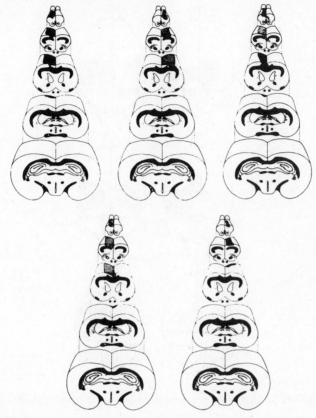

FIGURE 4. Sites of unilateral frontal lesions, drawn from serial sections.

some of those rats which showed no diminution of their responses after repeated immersions of the tail at 4° C, and the absence or presence of habituation was in no way related to the amount of cortical tissue removed, but only to the site of the lesions. It should be noted, however, that none of the lesions were large.

Effects of Lesions upon Established Habituation

After training to the experimental conditions over 14 days eight normal rats had their tails immersed six times daily for 10 min at a time in water at 4° C as in the experiments described above, but bilateral frontal lobe lesions were made immediately after the 10th series of such cold immersions. During the following 6 days the rats were placed vertically in the tubes with their tails at 31° C, as for preliminary training to the experimental conditions but without any cooling of their tails. On the 7th day after the operation the rats were again tested six times for 10 min with their tails at 4° C, and it was found

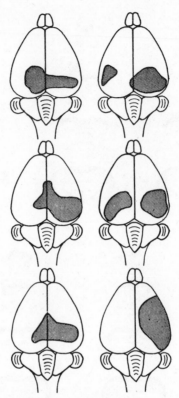

FIGURE 5. Sites of occipito-parietal lesions drawn from serial sections.

that the heart-rate response of two rats had returned to the same level as when the tail was first cooled, but in the other six the response remained low, which suggested that habituation had been lost in only two out of eight animals. The main results are given in Figure 6. Under the basic experimental conditions the heart rate did not increase significantly 7 days after bilateral frontal lobe lesions in any of these eight rats. Subsequent histological examination of the brains showed that the lesions were in the same regions and of a similar extent as bilateral frontal lesions shown in Figure 3.

Eight control rats were tested in the same way but without any operations. Habituation to immersions of the tails at 4° C closely resembled that shown in Figure 2A. Reduced responses of the heart rate to cooling of the tail were still observed 7 days or 14 days later, even though the tails had only been immersed at 31° C on the intervening days, there being only small and apparently random differences between the responses on the 10th day of daily immersions and after intervals of 7 or 14 days. This conformed with similar observations made on man (Glaser *et al.* 1959).

After habituation to the basic experimental conditions and to cooling of the tail, large lesions were applied to the cerebral cortex of two rats, without

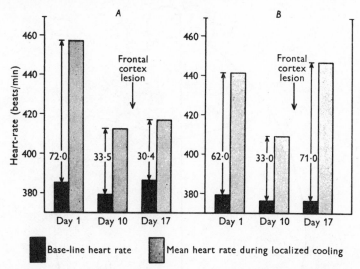

FIGURE 6. Effects of bilateral frontal cortical lesions applied after habituation to localized cooling. A. Mean results from six rats in which lesions did not alter the response of the heart rate to cooling of the tails. B. Mean of two rats in which 7 days after operation the response returned to its original level.

involving the frontal areas, but causing more extensive damage than any lesions shown in Figures 3–5. Seven days after such operations the heart rates were raised both under the basic experimental conditions and with the tails at 4° C, which conformed with findings by Lashley and Wiley (1933) that large lesions of the brain can cause a loss of stored information, irrespective of the site of lesion.

Stimulation of the Brain

Figure 7 shows the points at which stimulating electrodes were applied to the cerebral cortex. After habituation had been carried out over 14 days, as in Figure 1, the tail was cooled six times at intervals of 10 min as in all other rats, but throughout the 2nd, 4th, and 6th immersions the brain was stimulated by square waves of 24 μA at frequencies of 0·5–30 impulses/sec with a duration of 0·9 m-sec. Figure 8 shows the mean results from eight rats in which electrical stimuli were applied to the frontal areas of the cerebral cortex (numbers 2–9 on Fig. 7), and in all these rats the responses to cooling were greatly reduced or abolished, both while the stimuli were applied and thereafter. While electrical stimuli were not being applied, the mean increase of the heart rate during cooling of the tail was 63 beats/min; with stimulation it fell to 5 beats/min. Twenty-four hours after electrical stimulation of the brain the responses to immersion of the tail were still very much smaller than on the 2nd day of immersions in control rats (Fig. 2*A*) or in the same rats without stimulation, the differences being so large and consistent that statistical assessment

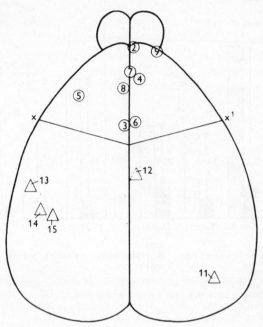

FIGURE 7. Sites of stimulating electrodes on the brain surface. x–x¹ shows the position of the fronto-parietal suture.

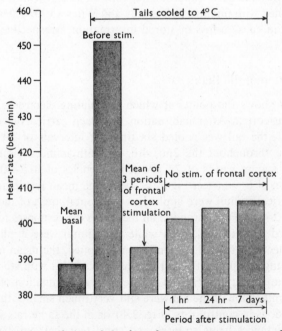

FIGURE 8. Effects of stimulation of the frontal cortex upon responses of the heart rate to cooling of the tail. Mean result of eight rats (numbers 2–9 in Figure 7).

of their significance was not appropriate (Fig. 8). For the next 5 days these animals were put vertically into the tubes with their tails at 31° C for 2½ hr daily, and 7 days after the electrical stimuli had been applied to the brain the responses of the heart rate to cooling of the tails were still almost as low as they had been during electrical stimulation.

Stimulation of the brain surface in the occipito-parietal region (Fig. 7, numbers 11–15) had no effect on the responses of the heart rate to cooling of the tail, either during stimulation or thereafter, and, if anything, stimulation was accompanied by a greater response of the heart rate to cooling.

Stimulation of the frontal areas at up to 30 impulses/sec under the basic experimental conditions while the tails were at 31° C did not alter the heart rate to any relevant extent. When the frontal cortex was stimulated during immersions of the tail at 4° C at 100 impulses/sec, no effect on the heart rate was observed either during stimulation or subsequently, which might have been due to a Wedensky inhibition.

Discussion

Validity of the Results

In the present experiment there were two habituations, one to the experimental conditions, the other to cooling of the rats' tails at 4° C. The former depended on a complex stimulus which consisted of the rats being placed in the vertical position inside tubes with their tails immersed to a constant level at a neutral temperature and with leads clipped to indwelling electrodes, and it included a small amount of constant noise from apparatus. The second was to a single precise stimulus caused by cooling of the tail. Responses of the heart rate to cooling of the tail were related to base-line readings obtained under identical conditions on the same day (Figs. 2, 6, 8) but habituation to the experimental conditions was expressed in terms of the actual heart rates observed (Fig. 1), as in rats any attempt to measure the heart rate will inevitably alter it. The normal heart rate of rats is not known. It was given as 328 beats/min with a range of 261–600 (*Handbook,* 1956a) and as 460 beats/min at a body temperature of 37–39° C (*Handbook,* 1956b).

Oestrus, which takes place every 4–5 days, was an uncontrolled variable and it may have contributed to fluctuations of the heart rate, but its effects were randomly distributed, so that it could not have invalidated the results, whereas the use of male rats could have introduced errors because of mild trauma to the scrotum by the tubes. Since analysis of variance showed that there were no interactions other than irregular daily fluctuations of the basic heart rates of individual rats which influenced the results, and since the design of the experiment ensured that all possible causes of error should either be excluded or randomly distributed, significant changes of the responses could only have been due to previous applications of the stimuli.

The fact that removal or stimulation of the cerebral cortex in the frontal areas had any effect on habituation must have been due to those particular procedures, since the removal or stimulation of other cortical areas had no such effect. Immediate post-operative disabilities could not have played any part, because these would have been the same in all operations on adjacent parts of the brain and because at least 7 days were allowed to elapse before any data were collected after any operation. However, the loss of habituation observed in two rats after large lesions not involving the frontal areas shows that conclusions based on extensive damage to the brain could be misleading in the context of the present experiment.

The question was considered whether it could be concluded that rats with bilateral frontal lesions did not become habituated to immersions of their tails at 4° C because these rats had higher initial heart rates under the basic experimental conditions and smaller responses to localized cooling than other rats. However, the actual heart rates during cooling of the tails were higher in rats with bilateral frontal lesions at the end of the experiment than in other animals at the beginning, and presumably baroreceptor reflexes had come into play while the tails were being immersed at 4° C; these reflexes would have prevented as great a relative increase of the heart rate as if the initial heart rate had been lower. The results can only mean that rats with bilateral frontal lesions responded to localized cooling and that they showed no signs of habituation.

The possibility that the diminution of responses to localized cooling of the tail might have been due to some adaptation of peripheral receptors seemed a remote one, because successive immersions at 4° C on the same day produced no consistent change of response, not even by analysis of variance, and this possibility has been eliminated in a separate investigation of nerve fibres in the rat's tail (J. P. Griffin and Ingrid Witt, unpublished). It is unlikely that the diminution of response observed after repeated cooling (Fig. 2*A, C, D*) was related to a change of blood flow through the skin of the tail, because the skin temperature did not change nor were there any obvious histological changes in the tails. The normal resting oxygen consumption of rats with bilateral frontal lesions (Table 1), and their normal growth and intake of water, make it seem unlikely that the gradual diminution of responses was due to some primary changes of the endocrine system, and it seems even more unlikely that such endocrine changes should have been prevented or abolished by bilateral frontal lesions and accelerated by stimulation of the frontal areas.

The Frontal Areas

It is evident from these findings that in rats the frontal areas of the cerebral cortex play a specific part in controlling the intensity of responses, both by immediate effects and by habituation. The fact that rats with bilateral frontal lesions failed to become habituated either to the experimental conditions or to immersions of the tails at 4° C, although unoperated controls and operated rats in which at least one side of the frontal area was intact showed normal habituations, suggests that the relationship between the frontal areas and habituation is not limited to localized nociceptive stimuli but includes the complex adjustments to the experimental conditions (Table 1, Fig. 2). The specific influence of the frontal cortex on the level of responses was further shown by the findings that stimulation of this area, but not of other parts of the brain surface, depressed the responses to localized cooling and accelerated habituation. The present results have thus confirmed and expanded earlier circumstantial evidence that "not only the responses but also habituation of these responses can be modified by the cerebral cortex" (Glaser, 1958). These findings are also in good agreement with those obtained in a different context by Brutkowski, Konorski, Lawicka, Stepien and Stepien (1956) and Lawicka (1957), who observed a loss of inhibitory conditioned reflexes in dogs after bilateral frontal lobectomies.

Previous experiments in which one hand was habituated to cold (Glaser and Whittow, 1957) or to heat and cold (Glaser *et al.* 1959) and in which responses of the heart rate were studied, suggested the possibility that habituation may have some functional localization in the brain, and the present experiments have shown that comparatively small areas of the frontal cortex can have an important influence upon habituation; but it does not follow that the frontal areas of the brain contain a kind of "habituation centre."

The Nature of Habituation

Habituation undoubtedly adjusts the level of responses in intact higher organisms according to previous experience of the appropriate stimuli, but the intensity of responses does not depend on habituation alone. Even if the stimulus is constant and the state of habituation unchanging, the magnitude of the appropriate responses can be modified by arousal from other stimuli arriving at about the same time (Glaser *et al.* 1959). It is known that arousal depends both on the brain-stem reticular formation and on the cerebral cortex (Hagbarth and Kerr, 1954; Galambos, 1956; Hernández-Peón *et al.* 1956; Dawson, 1958), and the present experiments have shown that habituation depends on the frontal areas of the brain. It would seem, therefore, that the cerebral cortex and the brain-stem reticular formation act together in adjusting the level of responses according to the intensity of present stimuli and according to stored information about previous stimuli. Habituation would appear to be that part of this mechanism which depends on stored information, but the fact that habituation was not necessarily lost after bilateral damage to the frontal areas (Fig. 6) probably means that the frontal areas are needed only to establish a change of response, not to maintain habituation.

It has been suggested that the processes which bring about habituation may take place at the central nervous synapses (Glaser and Whittow, 1957; Glaser, 1958). Learning in *Octopus* may depend on the fact that distinct sets of neurones "become so connected as to produce response in different directions" (Young, 1960), and it seems reasonable to assume that this could also happen in conditioning (Konorski, 1948). Changes of synaptic conduction are thus common to learning, conditioning and habituation (Glaser, 1958), but these three phenomena are not identical. In physiological terms, learning is the acquisition of a new response, or a qualitative change of an existing response, or an inhibition or facilitation of an existing response by a new stimulus; conditioning is the transfer of an existing response to a new stimulus; and habituation is a gradual quantitative change of response which may lead to a loss of response but excludes any change of stimulus and any qualitative change of response. Thus learning and conditioning imply mainly the forming of fresh neuronal circuits, whereas habituation involves mainly the inhibition of existing pathways. Inhibition in the central nervous system may arise from two distinct processes, post-synaptic inhibition due to a specific chemical transmitter and presynaptic inhibition due to a diminution in the size and number of afferent impulses (Eccles, 1961), but the evidence does not allow a definite conclusion whether habituation is a post-synaptic inhibition gradually taking place at the internuncial neurones.

Summary

1. A method was developed for studying habituation in conscious rats. This involved first the habituation of rats to the experimental conditions and then electronic counting of their heart rates while a uniform cold stimulus was repeatedly applied to their tails.

2. Cooling of the tail was accompanied by an increase of the heart rate in normal rats and in rats with various lesions of the cerebral cortex.

3. In normal rats this increase became gradually and significantly smaller after repeated cooling over a period of 10 days, which was taken as evidence of habituation.

4. Small bilateral frontal lesions of the cerebral cortex prevented habituation to the experimental conditions and to cooling of the tail in each of 9 rats so treated, but an established habituation was abolished by such operations in only two out of eight rats.

5. Eleven rats with unilateral frontal lesions or with occipito-parietal lesions of the cerebral cortex showed normal habituation to the experimental conditions and to cooling of their tails.

6. Electrical stimulation of the frontal areas depressed the responses to cooling of the tails and accelerated habituation, but stimulation of other areas of the cortex had no such effect.

7. It was concluded that the frontal areas of the cerebral cortex are necessary for the achievement but not the maintenance of habituation and that these areas are part of an integrated system which adjusts the level of responses in intact animals.

Assessment of the sites of lesions and helpful advice by Dr K. Weinbren, help and advice over histological techniques by Dr A. Howe, help with the measurements of the oxygen consumption and investigations of tail tissue by Mr P. D. Lewis, and much technical help by Mr J. Rawlings, are gratefully acknowledged.

References

Brutkowski, S., Konorski, J., Lawicka, W., Stepien, I. and Stepien, L. (1956). The effect of the removal of frontal poles of the cerebral cortex on motor conditioned reflexes. *Acta Biol. exp., Varsovie,* **17,** 167–188.

Davis, J. E. and van Dyke, H. B. (1932). The measurement of the oxygen consumption of small animals. *J. biol. Chem.* **95,** 73–78.

Davis, R. C. (1934). Modifications of the galvanic reflex by daily repetition of a stimulus. *J. exp. Psychol.* **17,** 504–535.

Dawson, G. D. (1958). The central control of sensory inflow. *Proc. R. Soc. Med.* **51,** 531–535.

Eccles, J. (1961). The nature of central inhibition. *Proc. Roy. Soc.* B, **153,** 445–476.

Galambos, R. (1956). Suppression of auditory nerve activity by stimulation of efferent fibres to cochlea. *J. Neurophysiol.* **19,** 424–437.

Glaser, E. M. (1953). Experiments on the side-effects of drugs. *Brit. J. Pharmacol.* **8,** 187–192.

Glaser, E. M. (1958). Adaptation, learning and behaviour. *Lond. Hosp. Gazette,* **61,** Suppl. 2.

Glaser, E. M. and Griffin, J. P. (1961). Changes of habituation induced by lesions and stimulation of the brain. *J. Physiol.* **155,** 54–55P.

Glaser, E. M., Griffin, J. P. and Knight, D. (1960). Apparatus for recording the heart rate in conscious animals. *J. Physiol.* **153,** 37–38P.

Glaser, E. M., Hall, M. S. and Whittow, G. C. (1959). Habituation to heating and cooling of the same hand. *J. Physiol.* **146,** 152–164.

Glaser, E. M. and Lee, T. S. (1959). Habituation to sensory stimulation of the mouth and the inhibition of such habituation by chlorpromazine hydrochloride. *Clin. Sci.* **18,** 81–88.

Glaser, E. M. and Whittow, G. C. (1953). Evidence for a non-specific mechanism of habituation. *J. Physiol.* **122,** 43P.

Glaser, E. M. and Whittow, G. C. (1954). Experimental errors in clinical trials. *Clin. Sci.* **13,** 199–210.

Glaser, E. M. and Whittow, G. C. (1957). Retention in a warm environment of adaptation to localized cooling. *J. Physiol.* **136,** 98–111.

Glaser, E. M. and Yap, T. B. (1959). Effects of anaesthesia upon responses to repeated cooling. *J. Physiol.* **146,** 42–43P.

Hagbarth, K. E. and Kerr, D. I. B. (1954). Central influences on spinal afferent conduction. *J. Neurophysiol.* **17,** 295–307.

Hagbarth, K. E. and Kugelberg, E. (1958). Plasticity of the human abdominal skin reflex. *Brain,* **81,** 305–318.

Handbook of Biological Data (1956a). P. 277. Ohio: Wright air development center.

Handbook of Biological Data (1956b). P. 438. Ohio: Wright air development center.

Hernández-Peón, R., Scherrer, H. and Velasco, M. (1956). Central influences on afferent conduction in the somatic and visual pathways. *Acta neurol. latinoamer.* **2,** 8–22.

Humphrey, G. (1933). *The Nature of Learning.* London: Kegan Paul.

Klüver, H. and Barrera, E. (1953). A method for the combined staining of cells and fibres in the nervous system. *J. Neuropath.* **12,** 400–403.

Knoppers, A. T. (1942). La queue de rat, témoin de la régulation thermique. *Arch. neerl. Physiol.* **26,** 363–406.

Konorski, J. (1948). *Conditioned Reflexes and Neuron Organization,* transl. by Garry, S. Chap. V. Cambridge: University Press.

Lashley, K. S. and Wiley, L. E. (1933). Studies of cerebral function in learning. IX. Mass action in relation to the number of elements in the problem to be learned. *J. comp. Neurol.* **57,** 3–56.

Lawicka, W. (1957). The effect of the prefrontal lobotomy on the vocal conditioned reflexes in dogs. *Acta Biol. exp., Varsovie,* **17,** 317–325.

Scholander, T. (1960). Habituation of autonomic response elements under two conditions of alertness. *Acta physiol. scand.* **50,** 259–268.

Scholander, T. (1961). Habituation processes. *Ann. Acad. R. Sci. Upsal.* **5,** 1–34.

Sharpless, S. and Jasper, H. H. (1956). Habituation of the arousal reaction. *Brain,* **79,** 655–680.

Young, J. Z. (1960). Unit processes in the formation of representations in the memory of *Octopus. Proc. Roy. Soc.* B, **153,** 1–17.

"Attention" Units in the Auditory Cortex

DAVID H. HUBEL, CALVIN O. HENSON,
ALLEN RUPERT, AND ROBERT GALAMBOS

Reprinted from *Science,* May 8, 1959, Vol. 129, pp. 1279–1280.

Cortical units that seem to be sensitive to auditory stimuli only if the subject "pays attention" were encountered in a series of experiments carried out on the auditory cortex of seven cats. The recording technique has already been summarized (*1*) and was as follows. Animals were prepared under anesthesia, with a small hollow plastic peg screwed into the skull over the cortical site to be examined. Several days later this peg was used to hold a hydraulic micropositioner containing a tungsten microelectrode (*2*). At the end of each recording session the holder and electrode were removed, and the cat was returned to its cage. The cats were studied for many hours during each of four to six recording sessions carried out over a period of 7 to 14 days. In each recording session the units were examined for periods of up to several hours, during which time the cat was free to move its head, groom, sleep, and so on.

Electrode sites were verified by marking the brain through the lumen of the peg with India ink, perfusing the cat with 10-percent formalin, and removing and photographing the brain. In this series of experiments it was not possible to measure the depth of the electrode accurately at the time of recording. All units, however, were located 5 mm or less beneath the cortical surface. From previous work (2) it is known that the electrodes used are capable of recording both from cell bodies and from myelinated fibers, but it was not possible to distinguish one from the other in these studies. Loud-speakers located near the cat's head were used to deliver the auditory stimuli. The frequency range from 50 to 50,000 cy/sec was adequately covered.

The following extracts from the protocol illustrate the peculiar behavior of these cells.

Cat 17

This unit studied for 1 hr 35 min showed little spontaneous activity. It could not be reliably driven by clicks, tones, or noise from the loud-speaker on repeated tests, although a new tone or noise might evoke responses during the first few presentations. When the experimenter entered the experimental room he discovered that a variety of natural stimuli could evoke responses provided the cat appeared to be paying attention to them. The unit responded briskly, for example, to (i) voice, (ii) squeaks emitted by squeezing a toy rubber mouse [Fig. 1], (iii) scratching fingernail on table nearby, (iv) hissing, (v) tapping the table. It responded regularly and consistently to clicks from the loud-speaker whenever the experimenter pretended to tap the loud-speaker in rhythm with the clicks but without actually making any sound. Passively closing the cat's eyes with the fingers did not stop the response when it was present. Discharge rate seemed to vary with the intensity of the stimulus and response frequently outlasted the stimulus by periods of up to about one second.

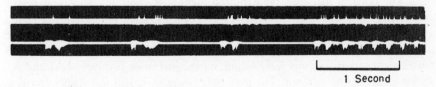

1 Second

FIGURE 1. Response of an auditory cortical unit in cat No. 17. Lower line shows response of a microphone located near the cat's ear; the deflections seen there were produced by squeaks emitted when a toy mouse was squeezed. The upper line shows the unit responding to the squeaks to which the animal was paying attention; this unit almost never responded to clicks, tones, or noise from a nearby loud-speaker.

Cat 18

This unit was spontaneously active but could not be driven by clicks, tones, or noise from the loud-speaker. Keys jingled by the experimenters outside the room in which the cat was isolated evoked responses when the animal looked toward the door, but not otherwise. The experimenter then entered the room, picked up a small piece of paper between each thumb and forefinger and held his hands to the right and left of the cat about 12 inches away from its ears. When the paper was rustled in the right hand no response occurred until the cat looked toward it, whereupon a large burst of firing occurred so long as the sound was produced. If now the paper in the left hand was rubbed, nothing happened until the cat turned its head in that direction, whereupon again the unit responded to the sound. If the noise was made to alternate between left and right hands, responses occurred only to the sound produced by the hand toward which the cat was looking. Holding the hands out of sight did not change the result: so long as the cat looked in the proper direction the responses occurred. The unit was studied in this way for many minutes.

Six units of the sort just described were seen in four cats. At least nine other units, somewhat less intensively studied, should probably also be included, for they responded poorly or not at all to clicks, tones, or noise from the loud-speakers but responded well to sounds produced near the animal. Since the total number of units thus far studied is more than 100, about 10 percent can therefore be called attention units. As for the remaining 90 percent, it is not our purpose to discuss the behavior of these units in detail here, but it should be pointed out that some of them responded reliably for long periods to stimuli presented by means of the loud-speakers, regardless of the behavioral state of the animal (alert, asleep, and so on). Furthermore, one well-studied unit (in cat No. 24) was exquisitely responsive to 53-kcy/sec sound, from which we infer that our failure to drive other units with tones was not due to failure to generate high-frequency sounds. Finally, it has proved impossible to discover the stimuli adequate for driving many of our cortical units, a fact we cannot readily explain.

The cortical loci thus far explored include A_1 and A_{11} and their rostral and inferior borders with adjacent cortex (Fig. 2). Five punctures (cats Nos. 13, 20, 22, and 24) in approximately the center of A_1 yielded no attention units, while three others (cats Nos. 13 and 24) did. In cats Nos. 17 and 18, where most attention units were found, cortex just in or just out of A_1 and A_{11} seems to have been entered. The material, however, is still too scanty for us to settle the question of just where attention units occur in and near the auditory cortex.

We have in four punctures (three cats) encountered both attention units and conventional responders in a single electrode penetration. In three separate penetrations in cat No. 17, however, we encountered only attention units, or units not driven by the loud-speaker stimuli. These facts would make it appear that attention units are both interspersed among conventional responders and collected in isolation apart from them, but, again, this problem cannot be considered as settled.

According to Erulkar, Rose, and Davies (3), 34 percent of the units

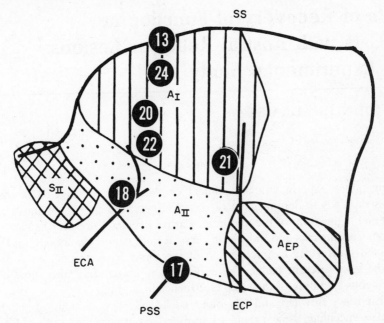

FIGURE 2. Schematic drawing of the left auditory cortex of the cat, showing the location of electrode tracks in seven cats. A_I, A_{II}, and A_{EP} are the main auditory cortical areas.

isolated in auditory cortex cannot be driven by sounds, and, in fact, only about 14 percent are reliably and securely activated by acoustic stimuli. The cats used by these workers were under light general anesthesia, and so it may be presumed that the attention units under discussion here were included in their class of nonresponders. It is not easy to understand why the auditory cortex, in the anesthetized or intact cat, should be populated with so many cells that fail to respond to auditory stimuli. Perhaps these cells become activated only when certain other conditions are simultaneously met. Thus, from our data one may conclude that the neural processes responsible for attention play an important role in determining whether or not a given acoustic stimulus proves adequate. Unfortunately attention is an elusive variable that no one has as yet been able to quantify. It may be that studies in which cortical unit activity is examined during the course of conditioning and learning will illuminate these matters.

References and Notes

1. D. H. Hubel, *Am. J. Ophthalmol.* **46,** 110 (1958).
2. ———, *Science* **125,** 549 (1957).
3. S. D. Erulkar, J. E. Rose, P. W. Davies, *Bull. Johns Hopkins Hosp.* **99,** 55 (1956).

Rate of Recovery of Functioning
in Cats with Rostral Reticular Lesions:
An Experimental Study

JOHN H. ADAMETZ

Reprinted from *Journal of Neurosurgery*.

Recent studies, experimental and clinical, emphasize that damage to the rostral brain stem leads to derangement of consciousness, the site of emphasis being the mesial tegmentum of the midbrain. Earlier Bremer [2] stressed the similarity between sleeping cats and those with cerveau isolé (midbrain transection) and attributed the former to interruption of the tonic drive propagated rostrally over the great afferent paths. The cerveau isolé preparation also showed the spontaneous spindling of the sleep electroencephalogram.

Lindsley, Bowden and Magoun [8] added selective sections of the lemniscus to encéphale isolé (acute Cl transection) preparations. This did not convert the activation tracing characteristic of the encéphale isolé to the cerveau isolé type. However, lesions that instead destroyed sub- and hypothalamus from optic chiasm to mammillary bodies or anterior midbrain did produce a sleep tracing. Additionally, Lindsley *et al.*[9] studied the effects of chronic lesions. In animals with lesions in the ponto-midbrain tegmentum, midbrain tegmentum, hypothalamus, and junction between hypothalamus and thalamus, the common behavioral result (variable in degree depending upon site and extent of the lesion) was a postoperative somnolence or lethargy in which the animal displayed little or no spontaneous activity of a purposive sort, and seemed unaware of ordinary environmental stimuli. The animal with a midbrain tegmental lesion blocking much or all of the rostral end of the reticular activating system lay on its side with eyes closed as if deeply asleep during its 21-day survival period. By contrast, in 2 animals in which the periaqueductal gray was injured an approximation of normal sleeping-waking behavior was regained. Two others, with lateral mesencephalic lesions which spared the mesial tegmentum, became able to stand and walk again and showed activation of the electroencephalographic tracing. Experiments on 9 monkeys reported by French and Magoun [6] appeared generally to confirm these results so far as destruction of the reticular activating system and the associated behavioral deficits are concerned.

Cairns [3] concluded from an extensive clinical study that brain-stem lesions occasion loss of crude consciousness. Of particular interest to the locale of the present investigation is the condition of hypersomnia wherein sleep continues but can be broken into by brief arousals produced by stimulation. A variant called *akinetic mutism* (Cairns *et al.*[4]) shows loss of spontaneous and of most other voluntary movements but is associated with the appearance of alertness because of ocular movement and fixation in response to the movement of objects or to sound. Jefferson [7] reported upon 6 cases in which there were disturbances of consciousness in conjunction with signs indicative of disorder of the midbrain. He concluded that obscuration of consciousness in variable degree was caused by encroachment of the lesions upon the reticular activating system. There were no pathological controls. French [5] found that in 3 of 5 cases in which there were profound alterations of consciousness the lesions were so situated as to destroy the reticular activating system. Penfield,[10] commencing in 1938, has come to consider the reticular substance of the brain stem as the core of his centrencephalic system.

The experiments reported herein were designed to establish whether the procedures involved in producing brain-stem lesions and in the aftercare of the animals contribute significantly to the behavioral results. Riese [11] in his *Principles of Neurology* generalizes as follows: "In the initial stage many more regions are functionless than in the residual stage, and this explains the unanimous observation that the initial defects are much more severe" (p. 119). This suggests the importance of comparing lesions of the same size (1) produced at a single sitting and (2) by step-wise accumulation. Aftercare of the animals was directed primarily toward securing the maximal possible survival period and secondarily toward encouraging self-feeding and self-care.

Method

For the more definitive experiments the cats were grouped for age and size. After preoperative still and motion-picture photography the animals of a group were divided into two sets of 3 each. In one set, a lesion (or lesions) of the desired size and position was placed at a single sitting; in the other set lesions totalling the planned size were placed step-wise in 2 or more stages, 1 to 3 weeks apart. When 2 stages were used to place bilateral lesions in the mesial tegmentum of the midbrain, each such stage was controlled by a set of 3 animals in which bilateral lesions of the same size were placed at a single sitting. The same operator set the Horsley-Clarke coordinates in each instance and the lesions were produced by a uniform technique.

Surital was used for anesthesia (1 cc./kg., intrathoracic). The lesions were made with cathodal current using a #7 milliner's steel sewing needle with tip exposure of 2–10 mm., depending upon the depth of the lesion desired. The current passed was ordinarily 4.8 MA., 50–70 sec., for each placement. For lesions localized to the mesial tegmentum a longitudinal row of electrolyses was usually placed 3 mm. from the midline. They were closely spaced enough to coalesce into a single lesion 2–3 mm. wide, 1 cm. long and 5 mm. in depth. Additionally corresponding bilateral mesial reticular lesions were placed at transverse plane A + 4 in each of several cats.

To approximate a uniform recovery rate as closely as possible all animals of a group were fed and cared for together, tube feedings always being given routinely to those animals temporarily or permanently unable to feed themselves. Antibiotics also were given routinely. Interim photography was done as recovery progressed.

After allowing ample time for recovery, or upon the death of an animal, the brain stem was prepared by frozen serial sectioning, and the sections were stained either with thionine for cells or luxor-fast blue for myelin.

Results

1. Comparison of Recovery Rates with Bilateral Mesial Tegmental Lesions. Done at 1 and at 2 Sittings

In one series of 3 cats bilateral lesions of approximately 1 cm. A-P length were produced in the mesial tegmentum of the rostral midbrain by a 2-stage procedure; the 2nd stage followed the 1st by 3 weeks, permitting thorough recovery from the 1st (unilateral) lesion. Each stage was controlled by 3 other cats in which bilateral lesions as nearly identical as possible (within the range of variability of the method) were produced at a single sitting. The same design had been carried through in an earlier series but with incomplete results since 2 animals died during the postoperative period. Matched pairs of animals (1- and 2-stage) prepared in a similar fashion brought the total animals observed to 12 with 2-stage and 15 with 1-stage operations.

Of the 15 animals with bilateral 1-stage lesions (including all those done to provide running mates for 2-stage animals) only one survived for more than 32 days. Except for that one all remained comatose throughout the survival period, existing on the tube feedings provided. Figure 1 illustrates a cat that had been in coma 30 days at the time of the picture, and the position and extent of its tegmental lesions. Figure 2 contrasts 3 cats with 2-stage bilateral lesions (sitting) in contrast with 3 others (1-stage) all lying upon their sides in coma. It was taken on the 1st postoperative day following the completion of the 2nd stage on the sitting cats.

The exceptional animal remained comatose until the 35th postoperative day and then commenced to take liquid food from a dish and to evidence other interest in its surroundings. From then on it gradually re-acquired the ability to stand and walk unaided. Before being killed on the 64th postoperative day it was moving about freely and purposively albeit clumsily. Its progression was sinuate and it did not always avoid obstacles placed in its way. This cat was observed to claw vigorously at a small cage containing mice, and it also caught mice quickly and purposively. Figure 3 illustrates the appearance of this animal upon the 59th day, and the size and position of its tegmental lesions. Those were as extensive as in any of the corresponding animals that died while still in coma.

In marked contrast to the last series, the 3 animals in which bilateral lesions of the same size had been produced in 2 stages, and 9 others became aware of their surroundings and able to feed themselves upon the 1st postoperative day following the placement of the 1st-stage lesion. Recovery of standing and walking was rapid and at the end of 3 weeks these animals were able to care for themselves in all respects. Nearly all 1st-stage animals showed cocking of the head with the occiput away from the side of the lesion. This usually disappeared after the 2nd stage when the symmetrical lesion was placed.

After the 2nd operation the animals again were able to eat unaided upon the 1st postoperative day, despite the fact that they now had an aggregate of lesions approximating those described above for the 1-stage comatose animals. From that time on their recovery progressed somewhat more slowly, but beyond comparison with the recovery rate of any animal in which bilateral lesions had been made at one sitting. Two months postoperatively several of these animals nearly approached normal except for movement upon horizontal ladders. Their inadequate placing reactions made them somewhat unsteady. They pursued mice, could jump a distance of several feet, and groomed themselves regularly. All were alert and constantly interested in their surroundings. At no time after the first few days was a significant disturbance of the normal waking-sleeping cycle observed: the animals slept at night and remained awake much of the day. They reacted quickly to noxious stimuli. Figure 2 illustrates 3 cats on the 1st postoperative day following the 2nd-stage operation (sitting) by comparison with 3 cats with the 1-stage operation (in coma). Figure 4 illustrates a close-up of Cat 48 after its 2nd-stage operation together with its tegmental lesion.*

One animal of this series died on the 5th postoperative day following a 2nd-stage (bilateral) lesion. To a few hours preceding its death its progress had been as satisfactory as that of any corresponding animal. It could stand and walk well and was rapidly regaining strength. Within a 4-hour period it became progressively more flaccid and unable to walk, its pupils dilating gradually and equally as it became less and less responsive. Necropsy revealed an extensive hemorrhage into the bilateral tegmental lesion, providing an obvious cause for the rapid deterioration in status that had ensued. Two animals with unilateral lesions were lost during recovery because they aspirated food with resultant pulmonary complications.

---

* Editor's note: Figures 1–7 have been deleted from the text of this article. The reader is referred to the original source for these illustrations.

2. Recovery Rate, One-Stage Bilateral Lesions in a Single Transverse Plane (A + 4)

Three animals were operated upon, all of which responded well, feeding themselves on the 1st postoperative day and thereafter recovering to an approximation of neurological normality. They demonstrate that more confined bilateral tegmental lesions need not produce coma when accomplished at 1 stage.

3. Recovery Rate with Multi-stage Electrolyses Designed to Completely Interrupt the Rostrally Directed Reticular Paths

Past investigations suggested this as another point of attack. The midbrain tegmentum caudal to the meso-diencephalic junction was destroyed as completely as possible by 6–8 electrolyses placed in a transverse row, one each at successive weekly procedures. The raphe was avoided to spare the periaqueductal gray. The destruction in this instance differed from that in the preceding in being more extensive at one transverse level, whereas the lesions described in section 1 destroyed a zone approximately 1 cm. lengthwise of the midbrain but were less extensive ventrally and in the transverse plane.

One such animal withstood 7 such lesions and 2 others 8 (Fig. 5). All were able to feed themselves and showed awareness of their surroundings after each of the procedures, although the ability to stand and walk, particularly on a smooth surface, declined progressively. Nevertheless all of the animals could still walk, although unsteadily, after the last operation. Except for the immediate postoperative period the waking-sleep cycle appeared undisturbed. Controls in which all electrolyses were placed at one sitting did not recover from coma and all were dead within 12 days (Fig. 6).

4. Spontaneously Developing Generalized Seizures in Chronic Animals

Each of 5 animals that had lived 2½ months postoperatively with mesial reticular lesions (11, 18, 20, 26, 33) had one known generalized seizure of 5–30 min. duration. In 3 animals the lesions had been placed unilaterally and in the other 2 bilaterally. One animal (18) had only a small unilateral lesion.

All seizures were of the tonic decerebrate type with opisthotonus. Clonic contractions were minimal. In all instances the animals became drowsy, listless and hypotonic immediately after the seizures. They also became increasingly difficult to arouse and died within 4 hours. Histological findings were unique only in indicating the variability in size and location of the lesions that could produce such seizures. Cats 11 and 26 had extensive bilateral mesial tegmental lesions. Cat 18 had a very small lesion outside the periaqueductal gray. Cats 20 and 33 also had a unilateral lesion but the size was significantly larger.

Three other animals are mentioned because the procedures were designed to occasion seizures but did not do so. Each of the 3 had been injected with aluminum hydroxide gel to fill a cavity formed by the usual bilateral electrolytic lesions. These were kept for several months with no seizures developing. One such animal was killed on the 35th postoperative day after the 2nd-stage operation. Fifteen days before that it had walked well (Fig. 7), and fed and groomed itself. Following this increasing spasticity developed in all extremities until at death it was unable to walk at all. However, it fed itself to the end and showed other evidences of continuing awareness. The bilateral lesions which in life were filled with alumina gel are remarkable for their size. They are also illustrated in Figure 7.

5. Periaqueductal Lesions

In 4 animals the lesions encroached upon the periaqueductal gray. One had involved the periaqueductal gray through an error in estimating the coordinates; the other 3 were provided intentionally as controls upon the mesial tegmental lesions described in section 1. All of these animals remained mute postoperatively although otherwise they recovered neurological normalcy with rapidity. In no instance was the mutism associated with akinesis, although one of them (11) was hyperkinetic.

The extension of all of these lesions into the periaqueductal gray was confirmed histologically.

Discussion

That brain-stem lesions show a high incidence of derangements of consciousness is attested to by both clinical and experimental studies. While presumably destruction of the reticular activating system is a primary factor in the production of coma by mesial tegmental lesions, other considerations have importance also. The experiments reported herein establish a shock factor (diaschisis), more enduring in the instance of bilateral lesions produced in 1 sitting than in that of corresponding lesions produced in 2 stages. The time the animal lives postoperatively is another important factor in the bilateral lesions placed at 1 sitting. In one such instance an animal remained comatose for 35 days—certainly not outside the possibility for return of consciousness in human midbrain injury—only to recover sufficiently to walk about, feed itself, and even to catch mice. Fourteen similar animals died in coma by the 32nd postoperative day.

While establishing a shock factor the above results do not provide any clear indication of how much of the cross-section of the tegmentum of the midbrain needs to be destroyed by step-lesions to produce coma. Current theory would suggest that this would be determined quantitatively rather than qualitatively, since reticular units are now conceived to be nonspecific in their activation. Partial answers can be obtained by multi-stage procedures in which a new lesion at a single transverse level is made each week, seeking to interrupt the whole of the through traffic before the loss of the animal. These animals, too, survived well the destruction of a considerable area of the tegmentum, again reiterating the importance of the shock factor. No animal in which the same procedure was undertaken at a single sitting lasted more than 12 days.

The 5 animals with late postoperative development of seizures (3–4 months) showed rough similarities in pattern of the seizures to the tonic decerebrate state (clonic component, minimal) and exhibited postictal flaccidity. Such seizures caused a 100 per cent mortality within a few hours. It might be presumed that the total mortality resulted from the addition of a state of seizures to the devitalizing effect of a tegmental lesion of significant size. However, one such lesion (unilateral) had contracted to a scar of small size scarcely recognizable in usual frozen sections. Thus, the probable locus from which the seizure spread would seem to be the important determinant of mortality, and the postulation of a devitalizing effect an unnecessary addition. It also seems probable that the epileptogenic locus was in fact in the tegmentum; the only other source would have been the cortical scar resulting from the passage of the electrode used in making the brain-stem lesion.

In the 4 mute animals the lesion in each case involved the periaqueductal gray, although encroaching to a variable extent upon the neighboring tegmentum. Since the lesions were ordinarily smaller than those placed in the mesial tegmentum, recovery of functioning was prompt. All these animals were known to meow before surgery; they remained quiet thereafter. Besides the muteness at full recovery, 3 were otherwise normal and 1 was hyperkinetic. At no stage did a mute cat appear to be akinetic. This differs from the results of Bailey,[1] but his akinetic mutes were produced by a different method.

Summary

Eighty cats with mesial tegmental lesions of the rostral midbrain were used in comparing ability to withstand complete interruption of the reticular paths done (1) at a single sitting and (2) in stages. With one exception extensive bilateral lesions made at a single sitting led to coma from which the animals did not recover although they sometimes were carried as long as 32 days on tube feedings. The same lesions placed upon one side at a time with an interval of 3 weeks between led to relatively quick recovery from coma and an early return of motor function.

Cats did survive 1-stage bilateral mesial tegmental lesions placed in one transverse plane (A + 4) provided the lesions did not extend too far in depth or laterally. Single-stage extensive interruptions in a transverse plane invariably led to coma and eventual death (longest survival, 12 days). However, animals did survive multi-stage procedures in which at weekly intervals one or more lesions were placed in a transverse row across the tegmentum.

In these experiments mutism associates with aqueductal or near-aqueductal lesions although in our experience it was not linked with akinesia (Bailey).[1] One such mute cat was hyperkinetic.

Seizures (centrencephalic?) occurred in 5 cats. These were of the tonic decerebrate type with a minimum of clonic movement. All such cats died within 4 hours postictally.

Continuation studies indicate that not all seizures that develop in animals with tegmental lesions terminate fatally within a short period. We have since carried animals for several days following such seizures, and it is possible that through improved care some might ultimately recover.

References

1. Bailey, P. Alterations of behavior produced in cats by lesions in the brainstem. *J. nerv. ment. Dis.*, 1948, **107**: 336–339.
2. Bremer, F. Cerveau "isolé" et physiologie du sommeil. *C. R. Soc. Biol., Paris,* 1935, **118**: 1235–1241.
3. Cairns, H. Disturbances of consciousness with lesions of the brain-stem and diencephalon. *Brain,* 1952, **75**: 109–146.
4. Cairns, H., Oldfield, R. C., Pennybacker, J. B., and Whitteridge, D. Akinetic mutism with an epidermoid cyst of the 3rd ventricle. (With a report on the associated disturbance of brain potentials.) *Brain,* 1941, **64**: 273–290.
5. French, J. D. Brain lesions associated with prolonged unconsciousness. *Arch. Neurol. Psychiat., Chicago,* 1952, **68**: 727–740.
6. French, J. D., and Magoun, H. W. Effects of chronic lesions in central cephalic brain stem of monkeys. *Arch. Neurol. Psychiat., Chicago,* 1952, **68**: 591–604.
7. Jefferson, M. Altered consciousness associated with brain-stem lesions. *Brain,* 1952, **75**: 55–67.
8. Lindsley, D. B., Bowden, J. W., and Magoun, H. W. Effect upon the EEG of acute injury to the brain stem activating system. *Electroenceph. clin. Neurophysiol.*, 1949, **1**: 475–486.
9. Lindsley, D. B., Schreiner, L. H., Knowles, W. B., and Magoun, H. W. Behavioral and EEG changes following chronic brain stem lesions in the cat. *Electroenceph. clin. Neurophysiol.*, 1950, **2**: 483–498.
10. Penfield, W. The cerebral cortex in man. I. The cerebral cortex and consciousness. *Arch. Neurol. Psychiat., Chicago,* 1938, **40**: 417–442.
11. Riese, W. Principles of neurology in the light of history and their present use. *New York: Nervous and Mental Disease Monographs,* 1950, 177 pp.

A Neurohumoral Mechanism
of Reticulo-Cortical Activation

DOMINICK P. PURPURA

Reprinted from *American Journal of Physiology*, 1956, Vol. 186, pp. 250–254.

It has been recently demonstrated that high frequency stimulation of the brain stem reticular system in unanesthetized cats produces a change in electrical excitability of certain cortical elements which persists beyond the period of stimulation (1). This observation coupled with the finding that short periods of high frequency bulbar stimulation are capable of activating and sustaining three per second "spike and wave" discharges in sub-liminally strychninized cortex (2) has led to a reappraisal of the conclusion that extraneuronal factors play a role in the phenomenon of cortical activation accompanying behavioral arousal. This was originally suggested by Ingvar (3) who observed long latency effects in neuronally isolated cortical slabs following reticular stimulation. Although these effects on the isolated cortex were associated with changes in the general cerebral circulation, it was proposed that humoral effects could not be excluded. "Humoral" activation studies were extended by Bonvallet *et al.* (4) and Dell *et al.* (5), who concluded that adrenaline produced cortical activation indirectly through stimulation of certain adrenaline-sensitive reticular interneurons. It was also suggested by these workers that "sympathin" demonstrated by Vogt (6) to be concentrated in certain brain stem regions might be liberated *in situ* by reticular stimulation.

In an attempt to define more precisely the existence of a neurohumoral factor liberated during reticulo-cortical activation cross-perfusion experiments were performed in unanesthetized animals with common circulation. With this technique, direct effects on the cerebral circulation, a seemingly unavoidable concomitant of brain stem stimulation (7), have been avoided.

Methods

Experiments were performed on 24 adult cats (2.5–5K) selected in pairs of approximately equal body weight. Two cats were utilized for each experiment. Under initial ether anesthesia tracheal cannulae were introduced into both animals followed by bilateral craniectomies and preparation of both femoral arteries and veins for cannulation. Usually the bulbar extension of the brain stem was exposed only in the animal receiving the electrical stimulation. This was accomplished by enlargement of the foramen magnum and gentle suction of the overlying cerebellum thus exposing the entire floor of the fourth ventricle. This permitted displacement of the electrode for stimulation in the bulbar reticular system. Eight animals were sectioned at the atlanto-occipital junction ("encéphale isolé") to avoid general cardiovascular reflex complications and liberation of peripheral neurohumoral transmitters during stimulation of descending spinal autonomic system. After completion of all operative exposures and termination of ether, skin margins were infiltrated with novocaine. Both animals were placed on artificial respiration and paralyzed by means of a constant succinylcholine-chloride saline infusion. Differences in degree of aeration in both animals were controlled by employing a single respirator with double output connections to the tracheal cannulae. Following complete heparinization (10 mg/K, i.v.) four no. 15 polyethylene catheters were so arranged as to permit the blood from both femoral arteries of one animal to be shunted to the femoral veins of the other animal and vice versa. In this way complete intermixing of the total blood volume of both animals was effected within a few minutes as indicated by the ability to maintain neuromuscular paralysis with succinylcholine in both animals by infusion of one. Despite the creation of two arteriovenous shunts in both unanesthetized animals, the preparations remained in good condition for 5–6 hours. Failure of either animal to tolerate the double shunt was usually evident within a few minutes after opening them. When this occurred both animals were discarded from the experimental series.

Stimulation of the bulbar reticular formation was carried out with a 0.5 mm concentric electrode held in a micro-manipulator. Stimulus parameters were from 50–300 cps/sec., 5–20 v; .5–1.0 msec., square waves. Periods of stimulation ranged between 20–80 seconds. All electrocorticograms were recorded bipolarly with cotton wick chlorided silver electrodes utilizing a standard clinical eight channel Grass model III unit. One of the channels routinely served as a stimulation indicator marker. In a few instances EKG monitoring was utilized for recording possible changes in cardiac rate during stimulation.

Results

Activation of Intact Animals

The effect of electrical stimulation of the bulbar reticular formation of one animal, which produced a typical activation pattern (8), on the electrocortical activity of the second animal consisted in long-latency effects similar to those obtained in the first animal. An example of this is shown in Figure 1. (In this and all subsequent records *"A"* refers to the donor animal being electrically stimulated and *"B"* designates the recipient of the neurohumor.) Electrical stimulation of *A* (at first arrow, Fig. 1) resulted in an activation pattern which persisted throughout the 50-second period of stimulation. During this time no effect was detectable in the simultaneously recorded activity of *ani-*

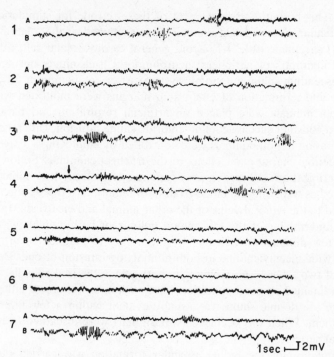

FIGURE 1. Simultaneous continuous electrocorticograms from *animals* A and B. Records obtained bipolarly from postsigmoid-ant. suprasylvian gyrus in A and postsigmoid-ant. lateral gyrus in B. At *first arrow* (1) stimulation of medial bulbar reticular formation was begun (10 V, 1 msec., 300/sec.) which ended at *second arrow* (4). Activation of *animal* B began in *row 5*, 65 sec. after beginning of stimulation.

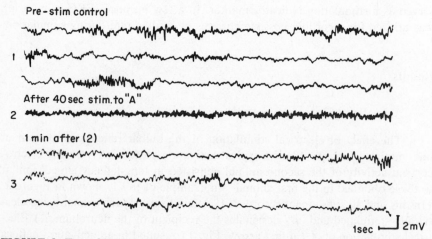

FIGURE 2. Examples of continuous record before stimulation (1); after 40 sec. of stimulation to *animal* A (2); and 1 min. after end of stimulation (3). Stimulus to A: 15 v., .5 msec., 300/sec. Note typical activation in (2).

mal B. A dramatic change in the character of this activity occurred about 65 seconds after onset of stimulation to A (line 5, Fig. 1). This activation pattern lasted 40 seconds then reverted to the pre-stimulation control (line 7).

Although the latency from the onset of stimulation of *animal A* to the beginning of activation of B was variable (30–80 sec.), from one pair of animals to the other, in any single pair this period was relatively constant (± 10 sec.). Latencies of from 20–70 seconds were reported by Ingvar (3) on isolated cortical slabs indicating that the circulation time through the recipient animal in the present experiments was not the major factor in the delayed effect.

To illustrate more clearly the nature of the humoral activation only the electrocorticogram of *animal B* is shown in Figure 2. This demonstrates the resting activity of B before stimulation of *animal A;* a sample of the change in this pattern after 40 seconds of stimulation of A; and the record 1 minute following stimulation.

It is important to point out that effects similar to those illustrated in Figures 1 and 2 depended on the initial level of excitability of both animals as indicated by the resting cortical activity. When a greater degree of cortical synchrony progressively developed in both animals, a decrease in electrical excitability of A and inability to obtain neurohumoral activation in B developed concomitantly.

Although it was unlikely that the long-latency changes induced in the recipient animal, B, on stimulation of *animal A,* might be due to cardio-vascu-

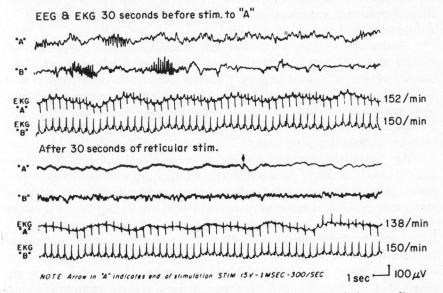

FIGURE 3. Simultaneous electrocorticograms of *animals* A and B and electrocardiograms of both animals. Bradycardia produced in *animal* A by stimulation (20 v, .5 msec., 300/ sec.) did not alter cardiac status of *animal B*.

lar alterations, EKG monitoring was carried out in a few experiments. Brady-cardia and tachycardia associated with pressor and depressor responses have been reported on electrical stimulation of brain stem regions co-extensive with the bulbar reticular formation (7). Examination of Figure 3 shows an example of the EEG's of animals *A* and *B* and their respective EKG's. It is of signifi-cance to point out that basal heart rates of both animals did not vary by more than 5% in intact and "encéphale isolé" preparations. After 30 seconds of stimulation to *A* marked flattening of activity occurred in *A* with activation of *B* as described above. Despite the slight bradycardia in *animal A* there was no change in the EKG status of *animal B*.

Neurohumoral Activation of Metrazol-Treated Cortex in Double "Encéphale Isolé" Preparations

It is commonly recognized that stimulation of the brain stem reticular for-mation may facilitate or inhibit paroxysmal activity induced by local applica-tion of dilute solutions of strychnine to the cortex (9). Effects of cortical activation on paroxysmal activity have been reported clinically (10). Brain stem stimulation was similarly shown by Ingvar to affect Metrazol activity in the neuronally isolated cortical slab. For this reason the effect of brain stem reticular stimulation of *animal A* on the Metrazol-treated cortex of *animal B* was studied in "encéphale isolé" cats in order to determine whether the neuro-humoral agent liberated on stimulation could reproduce these phenomena. This was confirmed as shown in Figures 4 and 5. These two figures illustrate the effect of neurohumoral activation of well developed Metrazol spiking (Fig. 4) and subliminal Metrazol activity (Fig. 5).

Reference to Figure 4 indicates that 30 minutes after the application of 3 drops of 5% Metrazol to the cortex of *B* intermittent spiking occurred be-tween resting synchronous activity. Reticular stimulation of *A* (first arrow) which lasted 75 seconds augmented the Metrazol-induced spiking to the point of maximal frequency after 65 seconds of stimulation. Below this (Fig. 4, *3*) 2 minutes after cessation of stimulation to *A*, spike activity markedly reduced to about the prestimulation level.

Of particular importance was the observation that although the amount and duration of action of the topically applied Metrazol was insufficient to pro-duce significant changes in the resting electrocortical activity of *A*, neurohu-moral activation oftentimes evoked paroxysmal activity to the point of sustained seizure discharges. This is demonstrated in Figure 5, which shows sustained seizure activity developing in *animal B* 60 seconds after stimulation of *animal A*. The sequence of events illustrated in Figures 4 and 5 could be readily repro-duced in the intact and "encéphale isolé" preparations. Less commonly it was observed that inhibition of well developed Metrazol activity occurred in *animal B* following reticular stimulation of *animal A*.

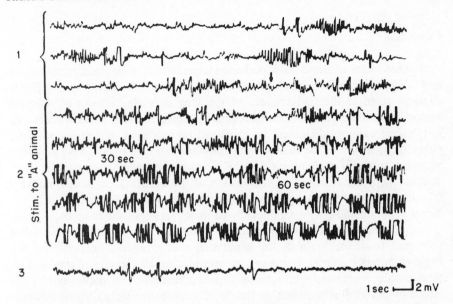

FIGURE 4. Electrocorticogram of *animal B* (postsigmoid-ant. lat. gyrus). Record begins 30 min. after application of 3 drops of 5% Metrazol to electrode sites. Stimulation of *animal A* (at first arrow) facilitated Metrazol treated cortex of B neurohumorally. Below this is a sample record 2 min. after end of reticular stimulation of *animal A*. Note in particular the activated character of the interspike activity after stimulation (3) as compared with the interspike activity prior to reticular stimulation of A (1).

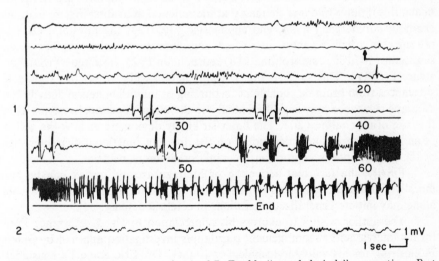

FIGURE 5. Electrocorticogram of *animal B*. Double "encephale isole" preparations. Postsigmoid-ant. lat. gyrus. Record began 2 min. after topical application of 3 drops of 5% Metrazol to B (subliminal). Note onset of spiking which developed into sustained seizure activity 60 sec. after stimulation of A. *Below*, basal activity 2 min. after end of stimulation.

Discussion

The results of these cross-perfusion experiments in unanesthetized intact and "encéphale isolé" cats provide additional evidence for neurohumoral factor at some stage in the maintenance of the long persisting effects of reticular system stimulation on electrocortical activity. Since the long latency effect (up to 80 sec.) cannot adequately be explained on the basis of circulation time, either the quantity of the neurohumor liberated must be regarded as attaining a certain optimum concentration in the blood of the recipient or certain intermediate steps are involved in elaboration of the agent(s). It is also unlikely that direct circulatory changes immediately consequent upon stimulation of the donor animal could play a significant role in activation of the recipient animal.

Stimulation of the bulbar reticular formation of one animal liberates a substance from the brain of the stimulated animal which, on perfusing the brain of another animal, is capable of reproducing all the electrographic features usually associated with reticulocortical activation. Uncomplicated by the effects of electrical stimulation on the tested animal (recipient), these observations may be interpreted as providing confirmation, in part, of Ingvar's findings on the neuronally isolated cortex (3).

Until biochemical studies now in progress reveal the nature of the humoral agent whose existence has been established by the present investigation, attempts to identify this neurohumor (or, "neurotropic" agent) (11) with the currently known brain constituents claimed to be neurohumoral are not justified at this time. While it is claimed that the reticular activating system neurons are both adrenergic (4, 5), and cholinergic (12, 13), the physiological significance of other recently discovered neurohumors remains obscure (e.g., serotonin (14, 15), cerebrotonin (16), encephalin (17), histamine (18), substance P (19)). This suggests that not only may a wide variety of extractable substances from brain be capable of facilitating or inhibiting neural activity but the same substance may act differentially on dissimilar functional systems as in the case of adrenaline (20). The latter strikingly demonstrates how the action of an agent is most likely dependent on the different functional characteristics of the postsynaptic receptors on the same or different neurons.

Finally, the fact that activation of Metrazol-treated cortex can be humorally facilitated raises the question as to what extent, if any, humoral agents alone may initiate generalized alterations in cerebral activity.

The author wishes to express his appreciation to Dr. J. Lawrence Pool for his interest and encouragement during this investigation and to Mr. Gidon F. Gestring for his valuable technical assistance. Dr. Eric Kandel's assistance in the laborious surgical procedures was especially welcomed.

References

1. Purpura, D. P. *Science* **123:** 804, 1956.
2. Purpura, D. P. *Ann. New York Acad. Sc.* In press, 1956.
3. Ingvar, D. *Acta physiol. scandinav.* **33:** 169, 1955.
4. Bonvallet, M., P. Dell and A. Hugelin. *Electroencephalog. & Clin. Neurophysiol.* **6:** 119, 1954.
5. Dell, P., M. Bonvallet and A. Hugelin. *Electroencephalog. & Clin. Neurophysiol.* **6:** 599, 1954.
6. Vogt, M. *J. Physiol.* (*London*) **123:** 451, 1954.
7. McQueen, J. D., K. M. Browne and E. A. Walker. *Neurology* **4:** 1, 1954.
8. Moruzzi, G. and H. W. Magoun. *Electroencephalog. & Clin. Neurophysiol.* **1:** 455, 1949.
9. Arduini, A. and C. G. Lairy-Bounes. *Electroencephalog. & Clin. Neurophysiol.* **4:** 503, 1952.
10. Li, C.-L., H. Jasper and L. Henderson. *Electroencephalog. & Clin. Neurophysiol.* **4:** 513, 1952.
11. Minz, B. *The Role of Humoral Agents in Nervous Activity.* Springfield: Thomas, 1955.
12. Rinaldi, F. and H. E. Himwich. *Arch. Neurol. & Psychiat.* **73:** 387, 1955.
13. Rinaldi, F. and H. E. Himwich. *Arch. Neurol. & Psychiat.* **73:** 396, 1955.
14. Amin, A. H., I. B. B. Crawford and J. H. Gaddum. Abstr. XIXth Int. Physio. Congr., p. 113, 1953.
15. Twarog, B. M. and I. H. Page. *Am. J. Physiol.* **175:** 157, 1953.
16. Taylor, R. D. and I. H. Page. *Am. J. Physiol.* **170:** 321, 1952.
17. Raab, W. and W. Giger. *Proc. Soc. Exper. Biol. N.Y.* **76:** 97, 1951.
18. Harris, G. W., D. Jacobson and G. Kahlson. *Ciba Foundation Colloquia on Endocrinology* **4:** 186, 1952.
19. Pernow, B. *Nature* (*London*) **171:** 746, 1953.
20. Bülbring, E., J. H. Burns and C. R. Skoglund. *J. Physiol.* **107:** 289, 1948.

Study Question for Part III

1. Consid[...] [...]nd who has
an antique clock[...] [...]g noise. At
first, you find th[...] [...]u no longer
attend to, or "h[...] [...]onversation
when suddenly y[...] [...]ped ticking.
The readings in [...] [...]for explaining this rather c[...] [...]ps in information processin[...] [...]e information flow from t[...] [...]nechanisms
in the brain. No[...] [...]nput. Consider whether th[...] [...]"active" or
"passive" proces[...] [...]context?).
Finally, see if yo[...] [...]and memory mechanisms.